Resistance Flexibility 1.0

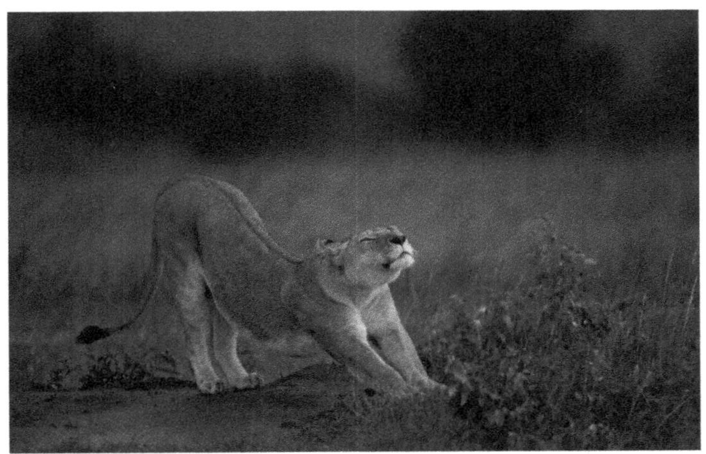

Bob Cooley

Director The Genius of Flexibility Centers in Santa Barbara, LA, NYC and Boston

Director of two 501 (3)(C) nonprofit corporations:

The Genius of Flexibility Research (Research on Fascia)

The *Types* Project (Research on Genetic Personality *Types* (GPT))

Director GPT Foundation Boston MA

Telemachus Press, LLC

Notice: Medical Disclaimer
Neither the Publisher nor the Author assumes any responsibility for any loss or injury and/or damage to persons or property arising out of or related to any use of the material contained in this book or web page associations. This book is not intended as a substitute for medical recommendations. Please consult your health care provider for medical advice. Rather it is to offer information to help you to cooperate with all your health care providers, to gain optimal health. Please note that it is the expressed concern of the writer that each person take responsibility for his or her health, and for any and all advice received when engaging a medical or health specialist.

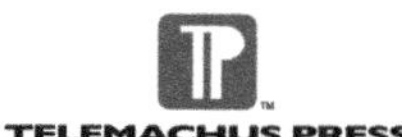

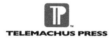

Telemachus Press, LLC
7652 Sawmill Road, Suite 304
Dublin, Ohio 43016
United States
Phone: (941) 504-5496
Email: http://www.telemachuspress.com/ContactUs.aspx

First Published by Telemachus Press 2016

Cover and Resistance Flexibility Stretch Photos by Michael Cuffe
MichaelCuffe.com and Warholian.com

Chapter Photos by Russ Spencer BisonFilms.com

ISBN: 978-1-942899-76-1 (eBook)
ISBN: 978-1-942899-77-8 (Paperback)

Library of Congress Control Number: 2016931397

10 9 8 7 6 5 4 3 2

2016.02.13

Dedication

To all my dear friends.

love

b

Special Thanks to Tom Longo, Luther Cowden, Dr. Christiane Northrup, Dr. Jean Claude Guimberteau, and Ratan Tata.

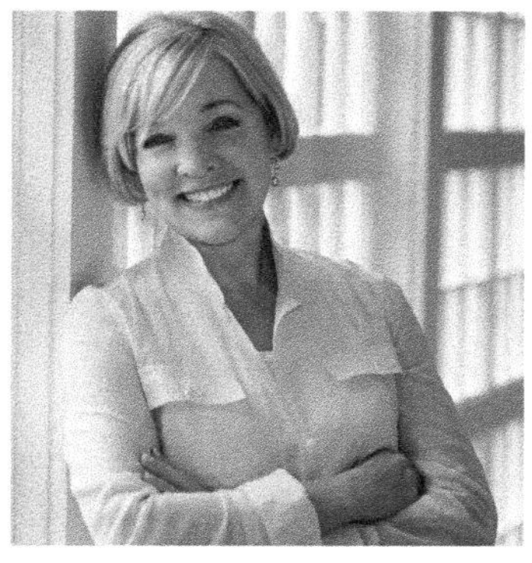

FOREWORD

DR. CHRISTIANE NORTHRUP

New York Times Bestselling author of Women's Bodies, Women's Wisdom, The Wisdom of Menopause, and Goddesses Never Age

A couple years ago I got an email telling me about Bob Cooley's work with fascia, and the fact his system of fascia restructuring—Resistance Flexibility had been scientifically validated by Dr. Jean-Claude Guimberteau in France.

I had long been fascinated by the fact that acupuncture meridians run in the fascia, and that the fascia itself is a crystalline structure that transmits energy nearly instantaneously from one part of the body is another. Acupuncture and Traditional Chinese Medicine had long been my first choice for medical care for me and my family. And bodywork of all kinds was and is a regular part of my life. I've had countless massages, foot reflexology sessions, and also numerous Rolfing sessions—all part of my ongoing healthcare.

As a physician, I had observed for years how the emotional events of our lives and the beliefs associated with them reside in our tissues and shape how we move and how our muscles and organs work. And that is why, when I was introduced to Bob Cooley's work, I knew right away that his Resistance Flexibility was hands down, the fastest way to change and heal the body that I had ever seen. I had the background to know an entirely new healthcare system when I observed it. This was it.

But Resistance Flexibility does far more than change muscles and joints. It also opens up new emotional, mental, and spiritual areas of life—parts of ourselves that we didn't even know existed. For example, Bob was able to identify dense fascia in my heart meridian that had been laid down in childhood from my relationship with my mother. He said that it gave me an "I'm not loveable" appearance—shoulders pulled in to protect my heart. Since shredding that fascia, I have experienced more happiness and joy in the last couple years than in the decades before that; a rather amazing development. Moreover the Dowager's hump that was developing on the back of my neck (from carrying the burdens of so many others) has gone away, and so has a niggling right hip problem that would no doubt, have led to a hip replacement had I not had Resistance Flexibility sessions.

I will be doing Resistance Flexibility for the rest of my life. This system is, hands down, the most practical way I know to remain ageless in body, mind, and spirit. Bravo Bob Cooley!

Christiane Northrup, MD — December 8, 2015

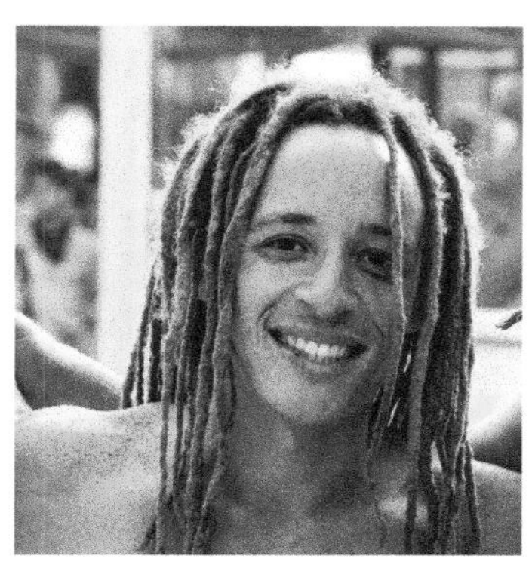

FOREWORD

LUTHER B. COWDEN

Director of Technology—TheGeniusofFlexibility.com
Elite Resistance Flexibility Trainer
LA, Santa Barbara, NYC, BOS

I'm excited for more people to learn about this new way to stretch. From my experience, Resistance Flexibility can create immediate improvements in the health of each individual and in turn upgrade the health of the entire planet. I've worked in just about every way that I know to make this information available to everyone including spending many years developing our website www.thegeniusofflexibility.com, self stretching, doing private individual sessions, teaching certifications, workshops, and classes.

As an avid fan of technology, I am very interested in using the latest tools as communication and educational platforms to bring out the best in the world. Be on the lookout for new changes and features on our website. Our goal is to use all available means to educate the world about Resistance Flexibility. This includes mobile apps in addition to our website. We plan to make future editions of this book available as an interactive app.

MY STORY

The moment I learned about Resistance Flexibility (RF), I knew that it was going to change my life and the world at large. I first heard about Bob Cooley and his work through a chance conversation with a stranger, in an airport on Christmas Eve of 2002. It wasn't the intriguing philosophy behind the 16 Genetic Personality Types or the new ideas about flexibility that moved me the most. It was simply a moment in time where life was telling me, "Listen up. This is something you need to know about."

Before too long, I spoke with Bob on the phone and was invited to attend a teacher training intensive. But I only wanted to establish a personal practice and wasn't interested in becoming a teacher. I was also a young college student, lacking the funds necessary to pay for the training, travel expenses, and accommodations. But, my instincts kept urging me to move forward, and so I did.

As my practice formed, I learned more about myself while continuously improving my health. I was excited to have finally found a form of physical exercise that worked for me. My digestion greatly improved. I became more grounded and less aloof, and could concentrate with ease. I slept soundly and experienced higher energy levels throughout the day. I started off as a skinny guy and soon developed a muscular physique. Changes like these continued to manifest and urged me to share this remarkable technique with others. Before long, I found that training others professionally was the best way to fully manifest my quickly growing passion for RF.

Resistance Flexibility has proven to be one of the most powerful gifts that I can share with others. It has been an honor to play a key role in the health of so many people by introducing them to this body of work. I'm particularly interested in how facilitating another person's development through assisted stretching brings people together, creating the most personal and unique form of interaction that I've ever experienced.

Over the years, I've worked with people from many walks of life. People simply looking to get in shape, severely injured individuals, professional athletes, high-end performers, and high-powered business people and educators like Oprah Winfrey. What I've witnessed with everyone, regardless of who they are, what they do, and where they are from, is that the body is something everyone can relate to. I've practiced Resistance Flexibility around the world and have seen it cut through regional and cultural divides, empowering each individual to become an authority of their own health, overcome their pain and discomfort, become more balanced, and develop into their best self. Resistance Flexibility has the power to help us put aside our differences and realize that we all have health challenges that require the assistance of others to resolve.

I'm grateful for Bob and his discoveries. I feel lucky to have him as a close friend, to have discovered this work, and to have followed my gut instinct to prioritize this practice and incorporate it into my life. My wish is that you also experience radical improvements in your health from this practice and let nothing stop you from continuously improving yourself. Below are ways for you to get involved and accelerate your development.

FOR YOU

USE THIS BOOK
RESISTANCE FLEXIBILITY 1.0

Use this book to discover the new basic principles for achieving true flexibility with Resistance Flexibility. RF teaches you how to remove dense fascia and scar tissue from your body and how this process develops you physically as well as psychologically, emotionally, and spiritually. Let the photos and descriptions in this book serve as a teaching aid so that you can put these principles into action through self or assisted stretching. In addition to this book, there are many other ways to get involved with Resistance Flexibility.

SUBSCRIBE
TO OUR WEBSITE'S VIDEO TRAINING ARCHIVE

Subscribe to The Genius of Flexibility's Training Archive at www.thegeniusofflexibility.com, which features over 200 (and growing) streaming instructional videos and photos of self and assisted stretching, full length classes/lectures, customizable exercise sequences, personalized flexibility tests, interactive muscular/meridian maps, online support forums, social features, and more.

VISIT
THE GENIUS OF FLEXIBILITY CENTERS SB, LA, NYC, BOS

Visit The Genius of Flexibility Center in Santa Barbara, Los Angeles, New York City, and/or Boston to experience RF firsthand.

Our location in Santa Barbara, CA is *the greenest building in town* and embodies our vision of an ideal work space: working within a structure that is ecologically sound so as to reflect the sustainability we create within a person's body. In addition, we have a new solar powered center in Los Angeles (Venice), a new center in New York City (SOHO), and a center in Boston (Copley Square).

Our centers offer certification trainings/weekend intensives, private sessions, classes, workshops, special events, and more. Contact us to come by one of our centers to observe, assist, and participate. There are many ways to get involved with Resistance Flexibility. Please let us know how we can assist you.

ATTEND
CERTIFICATION TRAININGS/WEEKEND INTENSIVES

Our trainings are designed to provide an entry-level education of all principles involved in Bob Cooley's Resistance Flexibility. They are open to all ages, abilities, and levels of experience. This is a great way to be introduced to RF for personal or professional gain.

These courses are physically demanding, but everyone works at his or her own pace. Variations are taught for every exercise allowing people of all ages and abilities to fully participate.

Trainings provide a place for participants to be introduced to our community. This growing community allows people to develop each other's health through assisted stretching and the sharing of perspective. Many people attend a weekend course with a friend so that they have someone to practice assisted stretching with.

SCHEDULE
PRIVATE SESSIONS
VIDEO CHAT PRIVATE SESSIONS

Our centers also offer private sessions. This is your time to work with highly skilled trainers for intensive and personalized flexibility training.

Visit our website to schedule online private sessions conducted via video chat. Get personalized assistance and instruction regardless of where you are in the world.

JOIN
OUR ONLINE COMMUNITY

We welcome you to our online community of Resistance Flexibility enthusiasts. Join the social forum on our website to ask questions and share your experience with others.

FIND AND CREATE
LOCAL COMMUNITY

Find a stretching partner and stretching group in your area. Simply type in your zip code on our website to get started.

STAY UPDATED

Stay up to speed on our latest news, offerings, and developments. Subscribe to our email newsletter at www.thegeniusofflexibility.com/newsletter

FOLLOW
OUR TRAINERS ON YOUTUBE—YOURGENIUSSHOW.COM

The distinguishing feature of The Genius of Flexibility's training programs when compared to other modalities is our priority on improving the health of the trainer. Resistance Flexibility places enormous and unprecedented physical demands on the practitioner. Our trainers are assisted in their stretching on a regular basis to remove this occupational stress and to develop them beyond their normal conditioning. The best measure of success for our trainers is not simply their level of skill when assisting others, but rather how developed they are themselves—physically, psychologically, emotionally, and spiritually. This ensures that the health of our team does not degrade at the expense of those we aim to help, which is a common pitfall in the healing field. We believe the trainer must first embody the changes possible through RF before they will be able to provide an optimal RF experience for others.

Follow our trainers online as we chronicle their development and feature status updates, video footage, and interviews.

Congratulations on putting forth the effort to develop yourself. I wish you the best and look forward to stretching with you.

Luther Bryan Cowden December 2015

The Genius of Flexibility
TheGeniusofFlexibility.com/luther
LutherCowden@TheGeniusofFlexibility.com

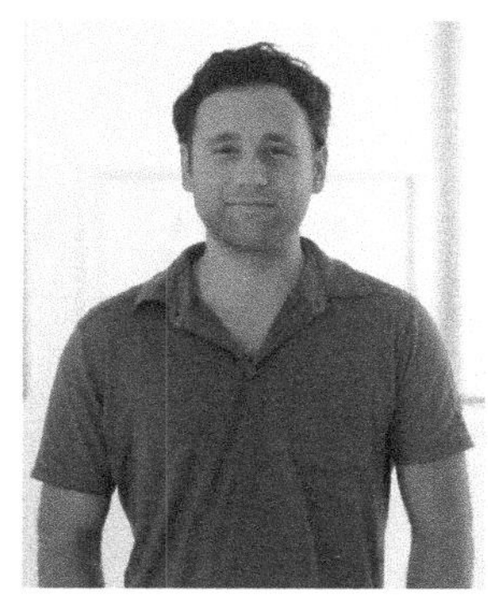

FOREWORD

NICK WARE

Elite Resistance Flexibility Trainer
SB LA
Health Hunter
Founder of HealthSafari.com

I met Bob Cooley in 2008 when I attended the grand opening of The Genius of Flexibility—Boston. I immediately recognized that Bob was everything my science professors had warned me about. Within the first three minutes of his talk, Bob had claimed that his stretching technology could help resolve physical problems, increase athletic performance and make people smarter, younger, more open-minded and better looking. Bold claims, given that there was no scientific evidence to back him up.

After Bob's talk, five people Resistance Flexibility trained my hamstrings for about an hour. I felt a sense of lightness and elasticity in my body that I'd never experienced. That afternoon, running the icy streets of Cambridge and Somerville, I set a new personal best for my 5K times—by 24 seconds. I stared at my watch. *Impossible.* That was my first experience with Resistance Flexibility. *What will yours be like?*

I was more interested in health and nutrition than I was in running. So, like an undercover scientist, I returned to the Center to investigate the health effects of Resistance Flexibility. I assisted Bob as he trained performers, professional athletes and people in search of anything that could help them get out of pain and step back into life. What I witnessed led me to withdraw my applications to medical school and instead study Resistance Flexibility.

I saw people transformed in the ways that Bob had claimed were possible. I experienced these upgrades for myself. I also watched unhealthy and diseased people get healthier by the day. I was enthralled. How was Resistance Flexibility helping people get healthy?

Bob explains, "Fifty percent of your health is based on your nutrition—the food, water and air that you ingest. But, the other fifty percent is based on the physical functioning of your internal immune system." This revolutionary idea will improve the way that people think about food and their health. It makes a lot of sense: We all know someone who eats the ideal diet, but struggles to get healthy. And we all know someone who eats a dreadful diet, but always looks and feels quite healthy.

One of Bob's greatest contributions is his identification of two meridians that are not included in Traditional Chinese Medicine. The Thymus and Appendix meridians are associated with overall health. So, if you want to improve your health, then you can Resistance Flexibility train the muscle groups associated with these meridians—the upper traps and the lats. People who struggle to look and feel healthy usually have a lot of dense fascia or scar tissue in one of these muscle groups. When the dense tissue is removed, their health skyrockets and Resistance Flexibility does just that.

As a Resistance Flexibility Trainer, I have been fortunate to help many people upgrade their health. When you remove dense fascia and scar tissue from the body, it causes the person to change their diet in ways that are beneficial for them. Each of these nutritional upgrades seems to come with a story. For example, a woman goes to her friend's annual chocolate party and discovers that she can't stand the taste of chocolate anymore—it's way too sweet! A teenager who wouldn't dream of eating green vegetables finds himself biting into a head of raw cabbage in the grocery store! A woman who was a vegan for twenty years has a recurring dream about eating beef. She can't stop dreaming about it, so she tries some steak and it gets rid of her chronic eczema. A man who has eaten meat for breakfast, lunch and dinner throughout his entire life starts drinking raw green vegetable juice. Even the best grass-fed filet mignon cannot give him the satisfaction that his green juice can. These stories go on and on; the point is that Resistance Flexibility helps people improve their nutrition *naturally*!

Our diets evolve as we do. Eating a highly regimented diet is a recipe for immune system distress and poor health. Getting healthy has a lot to do with listening to your body and letting your instincts direct you toward the foods that are best for you at this moment. A Holistic Health Coach, I assign people Resistance Flexibility exercises to help them contact these instincts and crave healthier foods. For example, if you want to get rid of sugar cravings, try doing the Pancreas exercises for 20 minutes a day. These exercises can help boost your production of digestive enzymes and cause you to experience sustained energy levels all day long. Therefore…no sugar cravings!

When Bob asked me to write a foreword for his book, I was greatly honored. Bob's discoveries have helped me upgrade my personal health in many ways. To name a few, I got rid of my lifelong seasonal allergies and my addiction to coffee. Beyond this, I see Bob's discovery and development of Resistance Flexibility as a significant contribution to humanity. His ideas have the potential to help billions of people live a healthier life. No special tools or expensive equipment is required- just a body and the desire to learn.

Previously, I mentioned that there were no scientific studies to validate Resistance Flexibility, but this is no longer the case. In 2011, Bob and I established The Genius of Flexibility, a non-profit organization dedicated to fascia and flexibility research. We have completed two pilot studies to date, both of which were presented at the International Fascia Research Congress. The first study demonstrated that Resistance Flexibility causes a 10x faster increase in hamstring length compared to all other modalities in the medical literature. The second, an endoscopic study conducted in collaboration with Dr. Jean-Claude Guimberteau of France, demonstrated that Resistance Flexibility causes an immediate and permanent change to the fascial structures of the body, making it the only non-invasive physical modality that has been proven to do so.

Everyone knows that if you want to get healthy, then ultimately you will have to eat a diet rich in organic green vegetables and healthy fats. But, what if there is something you can do that makes you *want* to eat the foods that are healthiest for you? In *Cooley Resistance Flexibility,* this is what Bob delivers. So, go ahead and transform your health! Start practicing these exercises for at least 30 minutes a day. You'll see what happens. Thank you, Bob!

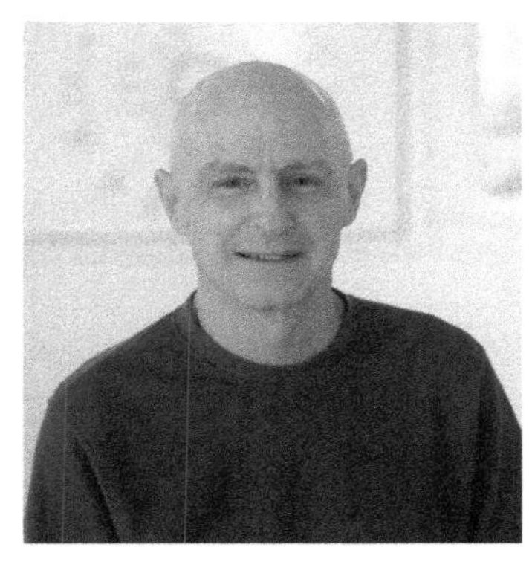

FOREWORD

BOB COOLEY

DIRECTOR THE GENIUS OF FLEXIBILITY CENTERS IN SANTA BARBARA, LA, NYC AND BOSTON

DIRECTOR OF TWO 501 (3)(C) NONPROFIT CORPORATIONS:

THE GENIUS OF FLEXIBILITY RESEARCH (RESEARCH ON FASCIA)

THE *TYPES* PROJECT (RESEARCH ON GENETIC PERSONALITY *TYPES*)

DIRECTOR GPT FOUNDATION

I really like the persons that everybody I know are becoming, and the person I am becoming. I have learned many tools that allow me to handle many different *types* of experiences. Most moments of the day, I am processing something new that was in need of my attention in order for me to grow: like being able to relax; this results in me being more socially available, or how I catch my resistance to most everything as an opportunity to overcome my fright and turn those feelings into stepping more into life. I love my awareness of life. There is so much life to have. Eat incredibly nutritious food. I wish myself and all others to be in life.

MY STORY

I survived a pedestrian automobile accident but my friend Pam didn't. With the enormous help from other people, I turned that tragedy into discovering and continuously developing Resistance Flexibility, and created the body-mind theory of the 16 Geniuses—Sixteen Genetic Personality *Types*.

The natural way to stretch, formally called pandiculation, is the way all animals stretch including us. Naturally allowing your body to tense and resist when you stretch dramatically upgrades all your myofascia tissues, as the fascia is restored towards optimal health. Stretching in this way helps to transform trauma into gifts. Everyone experiences being unsnagged by his or her traumas and lifted into a lightness in being. Resistance Flexibility is one of the best forms of preventative health care, and one of the future rehabilitative and regenerative therapies.

Oh Those Hamstrings—what else can I say. Everybody needs to Resistance Flexibility his or her lateral hamstrings. Begin now. Take a class, learn how on TheGeniusofFlexibility.com Video Training Archive of 200+ flexibility exercises with in depth explanations, hire one of our Certified Resistance Flexibility Trainers, and stretch your family and friends.

Change in spite of yourself with the help of others; healing only happens with the help of other people. Let me know how I can help.

WELCOME TO THE GENIUS OF FLEXIBILITY CENTERS

The Genius of Flexibility Centers creates a traditional healing environment that includes group participation, transparency, group perspective, and where the healing of the healers is a priority.

It is important for people participating at the center to understand how classes and private sessions are conducted. Often the activities involved in healing are in stark contrast to the current corporate health practices where the medical practitioner isolates the client in a closed room, and only they treat the person.

During both classes and private sessions:

1. Other people in the room are asked to give their perspective, feelings and knowledge on the changes that have occurred for someone who has been assisted or after their self-stretch. The perspective of others honors and acknowledges the genius of others knowledge.

2. Everyone can be asked to participate to help assist another person. Resistance Flexibility training often requires many people to help generate the movement necessary to help someone.

3. All four aspects of a person are discussed which is essential to creating those parts of a person that have yet to be developed and which are the root causes of their health concerns.

4. Though time slots are arranged, often both the beginning and ending times are somewhat flexible in order to allow both the participants and the practitioners to accomplish the work that has been attempted to help everyone.

5. Everyone needs to embrace the valuable opportunity to learn from others experiences. Often other people are assisted during a private session or discussions occur that are of significant value to everyone.

AND YOUR GENIUS

SEE GENIUSSHOW.COM ON YOUTUBE

Watch the trainers as they get assisted week after week, and change in all ways. The trainers tell about all the ways a person can change their bodies physically: their posture, getting rid of low back, knee shoulder, elbow and wrist problems, performance upgrades; how their organs work better for digestion, elimination, respiration; how they can change psychologically: losing addictions, depression, avoidance, repression, obsessions, etc.; how they can mature emotionally: becoming better looking, increasing their intimacy, process their past, discover self worth, self affirm, etc; and develop spiritually: develop better judgment, integrity, peacefulness, and connections. Totally exciting.

MimiAmritt@TheGeniusofFlexibility.com
JohnBagasarian@TheGeniusofFlexibility.com
EricBeutner@TheGeniusofFlexibility.com
ScottBottoroff@TheGeniusofFlexibility.com
SamuelCamburn@TheGeniusofFlexibility.com
NoelChristensen@TheGeniusofFlexibility.com
KatConnors-Longo@TheGeniusofFlexibility.com
BobCooley@TheGeniusofFlexibility.com
BonnieCrotzer@TheGeniusofFlexibility.com
LutherCowden@TheGeniusofFlexibility.com
LucaCupery@TheGeniusofFlexibility.com
PeterDonovan@TheGeniusofFlexibility.com
EthanDupris@TheGeniusofFlexibility.com
EddieEllner@TheGeniusofFlexibility.com
PatrickGregston@TheGeniusofFlexibility.com
RichardGregston@TheGeniusofFlexibility.com
BerylHagenburg@TheGeniusofFlexibility.com
KajHoffman@TheGeniusofFlexibility.com
JohnKelly@TheGeniusofFlexibility.com
TomLongo@TheGeniusofFlexibility.com
KarenMason@TheGeniusofFlexibility.com
BrianMay@TheGeniusofFlexibility.com
AlexNolte@TheGeniusofFlexibility.com
RobObrien@TheGeniusofFlexibility.com
ChrisPearsall@TheGeniusofFlexibility.com
PatriciaPilot@TheGeniusofFlexibility.com
KateRabinowitz@TheGeniusofFlexibility.com
ChrisRenfrow@TheGeniusofFlexibility.com
NurhadeSouza@TheGeniusofFlexibility.com
TomasTedesco@TheGeniusofFlexibility.com
NickWare@TheGeniusofFlexibility.com

WHAT TO EXPECT?

Immediate upgrades in posture and skilled movement.

Replacing trauma with the gifts from healing.

Retracing events that produced your problems but with current perspectives.

Physiological upgrades: digestion, respiration, elimination, immunity, and sexual function.

Advancements in psychological wellness and prowess.

Developments in intelligence and intuition.

Acceleration in rate of change.

Increase in discernment, insight, shrewdness, and judgment.

Diversification of positive character traits.

Self and other clemency and exoneration.

Filling ignorance with knowledge.

Replacing bias with appreciation.

Eliminating the duality of good versus bad,
and replacing it with an understanding
that all good is an alchemizing of bad.

Love and respect,

Bob

BobCooley@TheGeniusofFlexibility.com

Resistance Flexibility 1.0—

Becoming Flexible In All Ways

TABLE OF CONTENTS

PART I: RESISTANCE FLEXIBILITY AND YOGA

Introduction to Resistance Flexibility and Resistance Flexibility Yoga

CHAPTER 1

THREE NEW FLEXIBILITY DISCOVERIES

Everyone's Introductory Session with Resistance Flexibility™

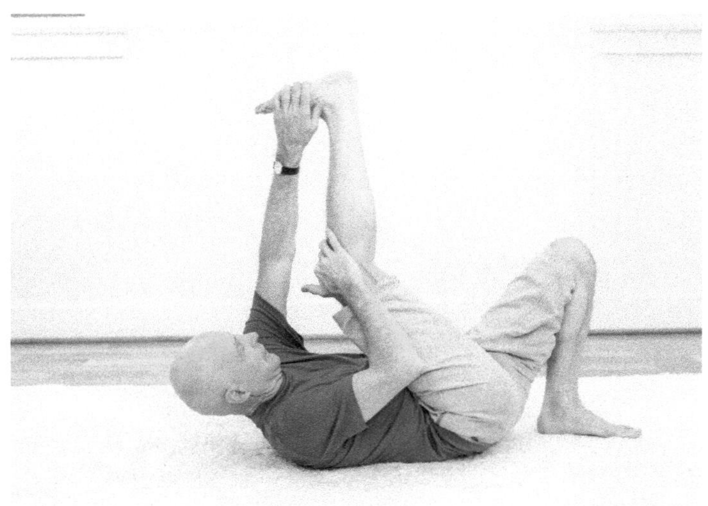

There is a natural way to stretch. I call this Resistance Flexibility™.

FLEXIBILITY PARADIGM SHIFTS—THREE NEW IDEAS

IDEA #1: When you stretch a muscle it naturally contracts, and the fascia that surrounds and roots into your muscles and other tissues resists. I call this Resistance Flexibility™. This is an intuitive way to stretch that prevents you from over-stretching and promotes natural health benefits. Defer to your body's wisdom, stretch naturally.

IDEA #2: This increase in true flexibility also results in an increase in the muscle's ability to shorten, rate of shortening, and acceleration.

IDEA #3: Balancing is the underlying principle for muscles, organs, and personality *types.*

Physical, psychological, emotional, and spiritual benefits result from stretching naturally using tension and resistance. The words everyone uses to describe these benefits created a new body-mind psychology I call THE 16 GENIUSES—*16 Genetic Personality Types.*

NEW IDEA #1—
RESISTANCE FLEXIBILITY™

Become flexible in all ways…

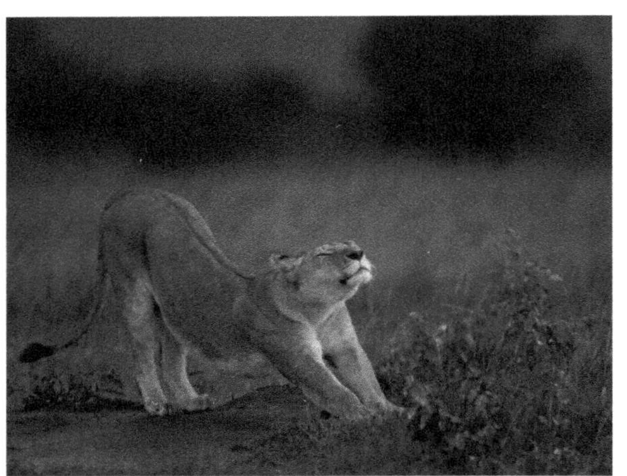

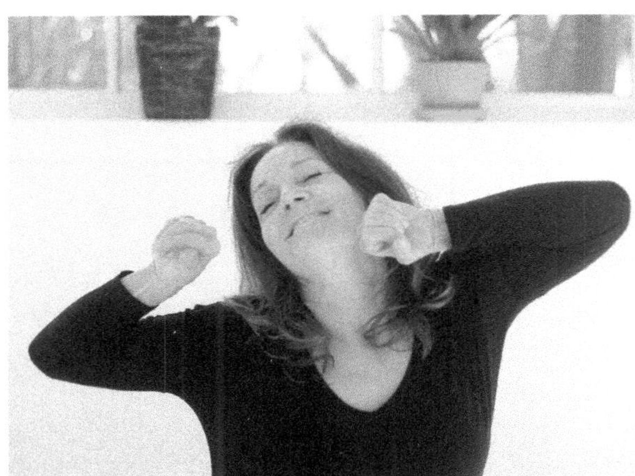

Like all animals, the moment you begin to lengthen a muscle to stretch it, the muscle naturally begins to contract and resist the stretch. You know that 'tension thing' the dogs and cats do as they reach forward and stretch? Or, when you get up in the morning before getting out of bed, how you lift your arms upward and then you do that same 'tension thing' while making that subtle grunting sound? Well, you're stretching. That's the way all animals stretch when you do that. It's called pandiculation—the act of stretching oneself. When you stretch, you lengthen, tense and resist simultaneously. I call this Resistance Flexibility™, and it is the natural way to stretch.

The tensing and contraction that happens naturally when the muscle is stretched is caused by the stretch reflex. The stretch reflex causes the muscle to tense the entire time the muscle is being stretched. The more you lengthen a muscle the greater the tensing. This is a natural thing every muscle does when it is stretched. Why?

The reason the muscle tenses when you stretch is because the fascia that is rooted into the muscle resists, twists ninety degrees and is instantly changed. Yes, your fascia is a 'cellophane-like layer' that surrounds and roots into all the other *types* of tissues in your body. It is reshaped and rehydrated when you stretch with resistance. How much is it changed? The fascia is permanently transfigured and renovated while removing excessive accumulated dense fascia and scar tissue (ADFST). The fascia is rehydrated, returning it to its original, healthy elastic state, thus freeing the muscles, joints, circulatory and lymphatic systems to work more optimally while psychologically removing trauma.

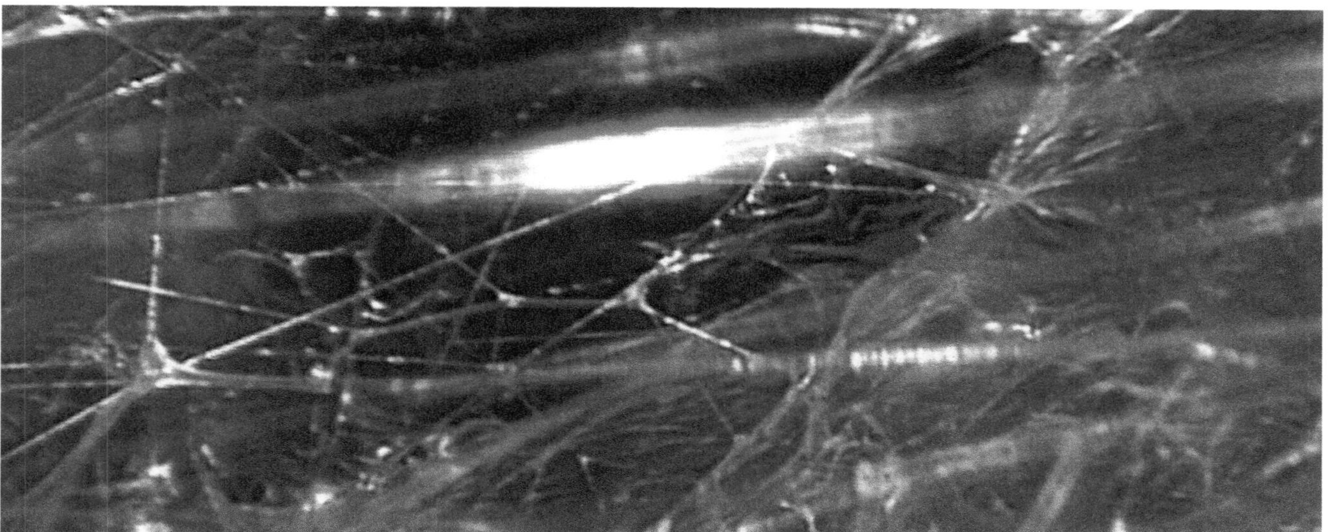

FASCIA (Photo by Dr. Jean Claude Guimberteau)

Endoscopic photo of inside the body at 25 X's magnification of the extracellular tissue that suspends the body by impregnating into all other *types* of tissue.

Every time you stretch, your body already has a built in natural mechanism that constantly upgrades your muscles and fascia. That is why you see a cat or dog stretch hundreds of times each day, where they naturally tense their muscles and resist while stretching. You may start stretching daily because you know how to stretch in a way that finally gives you the results you always imagined you would get from stretching. Ah, Resistance Flexibility.

This natural tensing and resisting I call Resistance Flexibility dramatically transfigures the fascia and strengthens your muscles resulting in immediate, cumulative, and permanent increases in flexibility and strength. There are additional unexpected benefits to stretching naturally. People practice Resistance Flexibility report they get concomitant physiological and psychological benefits while removing traumas as well has a redintegration (a return to wholeness). (See Chapter 6 more details).

You will need to corral and recruit tenseness from your entire body so it can be used in the target area you are stretching. Your whole body needs to be involved when you are focusing on a muscle group that you are stretching. Expect immediate, cumulative, and lasting results that from Resistance Flexibility. Every time you stretch you will achieve significant increases in flexibility and strength. Maximal tension is produced has the muscles are warmed up. Persistence and perseverance are necessary to remove accumulated dense fascia and scar tissue (ADFST), especially if it has been there for many years. Sometimes hundreds and hundreds, or even thousands of repetitions are necessary to remove scar tissue.

WARNING: If you interfere with your muscle's natural reflex to contract when you stretch, then you can overstretch your joint structures. Allow your muscles to tense and your fascia to resist when you stretch.

Diaries

"After I first began Resistance Flexibility training, I once awoke in in the middle of the night and found myself kicking my legs down into the mattress. Another night, I woke up in a stretch position (pigeon pose) and was once again kicking my feet, legs, and thighs down into the mattress. I was stretching in my sleep! It was as if my body was saying 'finally' to our new accomplishment of discovering how to truly stretch by resisting and generating tension. This new understanding took root and was so natural that it happened in my sleep, without conscious effort. I knew then that I had found a new way forward for being in my body, and there was no going back."
LutherCowden@TheGeniusofFlexibility.com Elite Resistance Flexibility Trainer

"Stretching with resistance is very different than the way most of us have become accustomed to stretching. If you haven't stretched this way before, you may feel some initial confusion about how to properly create the natural tension and resistance while moving your body during the stretch. You may also realize that this way of flexibility training feels vastly different than the stretching you have done in the past. When I was first introduced to this concept, I felt like it turned everything I knew about stretching upside down and inside out, but later I realized that this natural way to stretch was an intuitive and instinctual way to stretch, and that not tensing and resisting while stretching was actually counter intuitive. Be ready for a very new and different experience, and for profound and exciting changes."
NoëlChristensen@TheGeniusofFlexibility.com Resistance Flexibility Intern

"I remember when I was a child I would stretch and resist my movements in a natural and organic way. I haven't felt that feeling and the relief and freedom it brings until I found Resistance Flexibility. I am acutely aware of how the many years of neglecting that child-like kind of stretching has made it hard to reintegrate into my life as the natural thing it once was. It takes time! But it also feels so natural and familiar. The more I do Resistance Flexibility the more I regain genuine freedom in my body."
BerylHagenburg@TheGeniusofFlexibility.com Resistance Flexibility Intern

"I played a lot of sports, but I never stretched, because it didn't work, and it was uncomfortable. I knew my hamstrings were tight, but stretching didn't change a thing. Resistance Flexibility is totally different from traditional education about stretching. After my first time getting Resistance Flexibility trained, I was much faster, stronger, and I had more range of motion in every movement. I've taught athletes to practice Resistance Flexibility every day (especially their hamstrings) for performance increases, injury prevention, and longevity in your sport."
NickWare@TheGeniusofFlexibility.com Elite Resistance Flexibility Trainer

"Resistance Flexibility has dramatically changed my Yoga practice and teaching just by adding in the organic tensing and contracting of my muscles while doing yoga poses. I am beginning to tap into my true strength while no longer over stretching my joint structure. I am living in my body with less pain. I have a great understanding of the bio-mechanics happening while doing poses which has given me greater depth and breadth to my life and teaching."
KatConnor-Longo@TheGeniusofFlexibility.com Resistance Flexibility Intern

NEW IDEA #2—
MUSCLE SHORTENING IS DEPENDENT ON FLEXIBILITY

Flexibility is not the endgame. It is the ability of the muscle to shorten.
The ability of a muscle to shorten is determined by its flexibility.

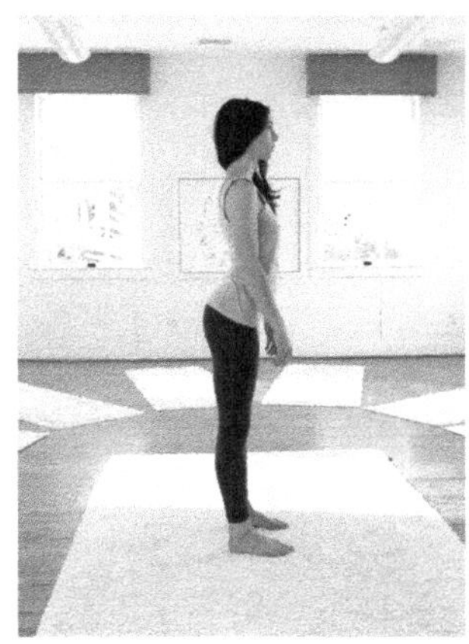

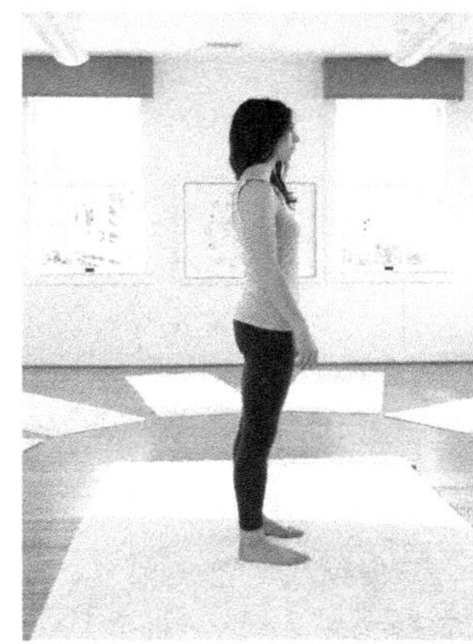

In Photo #1, Bonnie is demonstrating a person who has a pelvis that is too tilted forward which results in an excessive curve in her lower back and hyperextension in her knees. In Photo #2, Bonnie used Resistance Flexibility to increase the flexibility of her hamstring. This resulted in her hamstrings being able to contract and shorten which returns her pelvis to a natural level position thus eliminating the excessive curve in her lower back and hyperextended knees.

Once you learn the New Idea #1 about Resistance Flexibility you can get immediate, cumulative, and lasting increases in your flexibility. You then discover Idea #2 that as you increase your flexibility, you also simultaneously increase the capacity of the muscle to shorten. Surprisingly, the new increase in the muscle's capacity to lengthen also produces an equal ability for the muscle to shorten. The more optimally the muscle can shorten, the more optimally you can move. Your flexibility allows you to move and the muscle's capacity to shorten makes the movement. The more the muscle can stretch, the higher you can jump, twist or whatever way you need to move. The more flexible the muscle is, the more it can contract to move you in all eight directions.

The ability of a muscle to shorten

is directly proportional to its ability to stretch.

So when strengthening a muscle you need it to be able to shorten,

and that ability to shorten is dependent

on the flexibility of the muscle, because the muscle's flexibility

determines its ability to shorten.

Muscles don't just shorten more when they are more flexible, they also shorten faster, and their speed of shortening or acceleration increases. That means when you make a muscle more flexible it not only stretches further and shortens more, its speed and acceleration of shortening also increases. So for example, when you are more flexible, not only can you run faster, but also have 'gears to acceleration'! And the accuracy and repeatability of your movements improves.

Maximum Flexibility = Maximum Contraction

If the resting length of a muscle is this long:

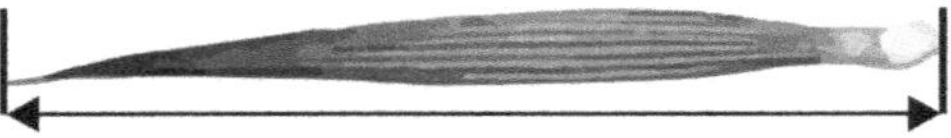

And if maximal flexibility length can be achieved:

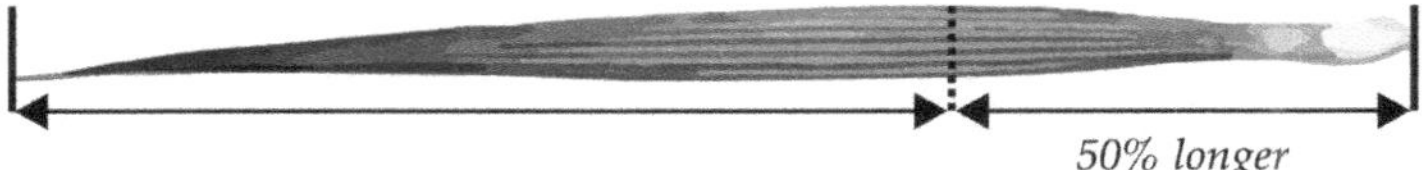

50% longer

Then this contraction shortening length is possible:

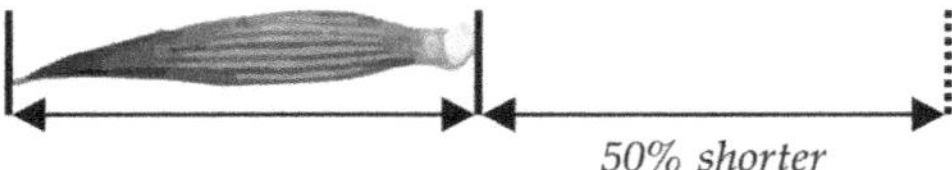

50% shorter

BUT,

Again, if the resting length of a muscle is this long:

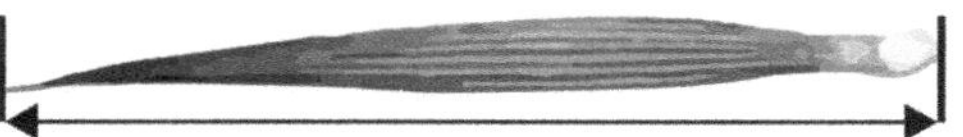

And sub-maximal flexibility is only 25% greater than resting length:

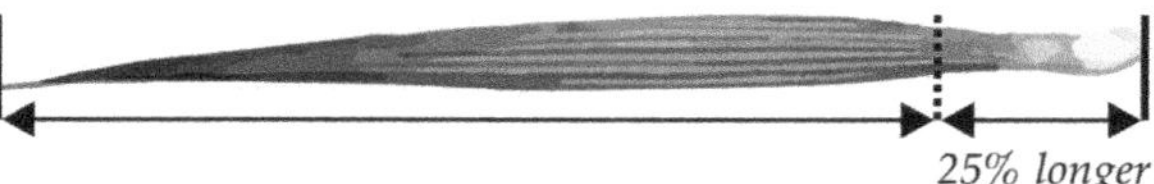

25% longer

Then only 25% shortening can occur:

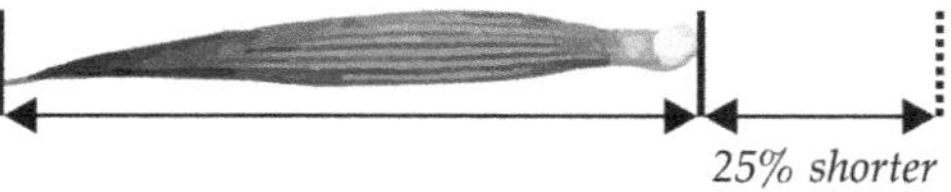

25% shorter

WARNING: A muscle can only be elongated as far as the muscle on the other side of your body can shorten. For example, when you want to strengthen your bicep your triceps need to lengthen, so if your triceps have the capacity to lengthen then you can fully strengthen your biceps, if not you can't. And when you want to stretch your biceps, you triceps need to shorten, so if your triceps have the capacity to shorten because they have sufficient flexibility, then you can fully stretch your biceps. In both cases, your triceps flexibility is the limiting factor.

Diaries

"A muscles ability to shorten is dependent on its flexibility was not something I knew. I thought like so many people that when you strength train a muscle that strengthening included an increase in the muscle's ability to shorten. But I discovered from Resistance Flexibility that only by increasing the true flexibility of a muscle by Resistance Flexibility training, do you get not only more flexibility but also surprisingly more capacity of muscles to shorten, and my muscles don't just shorten more but they shorten faster and with increased acceleration. As a result I am not only more flexible when I swim but also I swim faster."
TomLongo@TheGeniusofFlexibility.com Elite Resistance Flexibility Trainer

"This idea that a muscle's capacity to shorten is directly proportional to its ability to stretch is one of the concepts that is radically different from most peoples' ideas about stretching. It is the shortening capacity of the balancing muscle that is often the limiting factor for flexibility. We once worked with a yoga teacher who had trouble with double thigh quad stretch (in yoga called Supta Virasana). She thought it was her quads that were too tight that prevented her from lying back onto the ground, as they are the muscle groups that need to lengthen to allow lying onto your back. But we explained that the problem wasn't that her quads were too tight, instead that her medial hamstrings (the balancing muscle group to the quads) could not shorten sufficiently to allow her quads to stretch. So, we Resistance Flexibility trained her medial hamstrings for five minutes, and afterward, she could lie all the way back on the ground. I remember the look of surprise on her face as she experienced this change that happened in five minutes of assisted Resistance Flexibility versus decades of her trying through yoga. Flexibility can change at a much faster rate than most people are aware of. The more I practice Resistance Flexibility, the more satisfaction I get from being able to feel my muscles lengthen and shorten. This gives me more connection and access to my myofascial tissues. Instead of there being a lack of feeling in my muscles and then going into a super elongated positions to find sensation to stretch, I discover I have more sensation throughout my range of motion as the shortening capacity of my balancing muscles increase."
LutherCowden@TheGeniusofFlexibility.com Elite Resistance Flexibility Trainer

"It's counter-intuitive, mind-expanding, heart-opening and body-awakening to resist into the tight places in order to stretch them. This work will open you to all the ways you've been shut down. It will re-adjust the way you experience the world."
EddieEllner@TheGeniusofFlexibility.com Resistance Flexibility Intern

NEW IDEA # 3—
BALANCING IS THE FOUNDATION

Balancing muscle groups, organs, and personality types

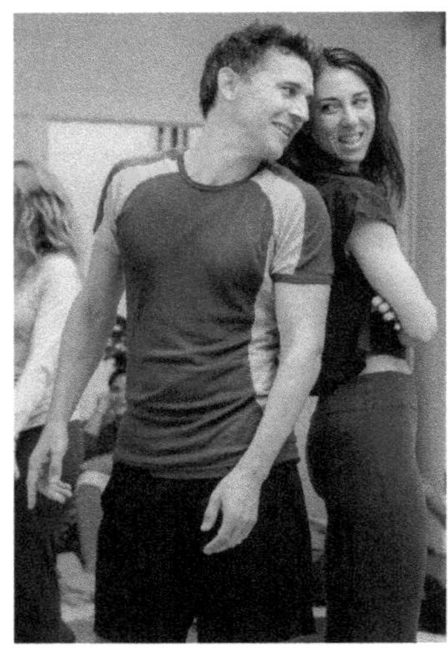

First you learned the New Idea #1 that muscles reflexly tense and resist when you stretch. Next, you learned Idea #2 that as the muscles become more flexible they can shorten more with greater speed and acceleration. Now you will discover the New Idea #3 that muscles on the opposite sides of the body have actions that balance. It is obvious to most everybody that you need to move in eight different directions in both your lower and upper body. Then it is not hard to imagine there must be eight different pairs of muscle groups in your lower and upper body that create each of these movements, and that these muscles work in pairs and balance each other's actions.

For example, muscles on one side of your body contract and move you forward, and the balancing muscles on the opposite side of your body move you backwards, or when muscles on one side of you make you jump, the muscles on the other side of you make you squat, etc. These actions balance. In traditional western terminology they call these pairs agonists and antagonists, but I like to call them balancing muscle groups because of their complementary natures.

The sixteen t*ypes* of stretches in Resistance Flexibility are ordered in pairs of balancing muscle groups. So stretch #1 and #2 balance, and #3 and #4 balance etc. Thus there are eight pairs of these balancing muscles groups.

Why is this balancing principle so important to realize? Because…

When you want to strengthen a muscle, the balancing muscle must be flexible enough to lengthen sufficiently to allow the movement. Most people think that when they get into a stretch that the inflexibility of the muscle groups they are stretching is the reason they cannot get further in range. This is true of course, but another reason why you cannot get into a greater range is because the balancing muscle isn't flexible enough to shorten sufficiently to pull you into the position to get a stretch. Therefore, whether you want to strengthen or stretch a muscle, the balancing muscle group is the limiting factor.

There is much more to this balancing idea. Not only do the muscles balance each other in action, in Traditional Chinese Medicine (TCM) each muscle group is concomitant with a specific organ and its balancing muscle group has a balancing organ, meaning those organs balance each other in their functions. For example, the Liver produces the bile and its balancing organ Gall Bladder stores the bile, or the Stomach prepares the food for digestion, and the Pancreas helps to provide the enzymes to digest it. Thus there are 8 pairs of balancing organs.

The hallmark discovery of Resistance Flexibility is that each of the 16 muscle groups is also concomitant with a genetic personality type (GPT). Each of the 16 *types* has differentiable high and low traits, and they also are in pairs that balance each other. What is conscious in one *type* is unconscious in its balancing *type*. For example, one *type* knows how to be devotional while their balancing *type* knows how to be free, or one *type* likes to work and their balancing types likes to have fun, etc.

Everything is balancing—the pairs of muscle groups and their actions, organ functions, and high GPT personality traits. For example, the muscle group on the outside of the lower body is concomitant with turning outward, the Gall Bladder, and with that *type's* high personality trait of devotion, while its balancing muscle group on the inside of the leg is concomitant with turning inward, the Liver, and with a *type's* high personality trait of freedom.

Balancing is the essence.

THE BALANCING ESSENCE

Muscle Groups, Organs, and Personality Types

1. Muscles Balance

All muscle groups on the opposite side of the body have actions that balance one another. The ability to both strengthen and stretch a muscle is dependent on the flexibility of their balancing muscle group.

2. Organs Balance Yin/Yang

All organs pair up to complement each other's physiological functions and have concomitant balancing tissues, seasons, time of day, kinetic patterns, etc.

3. Genetic Personality *Types* Balance

The 16 *types* have balancing high/low traits, and there are 8 Balancing *Types* for intimate relationships. Each *type* has an unconscious *type* that is identical to their balancing *type*.

Diaries

"I went to meet Bob in spring of 2013, and right away he sat me down in 'Badhakonasana' (bound angle pose) what Americans call Butterfly. My two bent legs knees went only half way down to the floor. Bob asked the question: 'Why don't your knees go all the way down to the floor?' He asked: 'What needs to be more flexible so your knees can go all the way to the ground?' Well of course I could feel just how tight my inner thighs and hips were. And he said: 'Yes, those muscles carry chronic tenseness but are tensing because the muscles on the outside back of your leg that balance those are not shortening enough. So your inner thighs are tense because they are getting over stretched and thus protecting your hip joints by tensing.' He continued: 'Those muscles on the outside back of your thighs need to be more flexible because their flexibility determines their ability to shorten, and if they can't shorten enough then you can't stretch your inner thigh muscles.' After I got past the embarrassment that I never thought of this myself, I celebrated the revelation. With people on both sides of my knees, and one person supporting my lower back, I pushed my knees outward and resisted as they brought my knees together to stretch the outside back of my legs, stretching those muscles them from their shortest range to their longest. After ten or so repeats, I started with my knees together and squeezed (resisted) as they opened my knees outward. Then the miracle happened, my knees went down to the ground! All of a sudden I liked the pose that had been a limiting frustration for many years. Ten minutes instead of 20 years."
KateRabinowitz@TheGeniusofFlexibility.com Resistance Flexibility Intern

"Proper balance of strength and stretch in balancing muscle group erases substitution and muscle imbalance which in turn results in suspension of the joint structures protecting the cartilage, avoids chronic pain, and increases quality of life. One muscle, organ, and personality doesn't work with out the balancing."
ChrisRenfrow@TheGeniusofFlexibility.com MSAOM, Elite Resistance Flexibility Trainer

"I have been studying and using different movement therapies for the last fifteen years and I believe Resistance Flexibility is the missing link to unwinding the restrictions in the body and creating new movement patterns and health. After finding the Resistance Flexibility community and participating in the assisted group stretches, I began to heal beyond what I ever imagined as possible. I began to learn about all the things that I had no idea about. I think Resistance Flexibility and the ever growing database of people learning together can greatly help heal the world."
SamuelCamburn@TheGeniusofFlexibility.com Elite Resistance Flexibility Intern

"The balance that is possible within the body, but is not often experienced by most people, is a reflection of what is possible in the world, but not yet experienced by the world at large. The forces on the other side that are seemingly against me are in fact there to support me, provided the relationship between the two sides can be explored, improved, and expressed in all ways. I experience a parallelity, intertwinedness, inseparableness, and interdependence between both muscle groups and two contrasting aspects of myself. Once worked through, this coordination of balance feels like an unshakeable foundation of support."
LutherCowden@TheGeniusofFlexibility.com Elite Resistance Flexibility Trainer

A NEW WAY TO HEALTH

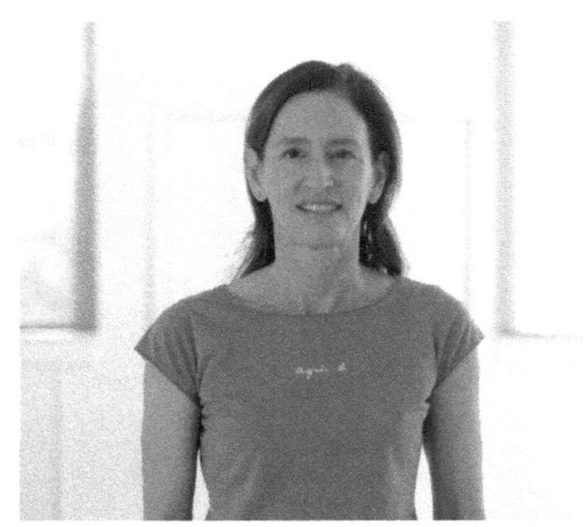

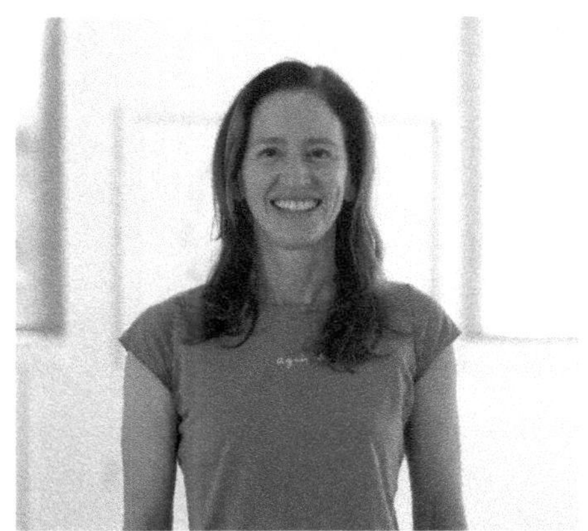

Unexpectedly, the three New Ideas resulted not just in dramatic increases in flexibility and capacity of muscles to shorten with acceleration, but facilitating predictable health in specific physiological systems, and in the development of personality *type* traits. I was totally clueless about any parallel association with my muscles and my organs, tissues, or personality. I simply thought about stretching as a physical thing, something that I used to get more flexible. But then I discovered with Resistance Flexibility I could set the stage for upgrades in my health in all ways.

Initially the more I naturally contracted and resisted when stretching, the more my health improved, but not just by physical structure. As each *type* of stretch increased my flexibility in one of the sixteen different groups of muscles, I experienced wellness benefits to specific organs and the *types* of tissues associated with those organs. This is well documented in Traditional Chinese Medicine (TCM), but I didn't know anything about TCM when I started stretching. I needed specific physiological health improvements because of my accident, not for just my muscles but also for my organs that were not in bad health after being struck by the car that was traveling so fast. My heart was malfunctioning, as was my bladder, digestion, sleep, and, lungs. I had become more sensitive to my organs because of my accident, so when I started to stretch many hours each day, it was obvious which organs were benefitted from different *types*. As I Resistance Flexibility trained, my organ functions simply got better and better and better.

As if that wasn't significant enough, I was also gaining personality trait developments from different *types* of stretches. For example, I was becoming better at relating, problem solving, social interactions, and developing spiritually. I wasn't expecting to gain social skills, or become better looking, or grow spiritually from stretching. Everyone who does Resistance Flexibility gains physical, thinking, emotional, and spiritual benefits.

Nothing quite like Resistance Flexibility.

CHAPTER 2

YOGA AND RESISTANCE FLEXIBILITY

Your brain is connected to your body but the light switch is your awareness.

THE NEW FACE OF YOGA

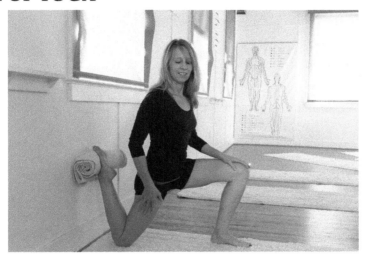

"A silent flexibility revolution is the next wave about to sweep across the world stage."

You can use the principles and practices of Resistance Flexibility to give you the ability to do all the yoga poses, especially the ones you could never do, no matter how many decades you've done yoga . The missing link, knowing to use tension and resistance while stretching, gives you the secret physical prowess to do all the yoga poses with physiological and psychological benefits. This will exceed anything you imagined you would benefit from your yoga or flexibility practice.

There is a new face when you practice Resistance Flexibility in your yoga. Because muscles naturally contract and resist when you stretch, you need to corral all the tension from your whole body to collect at the area you are isolating to stretch. Initially this shows up as your face, arms, legs and trunk expressing their chronic tenseness. As you learn more how to do Resistance Flexibility those other parts of you that are not being stretched send their tension contribution to the areas you are concentrating on to stretch. Afterwards, all the parts of you are more relaxed, and your face especially becomes more attractive because it is not carrying chronic tenseness—the new face of yoga.

Diaries

"I thought I knew yoga, having taught it for 18 years. I was wrong. The first Resistance Flexibility exercise I tried from Bob's book, I thought: 'Damn, this stuff works, I have to start from the beginning.' My classes went from 50 people to 10 as I struggled to assimilate the resistance principle into my yoga classes but it felt so right. I was an Old World Apprentice slow-learning a true skill at the hands of master tradesmen. Daily my self-concept and self-conceit was being torn apart, the ego death was brutal. I'm so grateful."
EddieEllner@TheGeniusofFlexibility.com Resistance Flexibility Intern

"After 40 years of practicing yoga in many different ways…from exploring as a teenager with relaxation and animal poses to a very ambitious undertaking of all the traditions from Iyengar to Ashtanga to Viniyoga…being with the master teachers in India and living the way of life. In relation to the body and the postures, after a certain point of 'attaining a posture,' I began to tighten and restrict more than stretch. My body was building up scar tissue in the joints, for example in the hips and shoulders and spine, I was becoming more stiff and in pain. From the overstretching (taking the muscle to its longest range and then pushing and pulling it from there) the buildup of scar tissue was a self-protective mechanism to keep me from injuring my joints. As I had practiced the poses for many years nothing was changing."
KateRabinowitz@TheGeniusofFlexibility.com Resistance Flexibility Intern

"What a relief it was for me to learn that there was a more natural way to process tenseness then by trying to control myself and force myself to relax. Instead I have learned how to naturally generate tension while stretching, which then 'spends' my chronic tenseness, turning it into something that helps me get a better and more satisfying stretch. This new knowledge of how to process tenseness in a new way, thus relieving me of the process of having to control myself, was by itself enough to help me feel more relaxed. Putting the concept into practice while stretching made the physical act of stretching all the more enjoyable and leaves me feeling more relaxed than ever before. The more truly relaxed I am, the better I feel and look.
LutherCowden@TheGeniusofFlexibility.com Elite Resistance Flexibility Trainer

"I am shocked at how much tenseness I chronically carry in my body and face! I have been massaged, exercised, meditated, but the only thing that relieves this chronic tenseness is generating tension during a stretch. The more tension I can generate when I stretch, the more that is released in my face and body. Everyone becomes better looking from removing this chronic tenseness by Resistance Flexibility."
BerylHagenburg@TheGeniusofFlexibility.com Resistance Flexibility Intern

"When I first was exposed to Resistance Flexibility, at a presentation by Bob Cooley, I was surprised by how much exertion was involved. Bob had people in the room pair up and do a simple arm stretch on each other. Afterwards my arms were pumped up and at the same time felt lighter and more connected to my body. The sensation was pleasant, and unfamiliar. I knew something new was happening in my arms."
PatrickGregston@TheGeniusofFlexibility.com Resistance Flexibility Intern

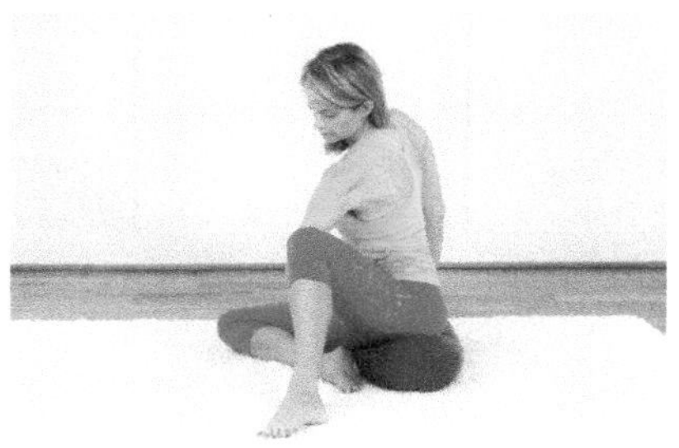

YOGA POSES ARE ARTISTIC CREATIONS

The classical yoga poses are works of art often by unknown artists.

I was never formally taught Yoga. Sure I looked at classic books on yoga, and immediately felt a deep respect for the lifetime commitments these special individuals had made. But I also needed tools for addressing my serious physiological and psychological traumas from early childhood and my automobile accident. I luckily got over some of my resistance to yoga, and one day in a yoga text I circled a bunch of what I thought looked like easy yoga poses. I tried to do them, but I could not do any of them—humiliating. I knew I was not very flexible but I didn't know I was that inflexible. Eeek! Instead I had to settle for five of the stretches that I had created for myself. I practiced them over and over and over again until I was flexible enough to develop others.

After creating my own stretches, a friend of mine came over to see them. She told me that after I stretched and ended in a final stretch position, that those positions were classical hatha poses. To configure my stretches I identified the necessity to exquisitely arrange my bones in precise rotational interrelationship. My hips had to turn one way, my thigh bone another, my lower leg, ankle and feet in others, etc. A unique combination of interrelated movements of my bones that were natural and comfortable for my body were essential. What I did to get into those final positions was not what people were saying to do when they taught yoga, but the end positions I created were yoga poses. I could have never have thought up those movements in spite of all the years I studied anatomy. I had to defer to my body and explore just how my bones wanted to be arranged in order to target specific muscle groups and unfold my yoga movements. I recognized that yoga positions are mapped in your body, and are waiting to be discovered.

I feel that everyone needs to practice flexibility exercises as if they are doing them for the first time. In the same way that I unknowingly recreated classical yoga poses—everyone can do this. It doesn't matter how you were taught to do yoga poses, recreate them…make them work for you…create your own natural versions. Find out how your bones and joints need to be organized relative to one another until you have a combination of arrangements that feel natural to you, and that position you to have great leverage for stretching specific muscles. You can be in repose to stretch or stretch isometrically or dynamically.

Diaries

"A friend of mine who's studied and taught yoga for 30 years was introduced to the resistance stretching of Bob Cooley and was so impressed she stopped teaching yoga and moved to Boston to study with Cooley full time. I realize my friend's decision was really a no brainer: the depth and potential of Cooley's work is profound: real flexibility training, the missing link in yoga and stretching. After a few weeks of awkwardly introducing resistance stretching into my own classes there really was no choice but to visit Cooley himself. The nine days I spent at his Boston studio confirmed the unprecedented value of his work. Simple movements, strong focus, big heart, big results.

"You'll recognize overlapping modalities in Cooley's work: yoga asana and Traditional Chinese Medicine as well as personality theories, and isometric exercise, but at it's heart Cooley's work embodies the heroic journey we all are taking to discover the essence of who we are. Bob is devoted to stretching people to their optimum physical, psychological, emotional, and spiritual health. At his studio, pro and Olympic athletes mingle with high schoolers, and senior citizens. There is no hierarchy, just a range of bodies seeking their maximum operational capacity. And there was heart, lots of it. There were many times that people paying good money interrupted their own session to help stretch others. It was more like a barn-raising, with each person's body as the barn, requiring the help of others to heal and complete itself. Cooley conducts a free flow sharing of insight and continuing education drawing perspective and wisdom from everyone in the situation not just from his own knowing. The emphasis is always on being open to going further with all parts of yourself."

EddieEllner@TheGeniusofFlexibility.com Resistance Flexibility Intern

"I tried a yoga class once, before I found Resistance Flexibility. I left the class feeling like a failure, as I was trying to fit my body into positions that I did not have true access to. I've learned through Resistance Flexibility that while each of the classical hatha yoga poses depict an ideal position, the value lies in where I'm at in relationship to that ideal. I love to get on the ground and defer to my body, moving in the ways that my body craves. As I continue to do this, I find every movement to be familiar and yet brand new at the same time. I may eventually find myself in the full expression of a classical hatha yoga pose, resisting and generating tension isometrically to get a stretch. Other times, I find myself going back to beginner style Resistance Flexibility movements, which allow for more natural movement of the muscle while stretching."

LutherCowden@TheGeniusofFlexibility.com Elite Resistance Flexibility Trainer

"I used to do yoga when I decided it was a good idea to get into shape and become more flexible. I started doing hatha yoga classes that were pretty basic, but always challenging. However, I found getting into many of the poses left me feeling confused and unsatisfied to a large degree. One of the great things I've been learned was to use Resistance Flexibility in these poses, and that allowed me to not only get into the poses safely, but get the most benefit from them. Using tension and resistance was the key to getting flexible in yoga. Knowing and utilizing what's happening with each limb, and the how those forces lead toward the next aspect of the pose has been not only clarifying physically, but also makes me appreciate the depth and sophistication of the yogic tradition that was developed thousands of years ago."

JohnBagdasarian@TheGeniusofFlexibility.com Resistance Flexibility Intern

THE BEST WAY TO TEST YOUR FLEXIBILITY

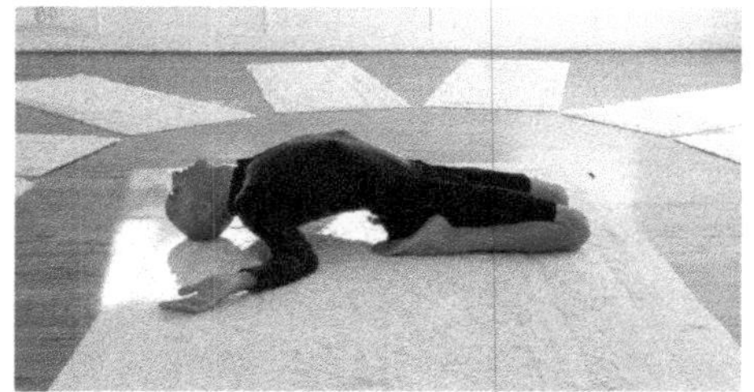
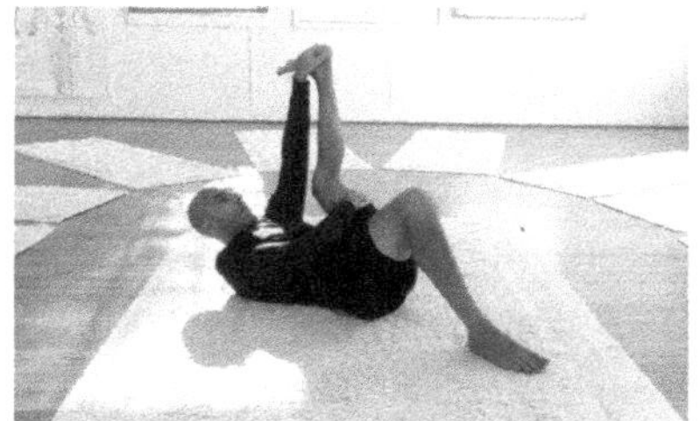
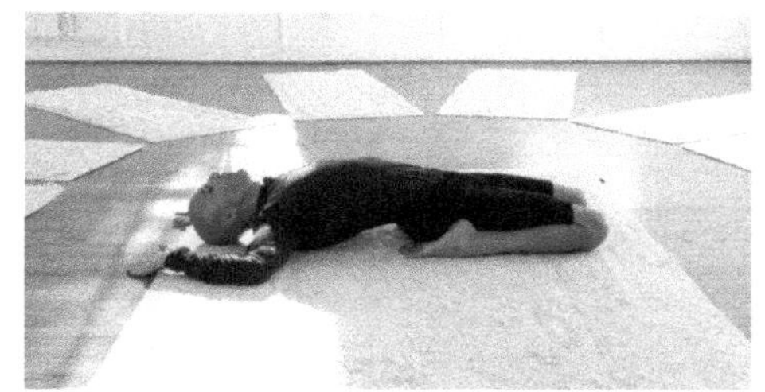

True flexibility versus range of motion (ROM).

In true flexibility the muscles are contracting while lengthening.

The best way to test your flexibility is not just by measuring your range of motion (ROM), but rather to measure the shortening capacity of the muscle. Why? Because when you simply measure your flexibility by your ROM, your bones can rotate substitutionally, and this presents false flexibility ranges. But also more importantly, because a muscle's ability to shorten is directly proportional to its ability to lengthen, you derive a truer measure of your flexibility by seeing how much the muscles can shortening where much less substitution occurs.

For example, when you do a forward bend, though your hamstrings obviously need to lengthen to decrease the distance of your hands down to the ground, your quads on the front of your hip need to shorten to help produce the forward bend. If your quads are not capable of shortening because they are not flexible enough, then you will not be able to get to closer to the ground even if your hamstrings can lengthen. So a forward bend is really a test of your quad flexibility!

The biggest limiting factor in any stretch position

is not the muscles that need to lengthen

but the capacity of the muscles that need to shorten

to bring you into the position.

Diaries

"What I find brilliant about Resistance Flexibility is the union of opposites that are facilitated by this practice. In one group, you have people who have extreme ranges of motion, which presents as extravagant movement or posture. But, people in this group often lack strength and integrity of movement in these ranges, and are often overextended in their joint structures, which leads to instability and potential injury. In an opposite group, you have people that have strength but are very limited in their range of motion, which is not ideal for movement either and can also lead to injury. The knowledge to differentiate r true flexibility and range of motion allows those in the first group to understand that they need to tense and resist while stretching and thus stay active throughout their range. This is where the gold is for them, and protects them from overstretching and injury while giving them true flexibility. Those in the second group can rest assured they aren't doomed to staying inflexible, because they can use their strength to get a great stretch by using their ability to contract the muscle through their current limited range of motion; which also results increases in true flexibility. Both groups gain much healthier myofascia tissues."
LutherCowden@TheGeniusofFlexibility.com Elite Resistance Flexibility Trainer

"True flexibility is your body's functional movement capacity. That means, it is not the simple range of motion that is your real flexibility, but instead your muscles ability to contract while elongating that is true flexibility. If you notice something is out of alignment during your movement there is no amount of thinking in your current state that will fix it, you have to give your body the ability to move freely by removing the ADFST, it has to be unwound…then your instincts take over and guide you in the right direction mindfully and effortlessly."
SamuelCamburn@TheGeniusofFlexibility.com Elite Resistance Flexibility Intern

"In the West, we have become conditioned to think that greater range of motion equals greater flexibility; that the farther we can coax our body to bend or reach, the better. This method can cause damage to our tendons, ligaments and joints due to over stretching. Instead, try keeping the contraction in the muscle while resisting. Your range may be less initially but you'll be on your way to true flexibility while keeping your joints healthy and happy."
Noël Christensen@TheGeniusofFlexibility.com Resistance Flexibility Intern

"I would have never imagined that people that appear to be so flexible are not necessarily flexible, the illusion fooled me. I have found from my own experiences now, that my flexibility shows up best when after Resistance Flexibility training a muscle group, I see just how much those muscles can shorten. That's the real test. Who would have ever guessed that a forward bend is a better measure of your quad flexibility and not your hamstring flexibility?"
TomLongo@TheGeniusofFlexibility.com Elite Resistance Flexibility Trainer

YOUR BRAIN AND BODY CONNECTION

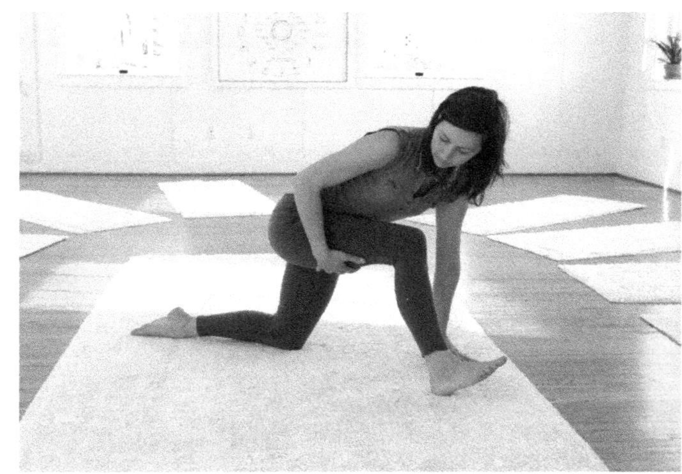

Your awareness guarantees that your brain knows what is happening in your body.

Everyone knows that their body is connected to their brain via their nervous system. And everyone knows that to turn on a light bulb, you have to switch on the light switch. Your brain is like that with your body. What's the light switch for your brain?

Your brain does not know that you are stretching a particular muscle unless you are aware of it! The light bulb doesn't simply turn on because its connected to the current, you obviously have to turn the switch on to get the light to turn on. The switch in you is your awareness for your brain. So when you pay attention to the area that you are stretching, it lights up, and then your brain knows about what is happening and can add its problem solving skills to help you get the best stretch.

Because your hands have many more receptors than your kinesthetic system inside your body, your brain can know much more about what you are stretching by touching those areas of your body. So when you stretch your hamstring, why not feel the back of your legs when you are stretching them? Or when you are being assisted by another person, why not feel those areas that they are stretching?

I found that a person that feels their hamstrings while they are stretching them can derive three times as fast a result than someone that doesn't!

Diaries

"When I stretch my hamstrings, my hand can feel so much better what is happening than me feeling inside my thigh kinesthetically. So I touch the back of my thigh when I stretch my hamstrings, and I'm convinced that I get faster results."
JohnKelly@TheGeniusofFlexibility.com Elite Resistance Flexibility Trainer

"I studied Feldenkrais and other somatic body techniques, and all of them point to the importance of being aware of yourself. I find that at any given moment when I stretch if I am not aware of the area that is getting stretched I don't achieve nearly the results as I do when I am aware. Now my awareness is not just about being with my body, it is also being aware of my instincts like fear, anger, anxiety and fright, about consciousness of other people's and my looks and desire, and about awareness of others lives and my own."
BobCooley@TheGeniusofFlexibility.com

"There have been many times when stretching where it is easy for me to detach from my body and simply rely on my natural resistance in order to continue making the required movements. This is nowhere close to as effective as having your focused attention on the connection to your nervous system. When detaching from the body and allowing natural resistance to take over, there is much less sensation of the stretching, as I have found myself relying on the scar tissue and ADFST to make the moment, which is not connected to the nervous system, thus taking away from the sensation of the stretch. So I have found for myself, time and time again, that when I keep my attention on my body, and the movement that it is doing, and the resistance that it is generating, I get loads more sensation. I no longer am "floating" through the stretch, but rather can now feel my body engaging and allowing more sensation to come into my body which even further exemplifies the stretch. The focus and connection to the nervous system is one of the many tricks that has helped me to find my body and the sensation of the stretches."
AlexNolte@TheGeniusofFlexibility.com

"The awareness piece is huge! It is a metaphor for our entire existence. Turning on the 'light switch' of awareness opens up an internal and external world that is always there, but that I had no way to access. Resistance Stretching is great because it gives you a concrete, reality-based thing to do: stretch your body. The more awareness I bring to my stretch, the more the more awareness I have in my life. I am more conscious of myself and the world around me—I find myself more aware of what I am doing while I am doing it and therefore more appropriate in my actions, rather than acting first and re-thinking it later. It really is true…you can't fix something that you are unaware of."
BerylHagenburg@TheGeniusofFlexibility.com Resistance Flexibility Intern

THE SECRET BEHIND RESISTANCE FLEXIBILITY

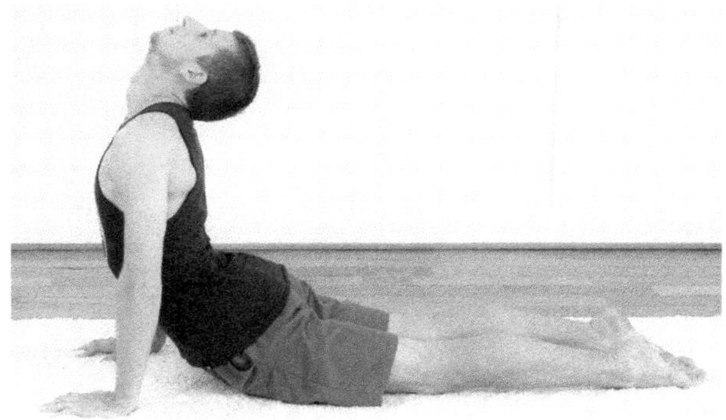

Be free with your attention.

Having a free attentional focus is explained as deciding to do something, and then that idea directs you to pay attention to things inside and outside yourself, and not you. It doesn't work for you to decide what to pay attention to unless the idea behind what you decided to do is directing you to do so. When you decide to do something, that idea guides you to collect the necessary information in the exactly the right order you need to learn things in order to master the thing you decided to do. At any moment when stretching, a person may be aware of the need to reposition, move, pay attention to certain things, breathe better, and awareness of energy.

In many physical, psychological, emotional, and spiritual practices, people are recommended to direct their attention. This simply doesn't work and greatly reduces the speed of learning. If you follow where your idea is directing you, you can master anything in three years. The Chinese call this: Learning the ten thousand things about any one thing. And little did they know that it takes precisely that number of molecules to pass from one axon to another to pass on a message.

The experiences you have with yourself and others when you stretch includes a vast arrange of thoughts and feelings that you may or may not understand initially but later often bring realizations.

Diaries

"For nearly ten years, I practiced yoga, and in nearly every posture, my sense of limit in my body was a spot on my left hip, right in the midst of my hip flexor. Even rotations on the other side of my body would seem to be limited by this other side sticky spot. Whatever the movement, I would be aware of this part of my body. When I learned RFST, I started experimenting with movements that would move this part of my tissue. After some time, I was able to identify the combination of flexion, adduction and rotation, and recruit others to help me achieve these movements with the forces required to change my fascia. Once this was known, and the people were helping me, it only took about 15 movements to break this free. The person leading the stretch could feel it letting go. The sensation was a sense of relief. However there was another side to this new condition. The next time I went to yoga, as I moved into the half moon pose standing on my left leg, instead of balancing on that left leg, my body pitched forward and I caught my fall with my arms. The muscles that normally would support standing on my left leg were weak, and untrained. I was totally surprised to realize that for years that same soft tissue impediment to all those other movements, was what I had been leaning on when doing half moon. It took a month of strengthening and learning to use those muscles to regain that posture. The path to a truly flexible body can be surprising."
PatrickGregson@TheGeniusofFlexibility.com Resistance Flexibility Intern

"RFST has been pivotal in helping me heal my concussions from Hockey hits and past car accidents. Has helped me greatly in getting my life back back and to my improve memory, being able to have thoughts come into my mind and instead of struggling to find the thought. I remembered feeling an underlying bother each day, always feeling charged and a little on edge from the event of the concussion. This would make my body tense up go into fight or flight mode feeling like Needed to defend myself even though I was no longer in the accident. This I experienced by not being able to handle normal daily stress as well and having reactions to people with escalation of anger. There was also an added feeling of being Pulled in a hundred different directions to micromanage many operations my Brain would be able to do on its own if not injured. Also From the worked I have experienced Improvement in energy and relief of headaches and pressure on the side of my skull, which was really uncomfortable. Also have had upgrades in vision, and helped relieving depression I experienced that from the shock post concussion. Have also notice my body more connected as a whole to recruit more accurate movement from head to toe with improved dexterity in especially in extremities. I Feel huge amounts of relief and happiness to have come upon Bob's amazing RFST over three ago and learning its invaluable trade in becoming an Elite trainer at the studio in Boston."
ScottBottoroff@TheGeniusofFlexibility.com Elite Resistance Flexibility Trainer

"When I first considered what Bob said about attentional focus asking what you want of your mind and then following where you attention goes I had to try it. I was stretching and so I asked to learn about stretching. Then watched where I was led and paid attention to that. That first time and each time I have done this I have been led off on a good adventure. This time my attention went to the relationship between meridians and types. I found myself thinking about it in my sleep. So instead of ignoring the input as a distraction when it woke me up I considered the ideas and wrote them down

and diagramed them. Pages covered with numbers sketches and diagrams. Days of talking with people about what these connections meant, inspirations coming at odd times while stretching. Maybe new ideas and understanding do not often come from the center of what you know and how you know to learn. As I just follow my focus I am led off to new considerations and approaches to issues. Like paying attention to your peripheral vision or the wisdom whispered in the corners of your mind that you had previously ignored. What I started learning on that adventure in following attention focus has become one of the corner stones of my understanding of stretching. More importantly I acquired new ways of learning and connections with how I and think and process information. The process of following attentional focus fires up my life with exciting personal journey. It is like listening to what is going on when I did not before."

EricBeutner@TheGeniusofFlexibility.com Elite Resistance Flexibility Trainer

"It is such a relief to able to use the unprocessed tension I have stored away in my body. This is what happens during an assisted Resistance Flexibility stretch. It is a truly liberating feeling to have the force I generate internally met by a group of trainers as they remove ADFT from my muscle tissue. The ability to fully engage in a stretch allows me to process the stress I have stored in my body. As the stress leaves my body my face becomes much more relaxed and more fully expressive at the same time. To my surprise I often look 10 years younger and so much more relaxed. Love it! My low back is much more stable and has much less pain since I have been doing Resistance Flexibility self stretches and assisted stretches. I believe it is because my lateral hamstring is able to lengthen and shorten more efficiently which is allowing me to move with greater easy. If you have back pain like I've had back pain (not being able to walk at times) and so many people I know have had back pain, then please pass the word along about what I've discovered through Resistance Flexibility. I had NO idea that the inflexibility of my hamstrings was causing my low back problems. Who would have guessed? I had done yoga and stretching most of my adult life but still had back pain. From my first assisted RF stretch, I got more flexibility than in all the years I was trying to relax my hamstring while stretching. I finally understand that it takes tension and resistance to remove my chronic tenseness and resistance from my hamstrings. It wasn't surprised that Resistance Flexibility worked to deter my back pain but it was how fast it worked that surprised me. Coming to Resistance Flexibility from yoga I realized in yoga my focus had been on end range of motion without strength. It wasn't until I started Resistance Flexibility that I realized that my true flexibility incorporated strength. I was over stretching my joints in my yoga practice. Now when I practice yoga I make sure I am tensing and contracting my muscles while exploring traditional Hatha yoga poses. I may not touch my ankle in triangle but I now have stability at my hip girdle."

KatConnor-Longo@TheGeniusofFlexibility.com Resistance Flexibility Intern

SUMMARY OF RESISTANCE FLEXIBILITY IN YOGA

1. Muscles naturally contract and fascia resists when stretching—called Resistance Flexibility.

2. Naturally contracting and resisting when stretching results in immediate, cumulative, and permanent increases in flexibility and strength because of the permanent architectural changes in the fascia.

4. Fascia is not innervated like you muscles so even though your fascia is generating enormous resistance when Resistance Flexibility training, there is Zero Pain.

3. Naturally contracting and resisting when stretching helps to prevent you from over stretching, helps to achieve better biomechanical efficiency and natural posture, and prevent injury.

5. Resistance Flexibility testing of 16 *types* of stretches can be used to help you evaluate your physiological, psychological, emotional, and spiritual developments. Resistance Flexibility affects every *type* of tissue in your body.

6. It takes a community of people to heal one another. Being assisted when stretching greatly accelerates your rate of improvements. Also the perspective offered by others watching the effects of your stretching can help to define all the parameters of health that are possible.

7. There is a natural way to breathe for everything. So learn to defer to your body's way of breathing and learn to give up old habitual ways of breathing that don't work.

CHAPTER 3

FASCIA AND RESISTANCE FLEXIBILITY

Fascia has 2-6 X's the resistive force compared

to the strength of the muscle

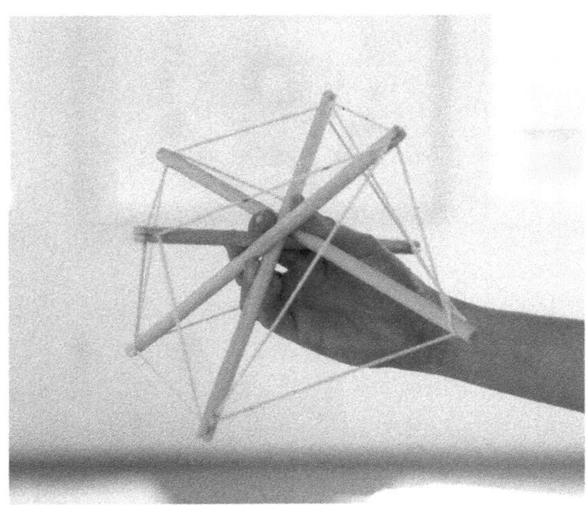

FASCIA

Fascia is like the soup stock

with muscles, tendons, skin, bones, ligaments, etc.

analogous to carrots, celery, potatoes, etc. within the soup.

And like the soup broth, the fascia penetrates into the vegetables

besides having its own layers.

Thus affecting the fascia dramatically affects all the other tissues.

You have your skin, a layer of fat, a thin layer of cellophane-like fascia, muscles, circulation, lymphatic vessels and nodes, nervous system, tendons, ligaments, joint capsules, cartilage, bones, fluid within the joints, and chemicals sourcing though your blood stream. And all those different *types* of tissues are separate EXCEPT the fascia isn't just separate. Based on Electron Microscopy, unlike all the other tissues that are more or less self-contained, the fascia roots into all the other tissues. The fascia roots into the muscles where the metabolism occurs, enters the ligaments, tendons, bone, joint capsules etc. The fascia connects everything, predates the nervous system, and has anti-gravity properties.

Diaries

"Learning about the fascia as a connective tissue that infiltrates all parts of the body from the organs, muscles, tendons and ligaments, bone, as well as the arterial anatomy has opened the door to an awareness of how the body works in both simple and complex ways. Understanding that this very essential material has such effect in our daily life has made it easier to converse and communicate about what I once thought to be difficult topics such as movement limitation, stuck areas in the body, or desires for physical improvements in strength and flexibility...which of course leads to more enjoyment and freedom in this exquisite and often challenging experience of living our life."
JohnBagdasarian@TheGeniusofFlexibility.com Resistance Flexibility Intern

"I've been practicing Resistance Flexibility for over a year and a half. I consider myself healthy and have always been active and fit. From years of Marathon running, I have accumulated much dense fascia in my legs. The other day I was being stretched by 2 Elite Trainers. We were on my left leg and doing some outside back of my leg (Bladder) stretches. They felt my resistance and we kept moving deeper into it. Upon their suggestion to "stay with it, and let go of the resistance," something shifted deep in my hip socket. I observed myself taking a deep breath in. It filled my whole body and I felt like I had never inhaled before! The feeling was new to me, very satisfying and emotionally fulfilling. I had experienced integrating into the emotional part of myself through a Bladder stretch! It's fantastic. I even see the change in my face...looking more beautiful! and it's STILL with Me! Really, I'm still with me!"
MimiAmrit@TheGeniusofFlexibility.com Resistance Flexibility Intern

"Fascia is not something that most anyone has ever heard about before they are introduced to Resistance Flexibility in their first session. When the trainer has a person strengthen their triceps, they can of course feel their muscle contract and shorten. But when they are told to allow their body to tense and resist naturally when the trainer did Resistance Flexibility on their triceps, they don't feel anything. But when they looked at the trainer trying to flex their elbow to stretch their triceps, the trainer can hardly do it. Now how does that make sense, most people think? Everyone learns very quickly that their fascia is generating the resistance when they stretch and not mostly their muscles, but the fascia is not giving them the kind of sensation they get from their muscles. Duh, is what a lot of people say when discovering this. For years, this is what everyone watches their dog do when they stretch everyday, many times a day. They just never have given it much thought. Their dog and cat were trying to teach they how to stretch."
BobCooley@TheGeniusofFlexibility.com

FASCIA AND FLEXIBILITY

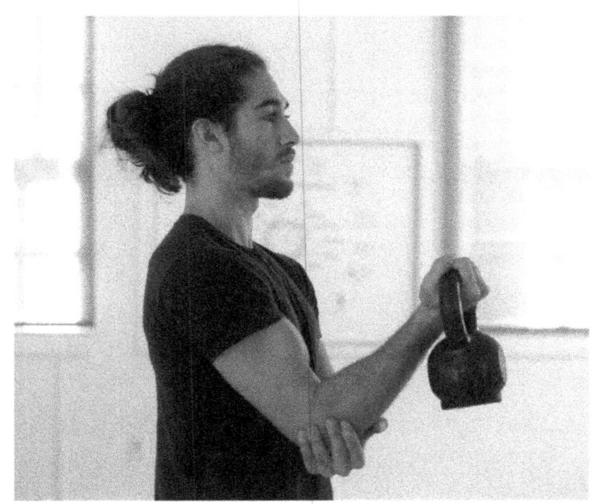

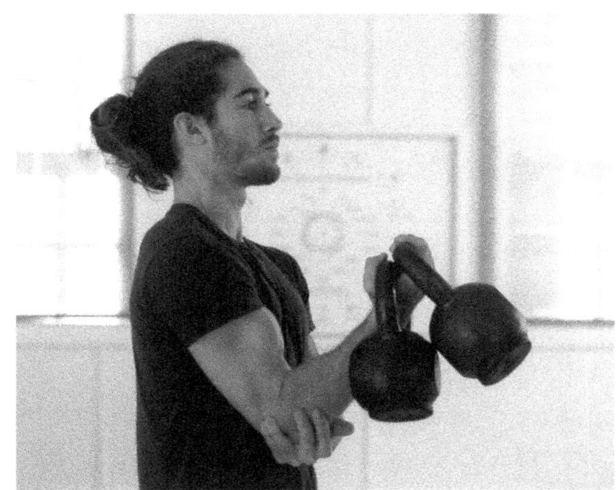

Photo 1: Brian is lifting the weight. Photo 2: But Brian can lower 2-6 X's the amount of weight he can lift. Why? Because the fascia when being stretched has 2-6X's the resistive force as the strength of the muscle.

Your fascia determines if your muscles can move you.

When you traditionally 'yank' on muscles when you stretch little happens to increase your flexibility, but when you defer to your body and allow your muscles to contract and tense, and your fascia resist while stretching like all other animals on the planet, you become immediately, cumulatively and permanently more flexible. Why?

Based on clinical trials, Resistance Flexibility in most of the medical literature is called excessive eccentric loading, the benefits include significant flexibility and strength gains, higher jumping, range of motions, improved balance while using low metabolic and cardiovascular costs. (See EEL ABSTRACTS CHAPTER 16)

While this muscular contraction naturally happens when you stretch, and because the fascia is rooted into the muscles, as the muscle lengthens the fascia is stretched in one of eight possible directions. This stretching of the fascia results in dramatic changes in its structure and consistency. The fascia regains its elasticity by becoming more hydrated, accumulated excess dense fascia and/or scar tissue (ADFST) is obliterated. And while the resistive force of the fascia when it is stretched is 2-6 X's the strength of the muscle itself, there is little to no sensation of the resistive force it is generating. Why?

Though your muscles, tendons, ligaments, joint capsule, etc. all produce sensation for people to feel when they are being stretched, the fascia is not the same. The fascia does not have the same receptors as the other tissue, so there is very little sensation when it is being affected. Because of this though the fascia and especially accumulated dense fascia and scar tissue (ADFST) has 2-6 X's the resistive force compared to the muscle's strength, there is little to no sensation, zero pain, and everyone is always surprised when they look at themselves in the mirror after stretching or being assisted and they see results they were not expecting.

Diaries

"The first light bulb that went off for me with this work was tensing a muscle as you lengthen the way animals do. I always felt animals were being physical way better then we were, or at least we have a lot to learn from them. I had moments of experiencing these phenomena on my own but could never articulate what or how I was doing it. I love the way my body feels when I move with resistance. And more so now I know what it's physiologically doing to my tissue by removing fascia."
Chris Pearsall@TheGeniusofFlexibility.com Resistance Flexibility Intern

"It is beyond remarkable that not until now has anyone I know of discovered that flexibility is mostly about the fascia needing to be repaired and not a joint or muscle issue, and the best way to do that is through natural stretching. I would probably never have discovered this is my life. Wow. What a life changer. I am not just more physically flexible, but I am as they told me I would be, becoming flexible in all ways."
TomLongo@TheGeniusofFlexibility.com Elite Resistance Flexibility Intern

"My first experience of this type of movement, contracting and then overcoming that contraction with force, was instantly a revelation. My limbs felt both lighter and more connected at the same time. The sensations of energy moving through my legs were like getting new, yet familiar information. The changes in mobility that happened with those first movements were exciting, as gaining just a bit of new mobility gave me the sense that if I could change this, I could accomplish anything."
PatrickGregston@TheGeniusofFlexibility.com Resistance Flexibility Intern

"Every time I go look in the mirror at what I think is going to be the changes from being assisted Resistance Flexibility trained, I am shocked. The changes are so much more dramatic. I experienced so little happening when being assisted even though I always see the assisters seriously struggling to move my legs, arms or trunk. But I stand up and the changes are always big changes not small changes. My bones have repositioned, my shape has changed, and my face is more relaxed. I mean it looks like I had cosmetic surgery, my face is totally smooth, with tight skin, my wrinkles have been removed and they were only working on the muscles in my arms, neck and shoulders. I also see the world differently, my perception has changed. I don't feel the same about people I see regularly. I'm more open, more accepting, and I have more objective perspective. And these results carry over into my life. They change the way I am being with people, the life decisions I make. Everything that was stopping me, things I was stuck on are freed."
TomLongo@TheGeniusofFlexibility.com Elite Resistance Flexibility Trainer

IT'S NOT MOSTLY ABOUT THE MUSCLE...

IT'S ABOUT THE FASCIA.

Flexibility: It's mostly about the fascia and not about the muscle.

Resistance flexibility is more of a subtractive technology.

Zero pain and stiffness from Resistance Flexibility techniques.

Totally unexpected concomitant benefits from Resistance Flexibility.

RF results in a reconstitution, transfiguration, reconstruction,

renovation, regeneration, vitalization, and transformation of the fascia.

Fascia is the web of life and holds your trauma and beliefs.

Your muscles move you, the joints ultimately determine your range of motion, but your fascia's health determines whether you can move all the parts in natural ways. When you remove damaged fascia, your joints have freedom of range of motion again, your muscles are no longer enjailed, and your circulation and lymphatic flow.

Your fascia unlike your muscles has considerably less nerves sending information to your brain about what is happening. The fascia and especially the scar tissue are not connected to your brain in the same way. There is almost no sensation when you stretch the fascia and scar tissue even though the resistive force is 2-6 X's the strength of your muscles!! And thus though you are using 2-6X's the force to stretch your fascia, their is zero pain! This 2-6 X's resistive force feels like nothing and is being generated by the natural resistive force of fascia when it is being stretched.

No sensation when stretching the fascia

yet 2-6 X's the strength of the muscle.

The cooperation between the muscle's strength and the fascia is essential to feel. The muscles need to be able to contract well enough so that the fascia that is rooted into the muscle can be transfigured when it is being stretched during a stretch. Without sufficient muscle contraction the fascia is not changed as well. So both the muscle and the fascia play their part in flexibility and depend on each other. Sometimes you need more strengthening of the muscle first, and sometimes you need to resistance flexibility train first. It's a cyclical relationship.

ACCUMULATED DENSE FASCIA AND SCAR TISSUE (ADFST)

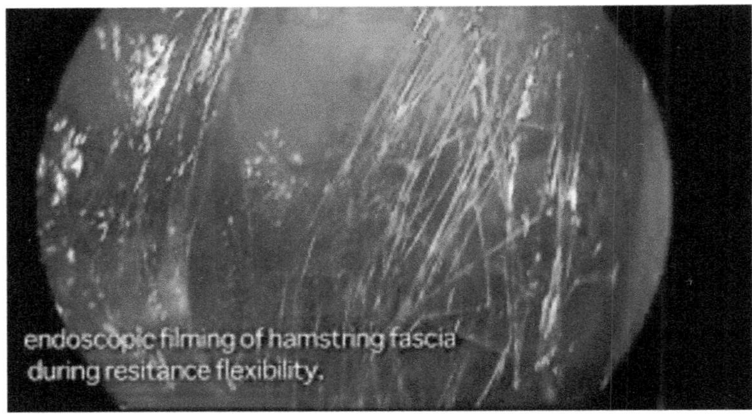
endoscopic filming of hamstring fascia
during resitance flexibility.

FASCIA (Photos by Dr. Jean Claude Guimberteau)

This 2-6 X's resistive force that the fascia and scar generates while stretching it is the amount of force necessary to return your fascia to its healthiest state. Simply yanking on your muscles or trying to get them to forcibly relax is counterproductive. And if you try to use this amount of force from outside your body in an attempt to change your fascia through deep tissue work, instead of that enormous amount of force being generated naturally from inside yourself by the fascia, you would not be able to tolerate the pain involved. Yet when you naturally resist while stretching that same force feels like nothing and painlessly transforms your fascia and increases your flexibility and the health of all the tissues in your body. All the other tissues that the fascia roots into are also changed. That means when you stretch naturally, you affect the health of all the other types of tissues in your body, your tendons, ligaments, circulatory system, lymphatic vessels and nodes, bones, etc. Your circulation increases, your tendons, ligaments and joint capsule become more springy and morphable, your lymphatic flow increases, your lymph nodes shine, your nerve linings are cleared, etc. WOW.

Once the tissues are warmed up, maximal tension and resistance are generated by the client while they are stretching or being stretched. It often requires 2-6 people to assist someone during resistance flexibility, especially to remove scar tissue within the myofascial structures.

There is ZERO PAIN during Resistance Flexibility training

and absolutely no discomfort in the joint structures.

Diaries

"It made sense to me that my physical flexibility would increase with Resistance Flexibility. I was surprised to find when playing music my memory got significantly better, as did the speed at which I learned new pieces."
KajHoffman@TheGeniusofFlexibility.com Resistance Flexibility Elite Intern

"As the overly dense fascial tissue is removed from my shoulders and back, the burdens and baggage that I've carried for my whole life get lifted away. I feel energized and strong. I stand tall because the world is full of possibilities. My eyes are open and I'm alive."
NickWare@TheGeniusofFlexibility.com Elite Resistance Flexibility Trainer

"When you apply the fact that fascia isn't connected to the nervous system in the same manner as muscle and other tissues, and add in the idea that your fascia is a physical place in your body that stores your history, then breaking down fascia will release those experiences when you stretch. For me, this meant a constant set of reminders of events from my past from benign incidents from childhood, including broken bones, to being dumped by grade school crushes that are in my fascia. Sometimes the release is dramatic, with tears and feelings from the events themselves, and other times just a fleeting physical sensation. Mostly however is a sense of wonder, that this event in my life has come to mind, and I am being released to live again in new ways."
PatrickGregston@TheGeniusofFlexibility.com Resistance Flexibility Intern

"Since being introduced to Resistance Flexibility, I've been much more curious about the nature and function of fascia. I had learned about it before, but never really got a grasp of its function and role. I've been especially fascinated by the connection I've noticed between the release of fascia in my body during Resistance Flexibility, and the release of stored memories, stories, and traumas from my past. Many times when I'm getting a deep stretch, and especially when I get brought to places I haven't been before in a stretch, I have seemingly random memories from my past and/or strong waves of feelings that come clearly to the surface. Sometimes these memories are immediate, sometimes they may take a day or two to surface. Because of experiences like this, I see my body much like water, or a crystal, holding and storing information from its surroundings and history since birth. Recently I was getting my left hip flexor stretched by 5 women when I was overcome, quite suddenly, with an intense wave of fear and flashes of a deeply buried abuse from my childhood. Having them there to hold space and bridge me into the reality of what was really happening at that moment was incredibly supportive and healing. I had done some work already with the trauma that came to light, but never was able to access it so clearly in my body or to release it in the way I felt I did that day. After I had an incredible sense of renewed freedom and strength that lasted for days."
Luca Cupery@TheGeniusofFlexibility.com Resistance Flexibility Intern

"Whether I am stretching someone or getting stretched, I am always amazed at the force involved. On the giving end, the person stretching has a vague look of effort, but we the stretches are wincing and using all of our might to move the ADFST in the target muscle group. On the receiving end, I feel the vagueness of a stretch that Bob talks about. It is more of a 'face-less' force. It feels like nothing."
BerylHagenburg@TheGeniusofFlexibility.com Resistance Flexibility Intern

TENSEGRITY MATRIX AND FASCIA

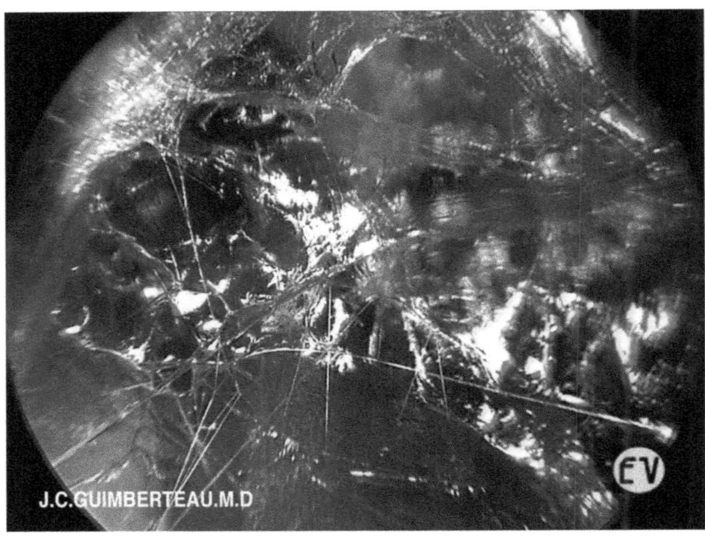

FASCIA (Photos by Dr. Jean Claude Guimberteau)

Cooley's tensegrity fascia model™ reflects the basis for the myofascial

training and rehabilitative therapeutic modality called Resistance Flexibility.

The model addresses the three-dimensional 8 permutational kinematic patterns

for the lower and upper body,

and addresses biomechanical principles for

balancing and opposing muscle groups,

and bilateral symmetrical balancing of muscles groups.

The *tensegrity* matrix of the fascia requires that the resistance flexibility movements be three-dimensional. There are 16 kinetic patterns used in RF, three-dimension movement patterns are utilized for 8 lower body and 8 upper body muscle groups. Flexion/Extension, Abduction/Adduction, Inward/Outward Rotation combinations are utilized. Individual muscle groups or whole groups of muscles can be stretched at the same time. Balancing muscle groups must always be included during the stretch of the target muscle group. These three dimensional kinematic patterns are concomitant with Meridian Muscle Groups (MMG) and Meridian pathways in Traditional Chinese Medicine (TCM).

Cooley's tensegrity fascia model™ is a polyhedron with fully triangulated surfaces including only four compressed struts (repulsion), and with prestressed tension members (attraction) with a right handed twist. This tensegrity model is formed because of the requirement of the fascia to be able to move three dimensionally with six degrees of freedom whose eight permutations established Cooley's 16 Kinematic Patterns™ for the lower and upper body.

Cooley's elastic model helps to explain the otherwise current chaotic description of fascia movement with a placable functioning unit for movement in eight directions. Vertices, tension elements, or compression elements may be shared so that this tensegrity unit can connect and create a chain of tensegrity units allowing for an infinite variety of shapes all acting as one in the myofascialskeletal system of contiguous muscle groups.

Dr Jean-Claude Guimberteau films confirm and illustrated books, present a groundbreaking work, and explain its significance for manual therapists and movement teachers, and its implications for what they do with patients and clients. They show the continuity of fibres throughout the body and how adjacent structures can move independently in different directions and at different speeds while maintaining the stability of the surrounding tissues. He has opened a window into a strange world of fibrillar chaos and unpredictable behavior, and has revealed the morphodynamic nature of the fibrils that constitute the connective tissue, as well as the fractal, non-linear behavior of these fibrils.

Dr Jean-Claude Guimberteau is co-founder of the *Institut Aquitain de la Main,* and past-President 2011-2012 of the French Society for Plastic and Reconstructive Surgery (SOFCPRE). He is the first person to film living human tissue through an endoscope in an attempt to understand the organization of living matter. He has developed his own concept of the multifibrillar structural organization of the body, of which the *microvacuole* is the basic functional unit. He has also developed a concept of global dynamics and continuous matter.

Dr Jean-Claude Guimberteau is the author of *Architecture of Human Living Fascia—The extracellular matrix and cells revealed through endoscopy.* See more at: http://www.handspringpublishing.com/our-authors/jean-claude-guimberteau/#sthash.pxvoGEmN.dpuf

Through endovivo.com he has published many videos on fascia: *Strolling under the skin, 2005; Skin excursion, 2008; Muscle Attitude, 2009; Interior Architectures, 2011; Skin, Scars and Stiffness, 2012; and Destination Tendon, 2012.*

OH THOSE HAMSTRINGS and LOW BACK PAIN NO MORE

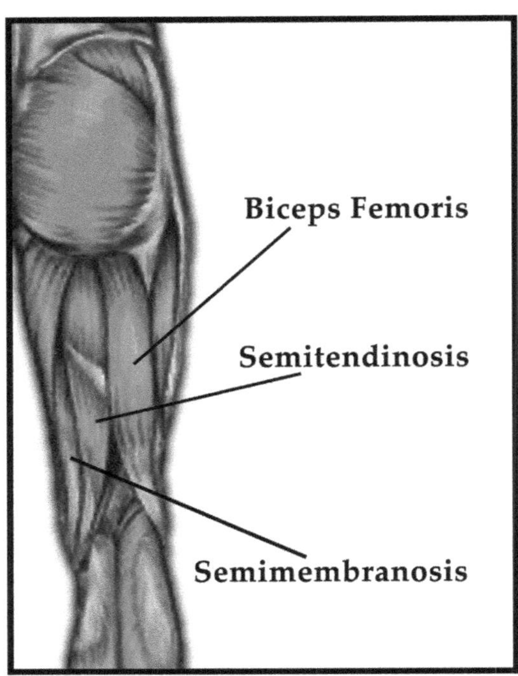

The largest amount of ADFST is in everyone's lateral hamstrings, regardless of age, sex, nationality, race, or preferences of any kind, based on international travel to more than twenty countries.

When everyone comes to our centers with their vast array of health concerns, regardless of what those concerns are, we always recommend for them to stretch their lateral hamstrings. It is an ongoing joke with everyone that knows Resistance Flexibility, that no matter what you have as a concern, Resistance Flexibility training your lateral hamstring will help.

Your hamstring are 3 in numbers, actually what I like to call 3 and 1/2 (the 1/2 being the short head of the Biceps Femoris). All the 3 big guys attach from the bottom of your pelvis and then two traverse to attach on the inside of your lower leg and one attaches on the outside of your lower leg. All three extend your pelvis, extend your thigh, and flex your lower leg. But the two on the inside also adduct your thigh or hip, and the one on the outside abducts your thigh or hip. And most importantly, the two on the inside inward rotate your thigh, and the one on the outside outward rotates your thigh. Their rotational action has big affects on your lower body.

Your three hamstring each affect different joints in you lower body. If your lateral hamstring that again has the most accumulated dense fascia and scar tissue (ADFT) in the human population of all muscles, has too much ADFST then your lower back is at risk. Why? Because the lateral hamstring when flexible extends your pelvis up onto your legs and allows your spine to stack on your pelvis. If your lateral hamstrings are too inflexible and weak, then you collapse in your lower back and this can produce lower back pain!

So the solution to most low back pain

is to increase the resistance flexibility and strength

of your lateral hamstrings.

Remember this, remember this, and tell everyone please.

Now, most people have never counted the number of repetitions or revolutions their legs make when riding their bike 5 or so miles but you can imagine that number is not a few hundred but in the thousands. So if you need to make this number of repetitions to ride a bike, you may be open to knowing that you may need to do thousands of hamstring stretches to win. We call that the 500 club for people that do 500 each day most days of the week.

Oh, and your two other hamstrings also have big affects. Your most medial hamstring determines how much rotation you have at your hip joint. So to avoid hip replacements, your medial hamstrings need to be flexible so that your fascia suspends your hip joint instead of compressing it. The compression can result in hip joint distress and destruction.

So the solution to your hip joint problems

is to increase the resistance flexibility and strength

of your medial hamstrings.

Dance and run to your hearts content. Tell everyone.

And your central hamstrings control your knees. So if you want to have great knees and avoid knee replacement, keep your central hamstring flexible and strong.

So the solution to your knee problems

is to increase the resistance flexibility and strength

of your central hamstrings.

Twist and untwist all you want. Tell everyone.

Diaries

"If you have back pain like I did and so many people I know have, then please let them know what I discovered—that my hamstring inflexibility was resulting in my low back problems. Who would have guessed? I had done yoga and stretching most of my adult life but still had back pain. When I found out about Resistance Flexibility and tried my first stretch, I got more flexible than in all the years I was trying to relax my hamstring while stretching. It only makes sense to me now that it takes tension and resistance to remove my chronic tenseness and resistance, like homeopathic theory. But it is not that it worked to get rid of my back pain, it is how fast it worked."
Anonymous

"When I first started stretching, I couldn't really discern if my hamstrings were stretching or not…I just couldn't feel anything for the most part. After a bit of consistent RF, I have come to feel what's it's like to actually 'feel' my tightness, rather than noticing or measuring by some outside context, and it's giving me greater insight into what I need to do to upgrade my physicality."
JohnBagdasarian@TheGeniusofFlexibility.com Resistance Flexibility Intern

"Before I started practicing Bob Cooley's Resistance Flexibility, I was continually perplexed and frustrated by my hamstrings. They always felt so stiff, like there was a deep, almost numbing cold stuck in the back of my legs. It seemed nothing I did would make a lasting change in the tightness in my body, even though all through my pre-professional and professional career I was the 'good' dancer; stretching and doing strength exercises while waiting for my turn in rehearsal, before and after warm-up class, in bed before going to sleep, fanatical really. I also practiced yoga almost everyday, had acupuncture sessions (which helped my energy a lot), received massage, all which gave temporary relief. After all this effort and care, I couldn't understand why my hamstrings and other parts of my body were still feeling so terrible. I knew when my knees started aching and my neck would throw out every other week that something had to give. At that moment, a friend lent me Bob's book. I did one stretch, adding resistance as I moved on the pathway of the muscle I was working, and I knew there was something to this!!! I immediately felt relief. I realized that previously my body naturally knew to resist at the end range of a stretch but that I was repeatedly over stretching and was much too hyper-mobile. Bob's discovery of contracting a muscle for the extent of its range changed everything for me. With a little help, my injuries from overusing my body for my entire life are now gone, just a few more tune ups to go. When dancing, the freedom in movement I am now blessed with translates into ultimate connection with audience, the divine, and myself. Time stops, I have everything and nothing all at once. And that is good."
BonnieCrotzer@TheGeniusofFlexibility.com Elite Resistance Flexibility Trainers

"Oh God, can you help me with my hamstrings? Seems like everyone's hamstring are the most inflexible things in the world. I have been trying to self Resistance Flexibility train my hamstrings and I like the results but having other people Resistance Flexibility assist me with my hamstrings is the best thing I have ever discovered. My low back doesn't hurt anymore, not just no pain, but I can jump higher, fold in half better, and I'm not sure yet, but I notice I am more conscious of being more honest and know how to emotionally defend myself better. I also make more money that is supposedly associated with my lateral hamstrings. Will confirm with you later about that. Thanks."
Anonymous

"I never EVER would have realized how much the problem of my hamstrings were contributing to much of my discomfort and pain. And not just for me, but for everyone!

"It seems funny but the ongoing joke is when in doubt, stretch your hamstrings! But it's amazing—the results I've seen in this area. My pelvis extends so my back pain completely dissipates. Miraculous. Not the idea, but the simplicity and completeness of it happens so quickly by using Resistance Flexibility."
ChrisPearsall@TheGeniusofFlexibility.com Resistance Flexibility Intern

"My quads and hamstrings were very tight always. I could never touch my toes. I would do hamstring stretches every day but almost nothing happened. However, not just conventional passive stretching, but when I learned to contract my hamstrings while stretching them as I resisted during the stretch everything changed. After awhile I could touch my toes, and I stood up straighter! But not only physical changes, I got physiological changes. I had more clarity of thought, I was so much more clear! I was able to problem solve things in my life, which I never had done before and I experienced this inner contentment that I had never experienced before. I had been excited in my life but this was different, it was coming from within! I know now the central hamstring represents the brain meridian! It was like I was in the Wizard of Oz and I was granted a brain for the first time. My quads were so tight that I could never sit on my feet without feeling that my knees would pop out and explode...the more I stretched and changed my quads the more access I had to them. Also I have more access to words that naturally flow from within me, where before I believed I had to go out and get them. I have more self-awareness. I was becoming more analytical instead of conceptual and my life is becoming easier! I had more tools and access to things I never knew existed. Bob and stretching with The Genius of Flexibility has changed my life in so many profound ways! I am hooked forever!"
RobObrien@TheGeniusofFlexibility.com Resistance Flexibility Intern

"As I self stretch and get assisted to remove the dense tissue in my hamstrings... I can feel the thawing and decompressing happen in my lower spine. I feel like a house that has been listing over from the foundation and little by little is getting propped up by my increasing the flexibility in my lateral hamstrings. I still have more to go, but it is remarkable to know how to directly experience the power my hamstrings have over my spine and how to heal myself by myself and with the help of others."
BerylHagenburg@TheGeniusofFlexibility.com Resistance Flexibility Intern

"For me, with Resistance Flexibility, I am able to bring that list of awareness from all of the muscles in my body, to my brain, it's quite amazing. It's like a beautiful gift you never expected to be greeted with. On top of that, the awareness has given me back my authority in my own body. It has also given me authority in my life. Resistance Flexibility is the signal most morphing body-work I have ever come in contact with. Before Resistance Flexibility, I had pain in my joint structures that I had learned to live with. I no longer have any pain in my joints, plus, I have overall muscle health and that is showing up for me as a more youthful body. I am 50 and I feel better than I did in my 20's. As my awareness increases it shows up in my organs as well. I am able to feel the effects of the foods I eat and how my organs are processing that food. I have felt an increase in energy flow inside my body. I have also received a greater awareness of the world and people around me. I am just scratching the surface of Resistance Flexibility and it has been quite life changing."
KarenMason@TheGeniusofFlexibility.com Resistance Flexibility Intern

"Stripping away layers of fascia and ADFST is similar to pruning a plant. When pruning a plant you strip away the brown, dead, unhealthy, vegetation, bringing more overall health to the entire plant. Life is then rerouted to the flourishing, parts of the plant. The brain of the plant is no longer confused, wasting time sending energy to useless dead growth. The plant can focus on bringing forward more health to the parts that are alive. Scar tissue and dense fascia can be stripped from the muscles as well, by using Resistance Flexibility. When the layers of fascia and scar tissue are stripped away, the health can increase in those areas. The muscles can become more hydrated and the organs and absorb more. With Resistance Flexibility, like the plant, the brain can focus on sending energy to the areas of the body and produce more health in those areas. The body then begins to flourish and become stronger and healthier. I have received outstanding results using Resistance Flexibility. I was able to remove scar tissue in my shoulders by getting assisted stretches. I have amazing range of motion (ROM) and I am experiencing so much comfort in my body, mush better sleep and better functioning of all my organs. I can feel the stripping away of constrictions in my body and also then that has reflected in stripping away constrictions in my life. What is happening for me on the inside has expanded to my outside life as well. The result is overwhelmingly satisfying and has given me a new relationship with my life."
KarenMason@TheGeniusofFlexibility.com Resistance Flexibility Intern

CHAPTER 4

TRAUMA AND SCAR TISSUE

Removing Scar Tissue, AND Replacing It With A Gift

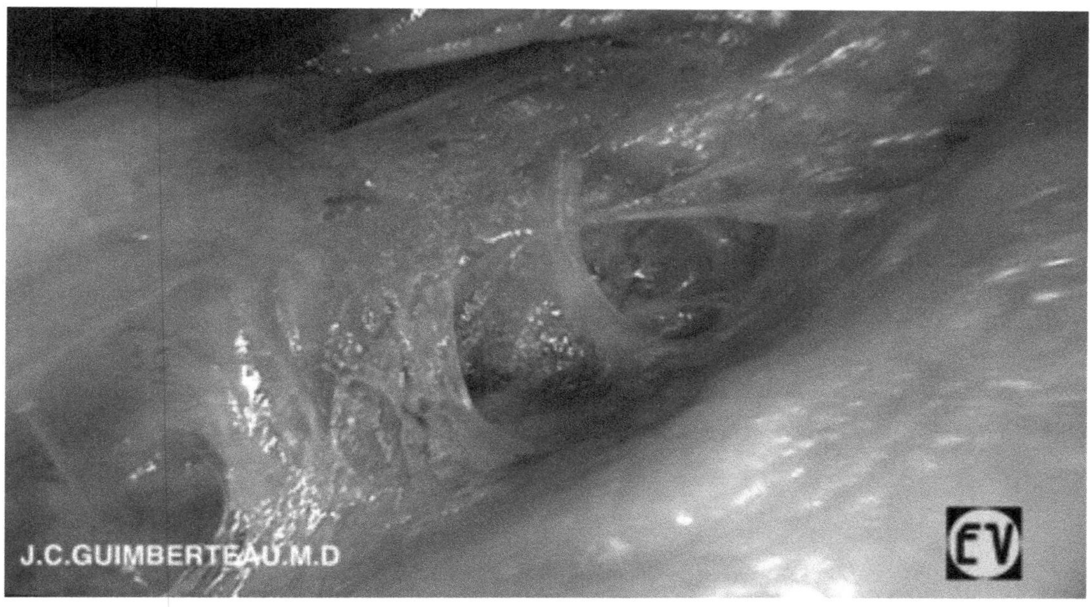

Scar Tissue (Photos by Dr. Jean Claude Guimberteau)

SCAR TISSUE

Obviously scar tissue does not have innervation, it is like a splinter in your skin, your nervous system does not grow new nerves to the scar tissue. Sure you can feel the splinter because of pain receptors in the surrounding tissues but you don't feel the splinter from nerves in it. The same is true for scar tissue.

The important thing about scar tissue is that its tensile strength, its ability to resist elongation, far exceeds the tensile strength of your ligaments, tendons, and joint capsules. So when you remove the scar tissue naturally by Resistance Flexibility, you will have no direct sensation of it being removed except for feelings from its surrounding tissues. A vague feeling of that area being stretched through the other tissues.

The forces that the person's tension and resistance creates during the resistance flexibility greatly exceed the forces that could ever be tolerated if those forces were administered from outside the person such as during deep tissue massage or Rolfing. Resistance Flexibility is a way to generate the extreme forces necessary to remove accumulated dense fascia and scar tissue (ADFST).

THE AMOUNT OF FORCE NECESSARY TO CHANGE THE FASCIA CANNOT BE TOLERATED IF ADMINISTERED FROM OUTSIDE THE PERSON IN DEEP MASSAGE OR ROLFING, BUT CAN OCCUR WITH ZERO PAIN WITH RESISTANCE FLEXIBILITY.

What is Scar Tissue compared to accumulated dense fascia? Scar tissue has significantly more adhesions into any types of other tissues and can pervasively affect the health of those tissues. Scar tissue can multiply in not just myofascia tissue but in organs, circulatory systems, joint capsules, bones, etc. Accumulated dense fascia refers to normal fascia that has undergone trauma that has resulted in its natural elastic properties being negatively altered. Accumulated dense fascia can show up as a dehydration, disorientation, aberrations in form and function of the fascia.

Scar Tissue takes over the real estate for muscles and other tissues. The muscles, tendons, ligaments, etc. when invaded by scar tissue can no longer have room to move or function. Removal of the scar tissue results in immediate increases in circulation and lymphatic flow and the ability to build the strength of the muscles which otherwise have no room to expand.

Scar tissue can be in any of the 16 types of tissues. Some people have scar tissue more in their muscle others in their tendons, or circulation etc. But regardless of where it is, Resistance Flexibility can help to regenerate those different *types* of tissues. Remember the scar tissue has 2-6 X's the resistive force as the strength of the muscle. So the tensile strength of the fascia exceeds the other types of tissues.

Scar tissue feels like anti-life and when your remove it, you immediately feel more alive and step back into life again. But that's not all that happens. When you remove scar tissue, the part of you that was thwarted during its residence, can now develop with gusto. And this means, that some extraordinary talents or gifts develop.

Scar Tissue requires other people to transform it. Because the scar tissue redirects movement, when being assisted the assister needs to know when the joint is directing the movement and the natural structural limitations in movement or when the scar tissue has taken over and detours all you movements regardless of all your mental attempts to make the right movement. An Elite Resistance Flexibility Trainer can help you with your scar tissue.

Diaries

"I never realized how much of a role scar tissue played in a persons well being until I started seeing people with lots of scar tissue as Resistance Flexibility trained people. The amount of force it takes to move someone along a path with ADFST is insane. But what's impressive is how little effort they need to exert for us to move them; the scar tissue creates all the resistive force not the person effort. Understanding more about TCM also unlocks knowing how this would obviously greatly disrupt the flow of energy on its meridian pathway through the body."
ChrisPearsall@TheGeniusofFlexibility.com Resistance Flexibility Intern

"At age thirteen, my daughter suffered a serious injury in a surfing accident. The fin of her surfboard cut five inches across her thigh and three layers deep, down to the muscle. In the first few years following the accident it became clear that her leg was likely to give her trouble throughout her lifetime. The quadriceps muscle had atrophied significantly and was not able to build strength or mass despite many hours of physical activity. The area surrounding the scar was still numb to light touch and any pressure was unbearably painful. The scar tissue caused by the trauma limited the leg's ability to return to its full function, and I knew that over time the dysfunction of the muscle would create problems in other parts of her body. Based on my training and personal experience with Resistance Flexibility, I was able help my daughter avoid these problems in her future. Through a combination of self stretching, assisted stretching from friends and family, and help from The Genius of Flexibility Trainers, she was able to break down the accumulated dense fascia and internal scar tissue without the pain or discomfort typically associated with physical therapy. Her leg is now pain-free, flexible and strong—relieved of the fascia and trauma that bound it. In fact she recently joined her college's long-distance intramural running team."
NoëlChristensen@TheGeniusofFlexibility.com Resistance Flexibility Trainer

"A critical thing RF taught me is that often where I most need to stretch—where there is dense fascia and scar tissue is in my body—I have little or no sensation. I used to try to stretch places where I felt discomfort, but that often irritated things rather than helping relieve problems. After RF Trainers helped me to identify areas in my body that need flexibility, and helped me to learn how I can stretch those areas without overtaxing others, I am much better able to resolve physical issues and develop the way I want."
KajHoffman@TheGeniusofFlexibility.com Elite Resistance Flexibility Intern

"I would never had imagined that it would take four skilled people to lift my leg to remove the scar tissue in my hamstrings. Each time they repeated the stretch, I could feel the scar tissue thin and weaken, until finally I began to feel more of my hamstring muscles contracting while stretching. When I stood up, my leg was under my body, supporting me for the first time since I can remember. My lower back felt relieved of the chronic pressure I usually feel, and more of my feet supported me comfortably. I had no idea my hamstrings were the cause of my low back pain. More specifically, that my back pain was coming from a personal relationship being so abusive."
BobCooley@TheGeniusofFlexibility.com

FASCIA AND TRAUMA

FOUR *TYPES* OF TRAUMA

1. PHYSICAL - DIRECT INJURY OR REPETITIVE STRESS
2. THINKING - PSYCHOLOGICAL MISEDUCATION
3. EMOTIONAL - SOCIAL DEVALUATION, SEXUAL ABUSE, LOOK DEGRADATION
4. SPIRITUAL - INTERFERENCE WITH SOMEONES LIFE

Fascia is the most energy efficient material in your body,

but when traumatized becomes the greatest energy hog.

Accumulated dense fascia and scar tissue usually exist on the lateral and posterior aspects of the person, what in TCM are called the yang muscles. Muscles on the front and medial aspects of the person rarely have accumulated dense fascia and scar tissue but d=characteristically house chronic increase tenseness unless these myofascial tissues have been damaged through trauma.

Trauma occurs in four ways: physically, psychologically, emotionally, and spiritually. Physical trauma happens from acute accidents, from repetitive stress or physiological illness. Psychological trauma occurs from unhealthy influences. Emotional trauma/abuse occurs from negative social or intimate experiences. Spiritual trauma occurs from negative life events, interfering with the course of a person's life in negative ways. These four *types* of trauma can occur anywhere in your body but are best affected by Resistance Flexibility training the four muscle groups associated with one of the four types of trauma.

Predictable personality impairment occurs based on the location of the damage, as well as concomitant physiological dysfunction. Damaged tissue is experienced by the person as an inability to consciously tense those areas of their body, an inability to physically 'put everything they've got into what they are doing'. These damaged tissue place a 'ceiling' on athletic and artistic success and longevity. Highly trained RF professionals are necessary to produce success in the use of these techniques when extreme damage has occurred. Static movements create more dense fascia and scar tissue then dynamic movements. For example, a flute player usually has more damaged tissue than an athlete. The prolonged static isometric holding of the instrument develops intense scar tissue, which often over time leads to cartilage damage.

Diaries

"I have had the humble privilege to be with people as they are processing life trauma's. The fascia holds the life story, good and bad; and when one is being RF stretched 'stuff' can come up. People have talked with me about all sorts a things including sexual abuse. One friend in particular has had multiple sexual assaults happen to her. It was a big deal for her to even be touched at first. After processing some of that trauma with our help, she then said how good it felt to be touched and have healing hands on her.

"In extreme cases, Resistance Flexibility can be a life saver, there have been a few occasions where I have seen folks come off addictive substances, supported in dealing with death of a loved one, etc."
BonnieCrotzer@TheGeniusofFlexibility.com Elite Resistance Flexibility Trainer

"Being able to differentiate between all the types of trauma your body holds gives the rest of you access to the information, a library the size of galaxies that you didn't even know was there. I just turned 40 and have been doing Resistance Flexibility for almost three years and have been able to release years of tightly wound patterns, my body moves better than it ever has. This makes the difference between feeling a little worse every year of your life or being a part of the changes and feeling better as you gracefully age."
SamuelCamburn@TheGenusofFlexibility.com Resistance Flexibility Intern

"As I had my Kidney meridian muscle group resistance flexibility trained by Bob and other trainers, I experienced a release of a trauma deep within me that I had no memory of. Though it was a new experience for me, it somehow felt very natural. I directly experienced the manner in which fascia stores my life experience and in this case, blinds me from it. In retrospect, I find Resistance Flexibility to be the gentlest form of self-protection imaginable. We are protected from that which we are not yet ready to process. It is stored in our fascia and we don't know it is there. When it comes out we feel a portion of the discomfort, but it gets compressed in both feeling and time. It seems that the trauma comes out of us in an instant, just as it went into us. We are not bound by the time we had to store it. This is remarkable and challenges my innate beliefs about who I am. It seems I can access within me a place that transcends time, space, and matter."
BerylHagenburg@TheGeniusofFlexibility.com Resistance Flexibility Inter

"One of the most incredible aspects of Resistance Flexibility is the ability to remove traumas through stretching the physical body. These traumas are not always physical injuries; they can be emotional, spiritual, and analytical. All of this information is stored in the body, and will show up in your tissue accordingly. For instance, someone who was sexually abused as a child may have some issues with their moods. The mood issue will also show up as ADFST in the hip flexors, or Sexual meridian. Through stretching those muscle groups and removing the scar tissue from them, you can transmute the mood disorder issue into high self worth and good looks. This is healing at its finest: transmuting a low trait to a high one."
EthanDupuis@TheGeniusofFlexibility.com Resistance Flexibility Intern

DEPERSONALIZATION, TRAUMA AND FASCIA

Trauma results in a characteristic warping of time of space.

There is a characteristic depersonalization concomitant with damaged fascia—a warping of time and space. Where the person feels pain is *very rarely* the area of damaged tissue. The pain area is usually referred pain that is being caused by damaged tissue sometimes quite a distance from the symptom. There is a pervasive and suspicious lack of feeling of one's body in those areas of ADFST. Damaged tissue, once removed, creates immediate changes in one's experience and understanding of space and time. Anamnesis usually accompanies interfacing with the ADFST. Damaged tissue literally holds that part of the person back at the time that the damage occurred. Freeing the person from this damage, results in a significant amnesia affect, as that part of the person begins to 'catch up' to present time. For example, if a person has been involved in a traumatic event and is then released from this event through RF by removing considerable amounts of accumulated dense fascia and scar tissue, then they experience a reorientation in space and time. If their attention is on those parts of themselves that have been freed, they often do not know where they are, and what year it is, however while simultaneously knowing their present place and time. They may ask what the objects are in the room they are in, objects that were developed since those parts of them were damaged. They may ask what year it is, wonder where they have been during the time that passed, and what has happened to them since their accident. When the damaged tissue is removed, the person has a simultaneous dramatic increase in memories from their past.

DAMAGED TISSUE HOLDS THE PERSON AT THE TIME AND PLACE THAT THE DAMAGE OCCURRED. ONCE THAT DAMAGE IS RELEASED, THOSE PARTS OF THE PERSON TRAVEL FASTER THAN HOW CURRENT TIME IS MOVING, AND CATCH UP TO CURRENT TIME AND LOCATION. THIS IS THE WARPING EFFECT OF TIME AND SPACE ASSOCIATED WITH DAMAGED TISSUE. TRANSFIGURING ADFST BRINGS SIMULTANEOUS MEMORIES OF PAST EVENTS ASSOCIATED WITH THE ADFST.

The elimination of ADFST can result in predictable significant physiological upgrades as well as a freeing agent psychologically. The elimination of overly dense fascia and scar tissue within the myofascial structures become a freeing agent psychologically. Areas of the body map into the development of specific personality traits. Thus, when specific parts of a person are freed from RF, specific personality traits are freed and encouraged to develop. For example, central hamstrings bring increases in trust, responsibility, and desire for mastery.

Damaged fascia is concomitant with increases in lack of wakefulness, consciousness, aliveness, and mental clarity. A warping of body placement in space is pervasive: "I think my arm is there but when I look, it is not anywhere near where I thought it was."

Diaries

"Throughout the Resistance Flexibility that I have been assisted in, there have been numerous times as to when I get the "time warp" affect of scar tissue being removed. My biggest memory of this was after stretching out my Brain, Thymus and Lung meridians on the back extension machine. On Thanksgiving Day of my senior year of high school, I was playing Tight End in the last football game of the season, when suddenly I dropped to the ground and had a seizure right then and there. I was rushed to the hospital and tested positive for all sorts of injuries and concussions. Turned out I had a moderate/severe concussion from hitting the ground on my way down. I had almost no recollection of what had happened. But after doing the stretches previously described, I remember standing up and suddenly feeling as if I was on the football field again at the moment I was hit. Suddenly I had this third person perspective on an injury that I had little to no recollection of. I remembered being blind-sided and hit in my Solar Plexus by an opposing player's helmet on a cheap-shot dive, I remembered not being able to breath before passing out and seizing, I remember people rushing over and trying to hold my body down as I seized for precisely 17 seconds. All things that I had no recollection of before. No one had ever told me exactly what had happened as I had been away from the developing play. And all of a sudden I could feel my body starting to catch up to the place and time that I was currently in, making up for all of the lost time. My body felt completely relaxed and free in places I had no awareness of being tight and locked up."
AlexNolte@TheGeniusofFlexibility.com Resistance Flexibility Intern

"The look during the stretch is initially intense effort but turns into a greater understanding of everything that you know, didn't even know you didn't know, or have ever felt about your life. The accumulated dense fascia and/or scar tissue in your chest shoulder and neck that are connected to the face releases. You feel what it's like to be you with out the things that hold you back, and the look afterwards is a better looking face and body that has had accumulated traumas transformed into gifts."
SamuelCamburn@TheGeniusofFlexibility.com Resistance Flexibility Intern

"When you are in that moment of healing for someone, it can seem like time can stop. You have most times 4-5 sets of hands on a person, all led by a skilled trainer, who feels where the body wants to move to get a stretch, and also where the body doesn't want to move through scar tissue. I think back to a stretch I was involved in with one of my dear friends at the studio. He went through a trauma that had happened to him in what seemed like the womb. In that moment you could see him reliving a moment in his past. I watched him interface with that trauma, and as we continued to stretch and coax him, he came out of the moment. He had no recollection of the event, but afterwards no longer was so anxious and jittery around the women in the studio. It seems he had an unconscious reaction to them because of the trauma that had happened in the womb. It was amazing to see him blossom more from that moment. The ability to take people through to the other side of a deep trauma is extremely rewarding to be a part of, because at the end of the day we all want the best for ourselves as well as one another."
EthanDupuis@TheGeniusofFlexibility.com Resistance Flexibility Intern

CLINICAL TRIALS OF RESISTANCE FLEXIBILITY AND ADFST

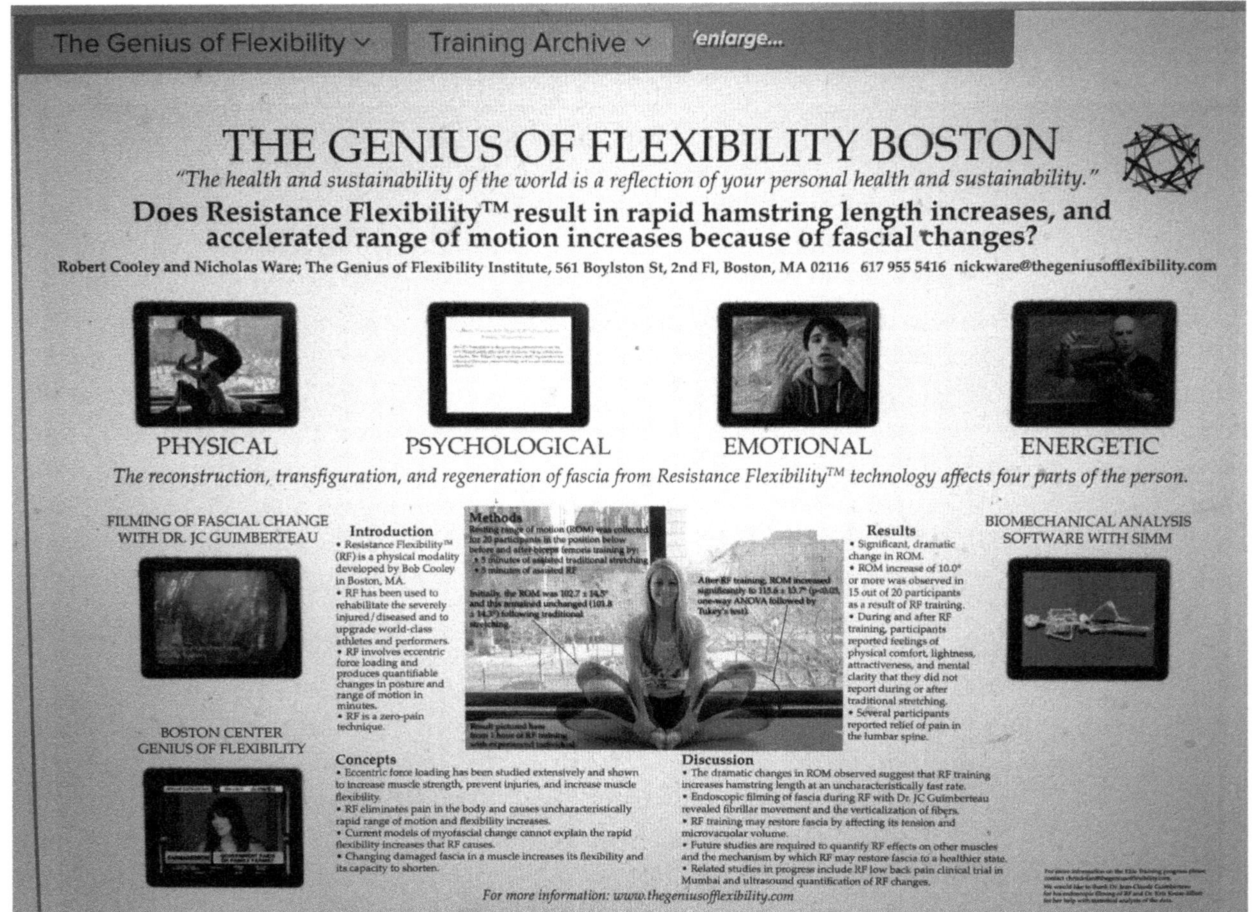

Significant biomechanical upgrades occur from Resistance Flexibility

In a clinical trial, Resistance Flexibility produced 10 Times the ROM improvements compared to any reported flexibility changes from any form of therapy reported in the medical literature. These data were presented at the Third International Fascia Congress in Vancouver, BC. Ultra sound and Endoscopic imagining verify the significant improvements in fascia from Resistance Flexibility. Nine other submissions were given to the 4th International Fascia Congress on Resistance Flexibility and fascia including topics on modeling of fascia, transfiguration of fascia, kinematic patterns, concomitances, personality trait development, low back pain elimination, rotator cuff rehabilitation, and concussions. See Chapter 16 for those abstracts.

Most remarkable with RF is the healing: regenerative, reconstitution, renovation, elimination of ADFST, and the recuperative benefits, and a youthification of the person. The person not only can move better than they ever have in their entire life, their looks improve and become younger, specific physiological upgrades occur; all these totaling a regeneration of myofascial tissues that are much younger in all ways compared to the person's age. Increases in elasticity, strength, suppleness, lightness, ranges of motion, reversal of aging, and longevity.

The extraordinary rate in which accumulated dense fascia and scar tissues (ADFST) can be repaired and returned to normal functioning using Resistance Flexibility exemplifies the health resiliency and psychological forgiveness of the human body.

THIRD INTERNATIONAL FASCIA CONGRESS
A poster presentation of our Clinical Abstract:

Does Resistance Flexibility result in rapid hamstring length increases and accelerated range of motion increases because of fascial changes?

Bob Cooley and Nick Ware. (See Appendix for Abstract Summary).

FOURTH INTERNATIONAL FASCIA CONGRESS
I received approval for four of my nine submissions to the 4th International Fascia Congress in December 2015. Here is a list of all nine submissions. (See Appendix for Abstract Summaries).

1 A TENSEGRITY IDEAL MODEL OF FASCIA™.docx

2 TRANSFIGURATION OF ACCUMULATED DENSE FASCIA AND SCAR TISSUE.docx

3 COOLEY 16 KINEMATIC PATTERN BIOMECHANIC MODEL™.docx

4 CONCOMITANCE OF TRADITIONAL CHINESE MEDICINE.docx

5 PSYCHOLOGICAL EFECTS FROM ACCUMULATED DENSE FASCIA AND SCAR TISSUE.docx

6 CONCOMITANCE OF GENETIC PERSONALITY TRAIT.docx

7 POTENTIAL LOW BACK PAIN ELIMINATION THROUGH RESISTANCE FLEXIBILITY™ OF BICEPS FEMORIS.docx

8 ROTATOR CUFF REHABILITATION AND PREVENTATION THROUGH RESISTANCE FLEXIBILITY™.docx

9 CONCUSSIONS, RF, and ADFST ELIMINATION.docx

CHAPTER 5

THE FOUR PARTS OF A STRETCH

The four parts of you reflect as the four parts of stretching

Four Parts of Cooley's Yoga & Resistance Flexibility

PHYSICAL

POSITIONING AND MOVING

Deferring to your body. Let your body show you how to position, reposition, and move to obtain the best stretch instead of just habitually moving.

THINKING

ATTENTION AND IDENTIFICATION

Deferring to you mind. You decide what idea you want to do and then the idea directs you to what to pay attention to—things either inside or out yourself, so you can learn how to do the thing you decided to do. Sensing what exactly is being stretched and the effect of the stretch instead of controlling your attention.

EMOTIONAL

USE OF TENSION AND RELAXATION

Deferring to your breathing. The muscles naturally generate tension when stretching. A person can be aware of the tension necessary to stretch a particular part of their body and will have to either reduce the amount of tenseness that is already present or increase the tension appropriate to the stretch instead of controlling your breathing.

SPIRITUAL

USE OF RESISTANCE OR YIELDING

Deferring to your spirit. The body naturally resists when stretching. This resistance is created by the fascia. A person may either need to resist more or reduce their resistance in order to get a stretch instead of controlling their energy.

"The whole is greater than the sum of the parts. Your body knows how to use all four of these parts when stretching. Let all four parts happen naturally."

FOUR PARTS OF FLEXIBILITY

Physical, Thinking, Emotional, and Spiritual

It is perhaps obvious to everyone that there are four parts of a person—the physical, thinking, emotional and spiritual. All traditional philosophies and spiritual traditions also identify these four parts of a person. It is also understandable that most people have developed some parts of themselves more than others. These four parts of a person are reflected in the same four aspects of flexibility.

After initially discovering Resistance Flexibility, I began to identify these four parts of each stretch: movements and positions, attention on what is happening breathing, and resistance. Positioning and moving naturally create the stretch, and allows me to adapt the position as I continued to get deeper and deeper into the stretch. Next I found myself identifying what was being stretched for example which muscle groups and which types of tissues were being targeted. Then I found that each position required me to breath in a specific way in order to generate sufficient tension and relaxation. And finally, how I needed to resist or yield when stretching.

This identification of the four parts of any stretch later turned into an understanding how each of these parts reflected as changes in my life. The physical part of stretch increased my instincts, the thinking part developed me psychologically, the breathing part matured me emotionally, and the resistance part changes my values. Let's look at these four parts in more depth.

1. PHYSICAL—POSITIONING AND MOVING

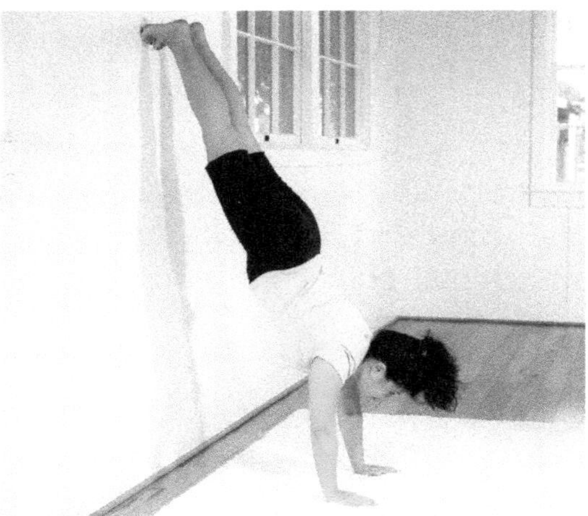

Chris's neck and head naturally want to arch upward. This head position 'fires off' reflexes that outward rotate her upper arms thus avoiding impingement in her shoulder joints. Defer to your body's wisdom.

Let your body show you how to position and reposition to obtain the best stretch. Defer to your body's instinctual way of abstract thinking and avoid moving in old habitual ways. Your body is already designed, so you don't have to design it, but just have to subtract what is stopping from moving. Your perception of the outside world changes as you stretch different parts of yourself.

Because your body can move in eight directions, there are eight different muscle groups in both your lower and upper body to move you in those directions. There are of course three pairs of directions: flexion and extension, abduction and adduction, and inward and outward rotation. These can be abbreviated as FL and EX, AB and AD, and IN and OU. The eight permutations of these create eight kinematic patterns or directions of movement:

FL/AB/IN and the balancing movement EX/AD/OU

FL/AB/OU and the balancing movement EX/AD/IN

FL/AD/IN and the balancing movement EX/AB/OU

FL/AD/OU and the balancing movement EX/AB/IN

Each one of these kinematic patterns is concomitant with one of the eight organ- meridian muscle groups in the lower and upper body:

GB and TH = FL/AB/IN and their balancing EX/AD/OU = LV and AP

ST and LI = FL/AB/OU and their balancing EX/AD/IN = PA and LU

KI and PE = FL/AD/IN and their balancing EX/AB/OU = BL and SK

SE and HE = FL/AD/OU and their balancing EX/AB/IN = BR and SI

Diaries

"One of the greatest gifts Resistance Flexibility is that it facilitated giving me a better relationship with my body. It's as if my body has been speaking to me throughout my life but I didn't know to listen or the language. Now I know how to defer to my body when stretching or doing any physical activity, and this facilitates effortless and natural physical expression."
LutherCowden@TheGeniusofFlexibility.com Elite Resistance Flexibility Trainer

"Learning to defer to my body's intelligence, and not impose ideas of 'correct' position and action on myself, has allowed me to have a much more satisfactorily stretch and achieve much better outcomes."
KajHoffman@TheGeniusofFlexibility.com Resistance Flexibility Intern

"Ever since childhood, accepting the physical limits of my body was always been frustrating. As years passed, whether in daily activities, training in weight lifting, running or swimming, or yoga, I would be acutely aware of what I couldn't do, how I wasn't matching the ideal forms. Once I had the concept of listening to my body, I instantly had much less emotion about it. I saw that these limits had physical causes, many of which were the results of my life's events and patterns. This enabled me to both accept how my body is, and feel empowered to start intentionally regenerating it. Transforming my frustration and the associated anxiety about how my body was aging, into a new relationship with my body, is liberating."
PatrickGregston@TheGeniusofFlexibility.com Resistance Flexibility Intern

"The idea of stretching yourself in respect to getting out of your comfort zone is a fairly mainstream concept, at least in western culture. However, we don't tend to do this from a physical standpoint as easily, and it leads to a place that settles for mediocre to poor levels of physical wellness and health. Stretching parts of the body you never thought to can lead to openings not only in your understanding of structural maladies, but also emotional and psychological areas that are challenging to face."
JohnBagdasarian@TheGeniusofFlexibility.com Resistance Flexibility Intern

"Becoming aware of the positioning and repositioning my body wants during a stretch has been one of the most empowering aspects of Resistance Flexibility for me so far. This part of stretching brings new life to my entire being and opens up a world of potential movement than I thought to imagine previously. It also makes stretching so much more enjoyable! Rather than simply trying to 'get it done' like many people feel about exercise, I now find satisfaction and pleasure during my stretches. This approach of deferring to my body while I stretch also gives me amazing perspective on how I am physically changing since the stretches are never the same."
BerylHagenburg@TheGeniusofFlexibility.com Resistance Flexibility Intern

2. THINKING—ATTENTION AND IDENTIFICATION

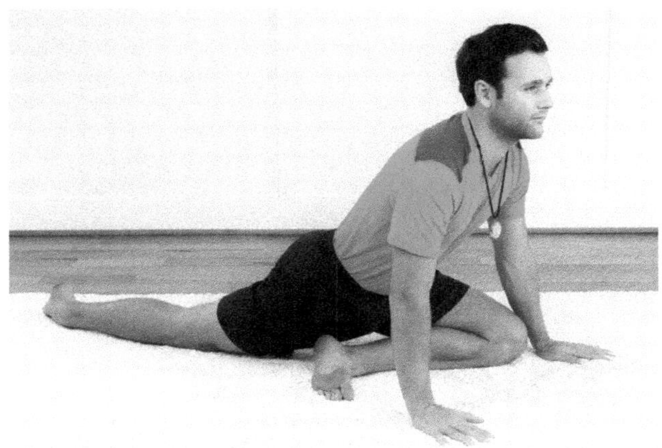

Nick told us his attention was on the muscles, and fascia stretching on the outside of his front leg, and the ligaments in his hips and ankles. He also found himself paying attention to an increase in ease in decision making, and his bodies ability to digest the good fats he ate earlier.

You decide what idea you want to do, and then the idea directs you to pay attention to things either inside or out yourself, so you can learn how to do the thing you decided to do. Sensing what exactly is being stretched and what things are associated with each *type* of stretch, allow you to know what each stretch can do for you and others. Each *type* of stretch affects the physiological function of a particular organ and a particular *type* of tissue in the body. There is personal content for each stretch. This personal content includes past memories associated with the positive or negative events in a different areas of the body. Your insight into yourself and others changes when you stretch different parts of yourself.

You will need to develop a new vocabulary to describe how each stretch affects you. Some of these new descriptors will include words for how your bones have repositioned, new posture and movements, changes in perception, the way you think, your looks, and new perspectives.

It is important to have a free attentional focus when learning anything. To do this means that you pay attention to whatever is coming up when you are learning something. Don't edit anything regardless of how irrelevant it seems. Many things that come up will make sense only in the future.

There are four ways of analytical thinking that everyone does: speculation, proving, problem solving, and understanding. The four groups of stretches develop these different ways of thinking.

Diaries

"As I started to practice Resistance Flexibility, my mind became more clear simply from training specific muscle groups and allowing my attention to be free. But, beyond that, the new authority I was giving to my mind to be free while stretching was priceless. I learned to naturally follow my attention while stretching, which taught me things about myself that I never would have learned had I tried to control my attention to manually attempt to clear my mind. I've been astonished as to what I've been able to learn about the internal functioning of my body and the bodies of others by allowing my attention to naturally be on the area that is either being stretched, or being affected by a stretch. Book studies can now compliment what I've learned about myself from these experiences, instead of me having to rely on book knowledge alone."
LutherCowden@TheGeniusofFlexibility.com Elite Resistance Flexibility Trainer

"The changes I have experienced in myself are amazing. Not only do I feel more movement and ability in my body from Resistance Flexibility, which has helped me recover form years of sports injuries, but I am digesting better, have better posture than I have ever had, I am thinking better, and best of all I am communicating and relating better with other people. Bob Cooley's Resistance Flexibility is the only work I have ever encountered that completely made sense to me."
RichardGregson@TheGeniusofFlexibility.com Resistance Flexibility Intern

"We are such a sophisticated creation and our wisdom relies among other details in union. My body cannot change unless my awareness supports it... When getting stretched or stretching myself, I have experienced that if my attention is not together with the stretch, then the change doesn't happen in its utmost way... By understanding the characteristics of my personality type and the other's types, I have bridged myself in different relationships with the same people."
NurhaDes@TheGeniusofFlexibility.com Resistance Flexibility Intern

"I have experienced personality traits that I had observed in other people but had not connected to within myself. I've found that from Resistance Flexibility, everyone develops psychologically in just the ways that were not yet developed. Some people need to be connected to and develop instinctual defense, others emotional ways of being, and others to develop perspective skills. After seeing many, many psychological traits being discovered for the first time by so many people, I began to accept that any personality trait that I wanted could be developed by practicing a particular type of stretch. I am knowing myself in ways that I never thought I was capable of being."
Bob Cooley@TheGeniusofFlexibility.com

"My philosophy on good and bad has forever changed. I use to have a model of good versus evil, but I have discovered that what is good comes from the transmutation of what is bad. So for example, when I am too anxious, if my attention stays outside on what I am attracted to, that is what my desires are directing me to pay attention to, and then my anxiety turns into excitement. The same is true for my depression that turns into creativity."
BobCooley@TheGeniusofFlexibility.com

3. EMOTIONAL—USE OF TENSION AND RELAXATION

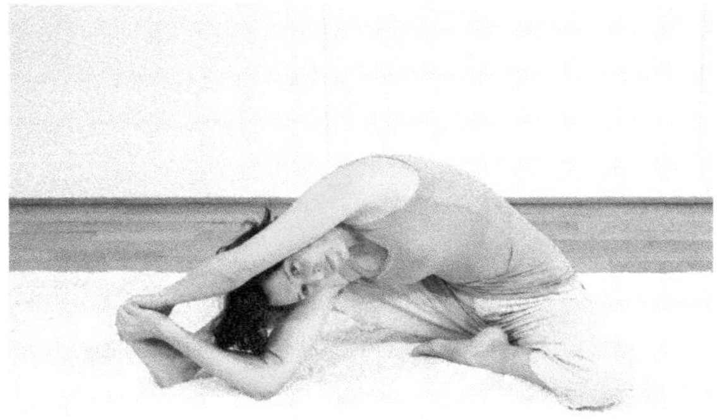

Petya became more conscious of feeling unstuck, freer emotionally. Her tendons were targeted in the stretch. Afterwards she was noticeably prettier which connected others to their feelings of self liking.

The emotional aspects of Resistance Flexibility include listening to you body so you can use just the right amount of tension and relaxation, how to breathe naturally, your looks and what they mean, and how to be more emotionally mature.

Muscles naturally generate tension when stretching. Everyone knows it takes tension before you relax when being intimate, and the same applies when stretching. A person can be aware of the tension necessary to stretch a particular part of their body and will have to either reduce the amount of tension that is occurring or increase that tension. There is an infinite ocean of tension that a person can resource when stretching, and allowing this to be natural is what you are looking for.

Your body knows how to show you how to breath, so you will have to learn from your body how to breath, and not try to tell your body how you think it should breathe. Your body has an involuntary way of breathing that is the foundation of your conscious breathing. Defer to how your body wants you to breath in new ways, and learn how to give up on old habitual breathing patterns. Learn to stay present with your stretching, and don't be distracted by a past event that wants you to reenact the ways you were breathing at that time.

Your face in particular is associated with your emotionality, and after you have had a great stretch your face is much more relaxed and better looking. Your looks have more meaning to others than you probably realized. There are generally four *types* of looks: beauty, image, sexy, and pretty/handsome. Each of these different *types* of looks has specific affects besides the person becoming more attractive. Each of these four different *types* of looks connects others to different parts of themselves. For example, when a person's beauty increases others become connected to increase feelings of self-affirmation. When a person's image increases, others become connected to increases in feelings of self-esteem. When a person's good looks (sexy) increase, this connects to feelings of their self-worth. And when someone's becomes more pretty or handsome, this connects others to feelings of self-liking. So developing better looks is a wonderful thing for everyone, but the affect those looks have on other people is very meaningful.

Staying conscious of the other people while stretching is essential for producing a great stretch. Without having your attention outside on others while stretching you cannot generate the necessary tension or relaxation. Stretching can increase your consciousness and help to connect you to your unconscious—which has the high/low traits of your balancing *type*.

Being conscious of what you like, learning to develop your feelings of what you like and dislike by expressing your attraction to others is the only way to mature emotionally. Similar to how one's thinking matures by taking your thoughts and putting them out there so that other people can mix in their insights, one's emotions have to be put out there so others responses can cause the chemical reaction that results in what everyone calls maturing emotionally. You can't emotionally mature inside yourself, maturing requires that you put your feelings of attraction out there so that other people have a way to attach to you and your emotions, and their responses is what matures you.

Often times, one aspect of a person can be in conflict with another part. For example, a person can find another person attractive yet think it is wrong for some reason. Stretching can teach a person to stay with their emotion and engage with what they are attracted to so that their attraction matures. Then their ideas of what is right are achieved naturally.

Intelligence is highly correlated with emotions. By increasing ones participation with their emotions, intelligence is accessed.

Diaries

"I am naturally predominantly aware of my breathing when I stretch. I have learned to allow myself to breathe normally. I breathe and resist a lot when I stretch. Learning to breath normally and yield to my resistance when necessary, has opened up the experience of the other aspects of stretching for me—the positioning, the internal sensation, and psychological content. This has allowed me to problem solve my own biomechanical problems, feel the alignment of my body, and my tissue in an entirely new way."
BerylHagenburg@TheGeniusofFlexibility.com Resistance Flexibility Intern

"I've always heard that breathing is an important part of stretching. But, it never made sense for me to force myself to breathe in and out manually. I gave it a shot anyway and practiced deep breathing techniques while stretching. I understood how this could be helpful, but I ended up feeling like it was an artificial attempt at producing something that should be happening naturally. As I began to stretch specific muscle groups in my body while deferring to my breath, I started to have experiences where my breathing was a direct reflection of my ability to 'be' with the part of myself that was emotionally undeveloped. As I continued to defer to my body, follow my attention, and breathe naturally, that part of me began to change at a rapid rate. I felt as if I was 'being breathed,' and a natural deep breathing occurred in a way and with emotional content that manual forcing of my breath could never match."
LutherCowden@TheGeniusofFlexibility.com Elite Resistance Flexibility Trainer

"Giving up the training to control my breathing, and discover how my body wanted to breathe brought new awareness of the rich flow of information available in paying attention to my body."
PatrickGregston@theGeniusofFlexibility.com Resistance Flexibility Intern

"Being introduced to using tension and resistance when stretching was only the beginning of my discoveries that followed. This in turn changed my breathing, and emotionality...an ability to go for what I wanted and not feel bound by habit. It gave me perspective on how I operate as an individual in social settings. I realized that being assisted was more than a physical need, it helps me emotionally, mentally, and spiritually."
KateRabinowitz@TheGeniusofFlexibility.com Resistance Flexibility Intern

"I had a really hard time not controlling my breath, and to allow my body to show me how to breath. My awareness of my breath is solely sufficient for my brain to be connected to how I am breathing, and then it changes my breathing. I don't need to think myself into breathing differently. I defer to my body to show me how to breathe instead of thinking I know better than my body. Deferring to body to show me how to breathe made me realize how much anxiety and how to change that into relaxation and satisfaction."
SamuelCamburn@TheGeniusofFlexibility.com Resistance Flexibility Intern

"Resistance Flexibility has helped me to regain ability to breath naturally and discover how that transforms my playing of music into a much more pleasurable flowing state."
KajHoffman@TheGeniusofFlexibility.com Elite Resistance Flexibility Intern

"For my entire life I have always spent much of my time noticing what is attractive, likeable, good-looking, beautiful, desirable and appealing in other people and also in objects. The more I do this, the more I get clarification on what I like and am attracted to. I hadn't realized it until Bob put it to words, but I am also aware of absorbing those qualities into myself that I find so desirable on the outside. So it would have to follow that I am projecting out all that I am able to absorb."
BerylHagenburg@theGeniusofFlexibility.com Resistance Flexibility Intern

"I think that adults have a false, or somewhat illusory sense of what emotional maturity actually means, much less how they can track it within themselves as we age…at least that shoe fits on me. The fun thing about getting feedback from others after a stretch is that you get perspective on things you couldn't possibly get on your own because you don't have a sufficient amount of information. This kind of feedback has given me great room to explore myself in the realm of how I am connecting with the outside world through my emotional body. I always thought of myself as emotional, but being told as a child that you're sensitive or moody, doesn't grant you a free pass to emotional relating in the world as we grow and change over the years. I can now see how I have been very much like a child, or a teenager in some of my ways of being that simply don't serve me as I am intending, and now have a more relaxed sense of how to perceive emotion in myself and others. I just feel more free and at ease with awkward moments of processing my experience, instead of pretending things aren't really effecting me and sweeping them under the carpet, because let's face it, nobody likes to go back and clean under that carpet. It's such a much more satisfying thing to be able to handle life when you aren't lying to yourself for self-protection or out fear of not knowing."
JohnBagasarian@TheGeniusofFlexibility.com Resistance Flexibility Intern

"All the sudden I was attracted to everyone! I almost couldn't believe the contrast of what I was doing before and what I saw now. Time slowed down and the density of the air seemed to increase between people, it was like information was being exchanged through breathing. I can see what is so special about each individual then allow myself to process the next feeling that comes up, jealously, envy, love, excitement and so on. When I let this process run its course I get to have more of that particular high trait and in return realize what is so special about myself. Imagine if every single person on the planet had the support to experience this."
SamuelCamburn@TheGeniusofFlexibility.com Resistance Flexibility Intern

"When you ask a type about their high traits or their 'intelligence,' they can connect you to that way of being instantly. It feels like a download- it is that powerful. It might be one of the fastest ways to change and develop. People are just waiting to give and share what they have in abundance. We just don't know what or how to ask! Learning about the types and their intelligence gives the question and allows you to receive the answer. I never cease to be amazed at how much I have misunderstood qualities associated with types other than my own. Everything becomes so much easier when you know the innately human way to do what you are trying to do. Did you know that a decision is made with the knowledge and anticipation that the decision will have to change as soon as you get more information on the topic? I never knew that- but now that I do I am so much freer to make a 'wrong' decisions."
ChrisRenfrow@TheGeniusofFlexibility.com Elite Resistance Flexibility Trainer

4. SPIRITUAL—USE OF RESISTANCE OR YIELDING

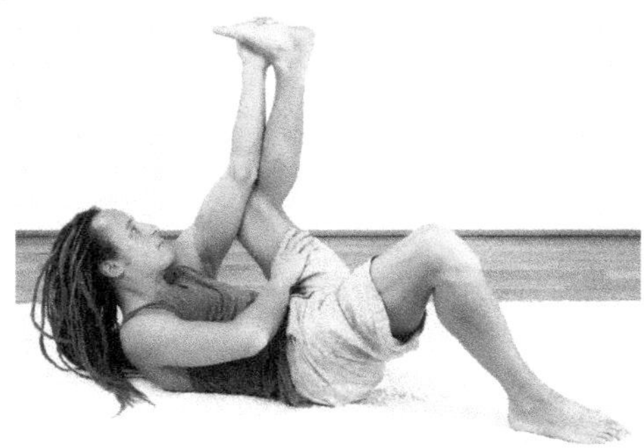

Luther became aware of getting more energy from doing this stretch. His perspective changed as he connected more to his life instead of being too martyrish.

Your body naturally uses resistance when stretching. Your fascia creates most of your resistance as it is transfigured during the stretch. Discover how much resistance is appropriate at any moment. Sometimes you are using too much resistance and need to yield, and other times you need to use more resistance.

The amount of energy that is necessary to perform each stretch and the energy that is liberated as you remove ADFST is remarkable. A person stretches and they and their life changes, and does everyone else's. A person's perspective changes as they become flexible. Energy awareness is a special aspect of stretching. Some parts of your body are more alive and some parts are less alive, some people call the later dead parts of themselves. As you do Resistance Flexibility on different areas, they come back alive, the awareness of those parts of your body are reconnected to, so now instead of you having to intentionally direct your attention to feel those parts, awareness from those parts naturally come up to you.

A person can be viewed as energetic container of every event that has happened to them. And you can connect to their life and learn from them by connecting to them energetically. Your awareness of other people's lives and your own is an essential aspect of stretching. As you stretch and watch other people stretch, you gain perspective on what a life can be.

Spirituality used to be confined to religious institutions, but no longer. Many spiritual traditions are now free to be experienced through many different mediums including lectures, workshops, on line trainings, videos, etc. Powerful virtues and spiritual values are available to everyone through the Internet.

Diaries

"I found Resistance Flexibility way back in 1993 when Bob was busy developing its core ideas and principles, but even then its transformative powers were obvious. I didn't come for personal change, I came for the stretching. I was doing a lot of personal growth work at the time through other modalities like Alanon and counseling, but I initially viewed these as separate from my stretching work with Bob. It took a while, but one day I finally realized how much faster I was changing, how much clearer I was about things in my life that usually confused me, and how I more easily overcame old obstacles by stretching. That's when I decided that Resistance Flexibility was one of the most powerful and valuable tools in my life."
TomLongo@TheGeniusofFlexibility.com Elite Resistance Flexibility Trainer

"The resistance that naturally shows up while stretching teaches me about the connection between the part of myself being stretched and my life. Resisting while stretching teaches me how to go up against that which is much larger than me and continuously try to hold my position even though the odds are against me. I also learn about the nature of my connection to that part of myself through resistance which then lets me know whether I should be resisting with an effort to 'stop' that force which is greater, or resist in a way where I yield to that which is greater, without giving up myself in the process."
LutherCowden@TheGeniusofFlexibility.com Elite Resistance Flexibility Trainer

"When the fascial glue keeping me in old trauma patterns gets stretched I feel like I'm going to die. In fact I am starting to live."
EddieEllner@TheGeniusofFlexibility.com Resistance Flexibility Intern

"There have been many times when stretching where it is easy for me to detach from my body and simply rely on my natural resistance in order to continue making the required movements. This is nowhere close to being as effective as having my focused attention on the connection to your nervous system. When detaching from the body and allowing natural resistance to take over, there is much less sensation of the stretching, as I have found myself relying on the scar tissue and ADFST to make the moment, which is not connected to the nervous system, thus taking away from the sensation of the stretch. So I have found for myself, time and time again, that when I keep my attention on my body, and the movement that it is doing, and the resistance that it is generating, I get loads more sensation. I no longer am "floating" through the stretch, but rather can now feel my body engaging and allowing more sensation to come into my body that even further exemplifies the stretch. The focus and connection to the nervous system is one of the many tricks that has helped me to find my body and the sensation of the stretches."

AlexNolte@TheGeniusofFlexibility.com Resistance Flexibility Intern

"I have experienced new virtues from Resistance Flexibility. I naturally gravitate to things that are good for me. But now I also learned about doing things based on principles, or integrity, or ethically. Having these additional spiritual tools for my life has broadened my perspective."
BobCooley@TheGeniusofFlexibility.com

"Resistance Flexibility always make me more aware of light and being light. I have entered into having much more awareness of how different everyone's energies are and what that means. My comparative perspective skills result in me being more objective without loosing my subjectivity, insights, or instincts about others. These spiritual developments are not something I would have ever imagined I would ever be aware of, much less that they could be developed by me stretching."
BobCooley@TheGeniusofFlexibility.com

"I have always wanted to have good judgment about others, but I never thought to ask others their judgment about me. Funny how something that I took to be so infinitely valuable, I had never thought to use for myself. Receiving perspective from others was not initially easy to handle, especially positive perspective, I thought negative would be difficult, but positive perspectives were harder for me. I found that when people give me positive perspectives, I have to handle my previously discounted attachments and knowledge of them."
Bob Cooley@TheGeniusofFlexibility.com

"Twenty years ago, if someone began talking to me about energy, I would think they were crazy. I had never had awareness of energy per se, but now I spend most of my time aware of the energetic connection with everything and myself. That's quite a leap. So when I meet people that have resistance to me talking about my energetic experiences, I have some knowledge of where they are coming from, so I don't act out of my reaction to them. I find that by having my reaction but not acting out of it, but simply paying attention to it, surprisingly both of us change."
Bob Cooley@TheGeniusofFlexibility.com

"When you are in that moment of healing for someone, it can seem like time can stop. You have most times 4-5 sets of hands on a person, all led by a skilled trainer, who feels where the body wants to move to get a stretch, and also where the body doesn't want to move through scar tissue. I think back to a stretch I was involved in with one of my dear friends at the studio. He went through a trauma that had happened to him in what seemed like the womb. In that moment you could see him reliving a moment in his past. I watched him interface with that trauma, and as we continued to stretch and coax him, he came out of the moment. He had no recollection of the event, but afterwards no longer was so anxious and jittery around the women in the studio. It seems he had an unconscious reaction to them because of the trauma that had happened in the womb. It was amazing to see him blossom more from that moment. The ability to take people through to the other side of a deep trauma is extremely rewarding to be a part of, because at the end of the day we all want the best for ourselves as well as one another."
EthanDupuis@TheGeniusofFlexibility.com Resistance Flexibility Intern

GAINING PERSPECTIVE FROM OTHERS, THE COMMUNITIY, AND HEALING

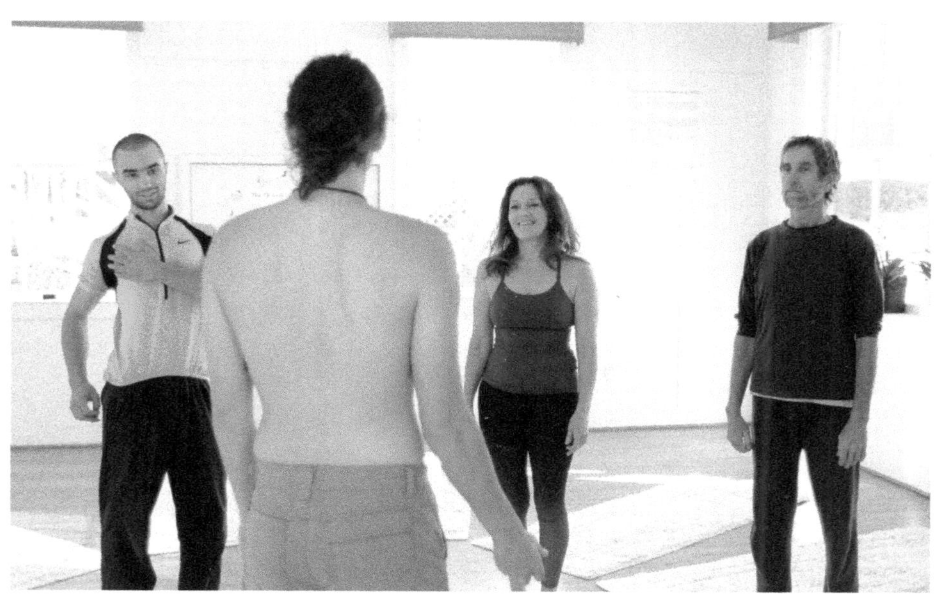

GETTING ASSISTED RESISTANCE FLEXIBILITY

Self-stretching is amazingly salubrious, but you will need other people to assist you in order to get the changes you want. You didn't make the clothes you wear, the car you drive, nor cut your own hair, etc., so why would you think you have to only stretch yourself and not like everything else have others help. Stretching needs you to depend on other people to help you, and they feel the same way towards you.

At all of our Genius of Flexibility Centers, when a client is being assisted by an Elite Trainer, the trainer may need additional assistance from other people, and some times many people. The clients and their trainers in the room often help for a couple of minutes to assist other clients or trainers.

The feedback an assister gives you to confirm or negate your interpretations of what you are feelings during and after being assisted is essential to learning how to know yourself and others. Often others find give a person perspective on different ideas about another person that are unknown to the person.

During and after a person is stretching, it is customary in our centers for other people in the room to give their perspective on the types of changes that have occurred for that person. This gives authority to everyone in the room, as everyone's perspectives provide a world of necessary information that no one person can give. The wealth of intuitive wisdom that comes from others is enriching beyond belief. Traditionally healing happens in a community setting not behind a closed door with one person. A group of people is necessary to heal everyone. This group approach to healing is a hallmark of Resistance Flexibility in all of our centers.

Diaries

"Having a community to bond with, transform with, and support each other to become the best version of oneself, is what we do. How else would you want to spend your time?"
ChrisRenfrow@TheGeniusofFlexibility.com MSAOM, Elite Resistance Flexibility Trainer

"The facilitation of another person's development through assisted stretching is the most unique form of human interaction that I've ever experienced. I get to have whatever thoughts and feelings I have about the person that I'm helping, whether that be negative or positive, while I assist a person through the parts of themselves that they are either struggling with or know nothing about. The exchange that happens between the person being assisted and the assisters is always new and evolving. The amount of force necessary to change accumulated dense fascia and scar tissue is beyond what most people would ever imagine. It's like building a great pyramid, except that a great person is being built instead."
LutherCowden@TheGeniusofFlexibility.com Elite Resistance Flexibility Trainer

"I have developed friends and community peer support through Resistance Flexibility that I always wanted but never found through practicing of yoga. To some extent I was trying to succeed in the yoga model of going into the 'cave' and healing myself, with occasional forays into the world for new ideas. And even when I tried to work with others in yoga, we lacked the foundational knowledge and techniques to be of much help to each other. With RF the model is community based and we need the help of each other other, and the depth of the knowledge and techniques allow us to help each other in much more effective ways. That assistance from others allows changes to occur much more quickly than I was able to achieve through my previous yoga practice. And it has also allowed me to change and develop in ways I previously had no idea how to begin to address."
KajHoffman@TheGeniusofFlexibility.com Elite Resistance Flexibility Trainer

"The force that is generated in the body from ADFST is unique! After getting assisted and assisting others 100s, if not 1000s of times—I always find that people are both surprised and unaware of the forces that are in their body from ADFST. If you don't get help from others and if you don't help people yourself, you will have no way of truly knowing about the fascia in your own body. You can't feel the full impact of its force through self-stretching because you can't resist yourself enough. You need others to receive your full resistance so you can learn about it. In the same way, when you feel the resistance and various qualities of tissue in another person, you gain tremendous perspective on your own body. Getting assisted and assisting others during a stretch is amazing and an honor. I have learned more about myself through the help and perspective of others than I ever imagined possible. Wouldn't the world be an amazing place if we could give one another the feedback and thoughts we are genuinely having. Imagine how fast we would evolve if we felt supported and were in a safe environment to hear how other people are viewing us. RFST is that environment and the human develop happens at a phenomenal speed."
BerylHagenburg@TheGeniusofFlexibility.com Resistance Flexibility Intern

"The experience of being assisted is as powerful as the stretch itself. To be taken beyond the threshold of possibility with care and kindness, to have your struggle, your story, your reactions witnessed is immeasurably healing."
EddieEllner@TheGeniusofFlexibility.com Resistance Flexibility Intern

"Self stretching has its place. Don't get me wrong. But getting assisted takes stretching to a whole new level. I couldn't have ever gotten results I've gotten without having one or multiple people helping assist me. But what it also does is open up new territory within myself to explore when I self-stretch. The more I get worked on, the more satisfying and productive it is for me to self-stretch. I quickly became aware that the amount of force we can generate within ourselves cannot at times be overcome others or myself. Sometimes it takes lots of people to assist me. It's also incredibly special and healing to work on each other rather than being in an isolated solo journey like other things I've tried."
ChrisPersall@TheGeniusofFlexibility.com Resistance Flexibility Intern

"When I first started trading stretching, I had an experience working with 3 other people that I will never forget. It illuminated a deeply healing aspect of this work that I didn't see coming. During the trade, were taking me into an intense hamstring stretch, my point of view contracted, my attention shrunk, and was pulled deep inside where I was primarily aware of the pain and personal suffering I was experiencing. After some time with this perspective, it's as if a veil lifted or a door opened. Suddenly, I was very aware of all of them out there, many arms and pairs of hands working hard to help me. My minds eye glimpsed the web of life coming together to help me. Recognizing the fact that these communities of people were willingly and happily offering their time and energy to move me in a way that would bring me greater freedom and ease in my life touched a deep place inside of me."
LucaCupery@TheGeniusofFlexibility.com Resistance Flexibility Intern

"I have developed friends and community peer support through Resistance Flexibility that I always wanted when practicing yoga. With Resistance Flexibility we need the help of each other, and the depth of knowledge and techniques allow us to help each other in very effective ways. That assistance from others has allowed changes to occur in me much more quickly than I was able to achieve through my previous yoga practice. And it has also allowed me to change and develop in ways I previously had no idea how to begin to address."
KajHoffman@TheGeniusofFlexibility.com Elite Resistance Flexibility Intern

"There is something simple and yet remarkable when there are multiple people assisting on one person being stretched. The totality of the energy being fed into one individual's needs is not an additional effect, but an exponential quality that exceeds quantification in a linear sense. I guess it's a bit like the old adage, the whole is greater than the sum of its parts."
JohnBagdasarian@TheGeniusofFlexibility.com Resistance Flexibility Intern

"The relationship with yourself is like any other relationship, you must listen to what your body is telling you, you have to form an intimate connection by bringing more awareness to all the little nuances that you need to thrive. Be exploratory in your movement with the excitement of a child learning everything for the first time and you will always find something new that lifts you to the next

level. In this nature you will show up to assisted stretching with the energy the group needs to connect with you. Exponential gains in development can happen within communities this way, everyone brings each other up. This can break too much of the 'fix me' mindset when healing or performing. The days that follow assisted stretching in a group offer some of the best opportunities to self stretch, all four part of yourself, physical, mental, emotional, and spiritual are provoked and loved and are ready for you to understand a little more.

"Group stretching is something we have all been looking for, it begins to complete something we have been trying to figure out from the beginning of our evolvement, and how we work. What's so special about everyone? what holds us back? Feeling into another body, sensing what they need, what you and the group need, being with everyone having their lives, and communicating together is the next age of development. The physical is the foundation and the restrictions in our body are connected to every block in the other three worlds. Releasing these patterns together and being able to see, hear, and feel how people are being differently with you can give you a lifetime of information. The more we do this the more we are comfortable speaking transparently about how we operate in the world. Sharing our internal dialogue is a key component in truly understanding what we need, what we are not getting, and what we know nothing about. This way of communicating strengthens everyone's beliefs and knowledge bases by a way of connecting them through intimate relationships. We can heal one another through communities of transparent communication."
Samuel Camburn@TheGeniusofFlexibility.com

"After Thursday I felt my wrists and hands even more, as they always feel folded in half and jammed into my body, while having heavy iron cuffs around the wrists, especially my left hand. I really wanted my hands and wrist and fingers to get stretched, since I always give people this experience and see there changes and relief with all types of trauma processed through the experience, I wanted this so bad! So I thought Chris would be a good person to give me this experience. As I went into session was very excited however noticed his mind was somewhere else, he said he had a lot on his mind. As I wanted him to be comfortable to do session with me. I really could see the love again that Chris puts in the stretch, which for me is so important to put me at ease, not everyone can do that is a special quality that I definitely need and is continuous theme of the week. Love the upgrades in dexterity in each finger creating more room in the joints so my fingers don't feel they are shoved into my hand so much. The wrists are starting to unlock, as this happens the thoughts of past abuse as I would continue to choose relationships that weren't healthy for me and even knowing it to be so, would go ahead and do it anyways, exposes some lack of self care and love on my part. Now I can just enjoy people more for who they are and how they're doing it different however the urge or charge of just wanting to be with them or to lust for them is not the only reason to do something. I also notice trauma of relationships start to come up out of my left hand, which had been trapped in my left wrist, which were making me feel not available to others and keeping me suspended in time of the trauma of the conclusion of the hurtful events of a past relationship that no longer is reality, however was holding on to it with such a tight grip, making me loose my own grip on myself. A ride I'm choosing no longer to take."
ChrisPearsall@TheGeniusofFlexibility.com   Resistance Flexibility Intern

"The first time I got stretched by a couple of interns, I had a profound experience. First of all, I was able to have a true experience of what the different muscle groups in my body were actually doing. I

didn't realize the amount of tension and holding I was doing in certain areas and the lack of strength that I had in others. I felt a greater awareness of my true flexibility and range as they assisted me through the stretches while I contracted and lengthened the different muscle groups. After having a daily yoga practice for 15 years, I thought I really knew my body well and was surprised at the new information I had access to with their assistance. One thing especially stood out. My left hip and leg was completely different from the right and there was a lot of 'stuff' in it. I had been having a little trouble and annoyance with my left hip, but nothing serious. When the interns started to work on it, I had an experience of accessing a 'black hole' there. It felt deep, dark, unending, and empty. A wave of intense fear surfaced in me at first. As they continued to be with me there, many old emotions and stories came to the surface.

"At first, I felt unsafe letting the feelings come up to be expressed. Then, I was moved by their steady and kind presence. I looked out and they seemed like angels, taking time and making efforts to help me. A little more came up during the session, but it was later that day and in the following days that I was really impacted by the effects of the stretch. I spent a long time letting tears pass, many of them with out any stories attached. It felt like really old layers of trauma had been stored in my body and were finally getting to come up and out. After spending some time journaling and getting rest, I felt a significant change in the way my hip felt and in the psychological weight I was carrying. Weeks later, I noticed the 'black hole' in my hip joint started to fill in and, although there is still a difference in my legs from left to right, they felt much more balanced."
LuceCupery@TheGeniusofFlexibility.com Resistance Flexibility Intern

"The perspective offered to the person being assisted is more valuable than gold. This opportunity provides people who are being assisted a well-deserved break from them having to problem solve themselves. Other people bring awareness to parts of the person being assisted that the person would have overlooked on their own, simply because those parts are changing and are too new for them to be fully aware of."
LutherCowden@TheGeniusofFlexibility.com Elite Resistance Flexibility Trainer

"From a personal experience with Cooley's Resistance Flexibility, the fascia tells the story of your life. Fascia holds the memories that your aware of and the ones your not, by using Resistance Flexibility as the doorway to the memories especially the ones your unaware it takes you back in time to experience/ event. Once your connected to the reality of the past it immediately takes you forward into your present life dissolving the part you did not remember and allowing you to live in real time."
ChrisRenfrow@TheGeniusofFlexibility.com MSAOM, Elite Resistance Flexibility Trainer

"I had major Resistance to being the focal point of attention and to be on the spot to give feedback initially when entering this world. It felt uncomfortable. My reaction to it was it seemed like an egocentric thing or that I wouldn't have the information people were expecting me to have. But I soon realized it's the fasted way to develop. We can't possibly have all the information or perspective ourselves so we have to defer to those we feel connected to who are also part of the experience and healing process. It's the best way to change. You gain immediate validation if you've felt something for so long and now you have people affirming those things for you. Of course the contrary may be the dismantling of beliefs you've had about yourself or others, which is perhaps for some way more valuable and humbling."
ChrisPersall@TheGeniusofFlexibility.com Resistance Flexibility Intern

"Resistance Flexibility has taught me I need others to help me identify my weaknesses, and that others can stretch me and help me grow in ways I can't possibly achieve, or at times even conceive of, on my own."
KajHoffman@theGeniusofFlexibility.com Elite Resistance Flexibility Intern

"We all have an internal reality. Hearing other people tell me what they can see after I have been stretching, informs that internal reality with their perspectives and sensibilities. Having my internal sense of what is happening be validated, or not, enriches the experience, helps me to connect with the actual changes happening in my body, often through ways I do not think or approach existence. I get to benefit from the intelligence and intuition of others. When these perspectives resonate with my internal reality, with my innate sense of who I am, my view of myself is enriched, fortified and less dependent on my rationalization and justification around my own insecurities."
PatrickGregston@theGeniusofFlexibility.com Resistance Flexibility Intern

"I have always thought that I had a pretty good grasp on what I was experiencing and how I was being perceived by the rest of the world. Little did I know that there are things that other people can see changing that I was not aware of. After the stretches, gaining the perspective from others helps ten-fold as it has many times helped bring my attention to places and changes in my body that I was not aware were happening. Rather than relying on my own perception of reality, the insight from others helps me to link into the full spectrum of reality, and the actuality of what other people are seeing me do, rather than what I think that they see me doing."
AlexNolte@TheGeniusofFlexibility.com Resistance Flexibility Intern

"Nothing is a substitute for stretching."

CHAPTER 6

FOUR *TYPES OF* BENEFITS FROM RESISTANCE FLEXIBILITY

Physical, psychological, emotional, and spiritual

> YOUR BODY REFLECTS YOUR HEALTH
>
> *It's about the food you eat and how flexible and strong you are.*
>
> *It's about your personal psychology.*
>
> *It's about your looks and intelligence*
>
> *And*
>
> *It's about the way you live.*

Physical, psychological, emotional, and spiritual concomitances

What is a concomitance between two things? A concomitant relationship between two things explicitly demands that one thing always bring with it the other...they have an inseparable relationship, not a casual relationship but a one-to-one relationship! A binding association between different *types* of stretches and their ability to access and produce specific physiological and psychological benefits is an example of *concomitance.*

When one thing is inseparably connected or associated to another thing,

there is said to be a concomitance between those two things.

Health has two wings: food and stretching. That's it. Simple. Nothing results in giving me greater physiological health then Resistance Flexibility. After my accident when I discovered how to naturally stretch, I created different stretches for my whole body. Those began and continue to upgrade my posture and movements in amazing ways. However the bigger surprise was that each of the sixteen different types of stretches returned me to having physiological health, and continues to upgrade my health. The Resistance Flexibility is what brought me to eating nutrient dense foods. One biodynamic orange satisfied me more than three non-organic oranges. Only organic foods feed me. I often fast instead of eating non-organic foods. Recovering from eating non -organic food is worse than being hungry for a while.

Each of the 16 *types* of stretches is concomitant with a group of contiguous muscle groups, meridian pathway, organ, *type* of tissue, physiological functions, and genetic personality *type.* These 16 *types* of stretches are in four groups: physical, thinking, emotional, and spiritual. Thus there are four *types* of benefits. Let's look more deeply into these *types* of benefits.

1.PHYSICAL / PHYSIOLOGICAL BENEFITS FROM RESISTANCE FLEXIBILITY

Posture, movements, alignment, organ, tissue, physiological systems, pain no more...

The 16 *types* of Resistance Flexibility exercises each specifically target all the muscles that you use to move in one of eight directions in your lower and upper body. By selecting any one *type* of the stretch, you are targeting a specific group of muscles and your different movements. For example, sufficiency in the flexibility and strength in various muscles in your lower body give you the ability to jump and squat, twist and untwist, turn in either direction, and to go forward or backward, or in your upper body to throw and catch, push and pull, open and close, and lift and lower. So the more sufficiency in flexibility and strength a person has in the specific muscle groups necessary to move in one of 8 ways in their lower or upper body, the more optimal the movements.

There is a concomitance between each of the 16 different muscle groups or *types* of Resistance Flexibility stretches and your physiological health according to Traditional Chinese Medicine (TCM) theory. Each of the 16 muscle groups is concomitant with and organ, its tissue *type,* and a physiological system. For example, the same muscles that give you the ability to jump also as concomitant with the health of your bladder and bones according to TCM theory, or the same muscles that you use to throw a ball are concomitant with the health of your lungs and the oxygenation of your blood according to TCM theory.

There is also physical concomitance between each of the 16 different muscle groups or *types* of Resistance Flexibility stretches and your ability to have naturally good posture. For example, sufficiency in the flexibility and strength in the muscles on the back of your scapula give you uprightness, while the muscles on the back outside of your legs stack you on top of your legs. The body naturally suspends and erects itself when there is sufficient flexibility and strength. No mental effort is necessary to remind or control oneself to have natural posture.

CONCOMITANCES EXAMPLES:
MUSCLE GROUP <—> ORGAN <—> TISSUE <—> GPT

Therefore for each group of muscles and *type* of stretch, there are concomitances posture and movements, physiological health, potential advancements of specific personality traits (GPT), and spiritual value development. Here are some examples:

1. MUSCLE: TENSOR FASCIA LATA
   ORGAN: GALLBLADDER AND FAT METABOLISM
   TISSUE: LIGAMENTS
   GPT: DECISION MAKING / DEPENDENCY

2. MUSCLE: VASTUS LATERALIS
   ORGAN: STOMACH AND DIGESTION
   TISSUE: MUSCLES
   GPT: SOBRIETY / ADDICTION

3. MUSCLE: TRICEPS
   ORGAN: INTERNAL IMMUNE (THYMUS) AND LYMPH NODES
   TISSUE: LYMPH NODES
   GPT: HEALING / MENTICIDAL

4. MUSCLE: INFRASPINATUS
   ORGAN: SMALL INTENSTINE AND ASSIMILATION OF PROTEINS
   TISSUE: CEREBRAL SPINAL FLUID
   GPT: CREATIVITY / DEPRESSION.

Diaries

"Resistance Flexibility has given me the experience of continuing to grow and successfully work out biomechanical issues in my body that had been stuck ever since I can remember, including through more than 20 years of dedicated yoga practice. I now regularly discover new ways of moving and being in my body, ways that are freer from old constricting and sometimes painful patterns, and are more and more effective and satisfying. Resistance Flexibility has given me a framework to better understand and appreciate the different ways people are being and functioning—physically, psychologically, and emotionally—in the world and in themselves. Resistance Flexibility has given me a way to see and feel into others' bodies to help them move and be in healthier, more satisfying ways."
KajHoffman@TheGeniusofFlexibility.com Elite Resistance Flexibility Trainer

"It never fails when someone comes out of a stretch they feel the lightness. Often times they note that the stretched limb feels healthy and alive and the un-stretched areas feel sick and dead. In my own life I now have a constant feeling of aging in the opposite direction or backwards. I feel like I am moving away from my premature age and toward my true age. I feel hopeful about my body in the future rather than anticipating its deterioration. I can only imagine feeling better and better than I ever have- even in my early youth. Once you experience Resistance Flexibility, you can't help but expect continual development on all levels. I now experience the infinite capacity and potential in my body that I once only credited with my spirit."
LutherCowden@TheGeniusofFlexibility.com Elite Resistance Flexibility Trainer

"It just makes sense to me that I shouldn't have to control my posture in order to have 'good' posture. I'm busy enough living my life as it is without having to think about how it is I'm standing or sitting. My posture should be a reflection of my health, and not a posture I'm trying to hold together for reasons of image or physical comfort. I like to look in the mirror and see the areas of my body where my posture could be better and then Resistance Flexibility train those areas to remove what is preventing me from having natural and effortless posture. It's quite remarkable to see someone come into The Genius of Flexibility Center slouching or hyperextending in their natural posture, and after a bit of Resistance Flexibility notice how their alignment is significantly changed without any pain or discomfort in the process…effort yes, but no pain or suffering. The individuals feel a lighter, more free sense of standing in their body, and sometimes it's as if they went back to their childhood when everything moved with ease and without thought or fear."
JohnBagasarian@TheGeniusofFlexibility.com Resistance Flexibility Intern

"Because muscle groups on the back of my scapula are associated with the Small Intestine in TCM theory, and Resistance Flexibility training these specific muscles stimulates an increase in the pressure of cerebral spinal fluid, my depressed posture changes into an ease of verticality up my back, after I have been doing the stretch for but a few minutes. Now I naturally sit up without having to think about it."
MimiAmrit@TheGeniusofFlexibility.com Resistance Flexibility Intern

"In doing so much dance, yoga, and Pilates my whole life, pre-Resistance Flexibility, I had always thought that to hold my body in a certain way, only required me applying an idea (such as, lift the lower

tummy to support your low back and extend the pelvis). But what if my body actually fails to have the biomechanics to 'keep my shoulders down?' As I am doing Resistance Flexibility and see the results of other folks getting Resistance Flexibility assistance, the posture becomes natural, its is amazing to see the same goals achieved in body alignment without any mental control, the body should comfortably have posture on its own. One friend of mine, after being assisted stretched for her hamstrings and back, she always exclaims, 'I have no choice but to stand up straight! My feet are planted and my shoulders are naturally back.'"
BonnieCrotzner@TheGeniusofFlexibility.com Elite Resistance Flexibility Trainer

"I have been a runner for over thirty years. When I was running competitively, I was taught to adjust my body in order to improve my posture and stride. Each time I ran, I learned to consciously stand more upright by straightening my spine and pulling back my shoulders. These imposed adjustments did not actually change my posture; instead they placed stress on other parts of my body as I tried to accommodate the ideal running form. A number of years ago, I began practicing Resistance Flexibility Strength Training. I also took some time off from running, fearing that the long-term effects were doing more harm than good. In time however, I felt so great from the resistance stretching that I was encouraged to start running again. As was my old habit, I attempted to adjust my running posture, but was surprised to find that my body was already naturally upright, with shoulders back and a straight spine. In disbelief, I checked my form week after week and found that the improvements stayed—my body had made a permanent and positive change."
NoëlChristensen@TheGeniusofFlexibility.com Resistance Flexibility Intern

"It's like magic! Every time I come out of a stretch I feel my alignment improve. My shoulders extend, my chest opens up, I feel supported from my truck, and my legs get straighter and feel well placed in the joint. For my entire life I would hold myself upright as I sat and stood. I barely ever find myself doing that now."
BerylHagenburg@TheGeniusofFlexibility.com Resistance Flexibility Intern

"Adding in the resistance flexibility really helped with my breathing and increasing energy, as I had really flexed shoulder girdle that was also twisted from playing hockey and taking some many shots, and skating in a bent over posture for 31 years. Found myself having anxiety or even panic attacks from having the front side of my body and chest being so tight and twisted. I find my posture to be so much more open and untwisted feeling with the ease to breathe feeling more alive and excited."
ScottBottorff@TheGeniusofFlexibility.com Elite Resistance Flexibility Trainer

"My initial reasons for doing Resistance Flexibility were simple, I wanted to stretch and feel better in my body. At the time I wasn't very focused on physical activities or athletics, I just wanted to feel better. Over time I got focused on the psychological and life improvements as these became quite obvious to me. The physical body changes sort of snuck up on me after that. At first I merely started being more present in my body, more aware of feeling the different parts of it, feeling specific joints and muscle groups and sensations, and I developed a sense of comfort and discomfort. Then I began feeling a need to do more strenuous physical activities, and I took up roller blading and swimming, though I wasn't very good at either at first. But then one day, suddenly it seemed although it had been developing over time, as I was rollerblading through the streets of Boston, I instinctively jumped up in the air and over a chain that

blocked my path. And it was as easy as that, yet before that moment I would always carefully go around such things so as to not risk injury. Swimming is a story for another time."
TomLongo@theGeniusofFlexibility.com Elite Resistance Flexibility Trainer

"Once I began to become a little fluent in the vocabulary and understandings of the Resistance Flexibility techniques, my daily experience shifted. Where I used to wake up and wonder, 'what's that' sensation, now I find that the sensations of a new day are usually from the work I am doing on my body. And anything that I find annoying, I can apply the technique, and disappear in a few minutes. I no longer suffer a crick in my neck, or a wonky knee through the day. I have gone from being concerned about doing certain things 'before I get old' to confident I can do what I love or want to do as long as I live."
PatrickGregston@TheGeniusofFlexibility.com Resistance Flexibility Intern

"I came to RF because of pain in my right knee, after trying many other alternative modalities which gave little, if any, relief. My knee pain is now largely gone, and in the process of addressing that, I have learned a lot about the ways in which my body goes out of balance that resulted in the pain. Now, with much better knowledge and tools than I ever had before, I am working on resolving those deeper patterns—such as scar tissue in my hamstrings, a torqued pelvis, and scoliosis—that set the stage for my knee problem.

"Resistance Flexibility has provided me with highly effective methods and knowledge for healing and developing in many ways. Through the Resistance Flexibility training and practice I learned, for the first time, how to stretch and be stretched really effectively—systematically, predictably, and reliably. I learned how intelligent and subtle real stretching and strength training could be. I found how deeply satisfying and therapeutic it is to be stretched by a supportive community of fellow practitioners. I learned how essential the assistance and perspective of others is to my wellbeing and growth."
KajHoffman@TheGeniusofFlexibility.com Elite Resistance Flexibility Trainer

"A first time client, had to park a long block away from the studio. She had to sit down half way along the block; she couldn't walk far due to lots of biomechanical and physiological issues. She texted me the next day after she got worked on. She didn't need to sit down on the way back to the car and she had gone out to take a MILE long walk the next day. Walking is her favorite thing."
BonnieCrotzner@TheGeniusofFlexibility.com Elite Resistance Flexibility Trainer

"It has been very helpful to know which particular muscle groups are responsible for particular movements. When I'm feeling challenged performing a particular physical activity, I can know which muscle groups to work on to facilitate better movement in that activity."
LutherCowden@TheGeniusofFlexibility.com Elite Resistance Flexibility Trainer

"Resistance Flexibility has helped me to understand all the movement patterns of the body, as well as how those movements interact with and affect each other. This has helped me to better identify and diagnose problems in my body and others, and too much better develop strategies for resolving them. RF has given me the opportunity to feel what it is like to really be in my body in a natural, instinctual way, and allow my body to move from that place rather than imposing limited ideas of how I am supposed to

move and position myself. RF has helped me to regain ability to breath naturally and discover how that transforms playing music into a much more pleasurable flowing state. RF has helped to increase my facility, speed, endurance, expressiveness, and pleasure when playing classical guitar and piano."
KajHoffman@TheGeniusofFlexibility.com Elite Resistance Flexibility Intern

"I am a body worker and have studied movement and helped people get better from injuries for 25 years. This information of how muscles stretch and shorten and balance in pairs has become the corner stone of my work, my understanding of how people move of how to analyze and treat injures of other people and myself. I have repeated this basic revolutionary information so many times to help people. And it works. Today at the farm stand my farmer Vera could not lift her arm because of shoulder pain. She was heading out for Christmas and wanted to play with her great grand children. So standing by the road we did 10 minutes of resistance stretching me pulling her arm down against her resistance. Laughing having fun and now Vera can lift her arm. Not a cure but impressive improvement in function and comfort. The thing is she understood the idea. Like many people, especially ones who have been moving all their lives, it made sense to her It just makes sense to your body. Because it is how our bodies work. When next I see her I expect to find she has taken the stretches I gave her and applied her own genius and commend sense and will show me a stretch and movement that is useful and innovative. Something that works for her."
EricBeutner@TheGeniusofFlexibility.com Elite Resistance Flexibility Trainer

"I have physical trauma in the form of a physiological illness in my lung, appendix, and thymus meridian muscle groups. As a child I ingested a toxin and because I never displayed an obvious negative reaction…the toxicity festered in my system without getting removed. When I get these muscle groups resistance stretched I feel like my head and chest could explode. The intensity of feeling requires all of my effort and stamina to complete the stretch. I don't really have any words to describe the level of effort it takes. The only things that I have found make it possible for me to muster this effort is the intent focus and support of those assisting me in the stretch, and my own desire to 'know' the feeling I have during the stretch and to also discover what is on the other side of it- or what it will turn into. The tissue force is so tremendous it requires a minimum of 3 people to move. Without fail, the stretching lasts for up to 45 minutes and I experience it as no more than 5 or 10 minutes. Time seems to warp and stop allowing me as much as I need to process this trauma out of my body."
BerylHagenburg@TheGeniusofFlexibility.com Resistance Flexibility Intern

"After resistance stretching, I felt like I regained access to the control panel of my health. My daily practice becomes more satisfying each time, each time I release a little more of the restricted patterns and learn more about what my body needs. If at any time throughout my day I get a signal from by body that something is out of alignment or about to flare up and restrict me, I know what to do to relieve it on the spot."
SamuelCamburn@TheGeniusofFlexibility.com Resistance Flexibility Intern

"I was diagnosed with Parkinson's disease in January of 2013 at the age of 49. Since September of 2015, I have been seeing Bob Cooley and his Santa Barbara team for Resistance Flexibility. Even though Parkinson's is known solely as an incurable, progressively degenerative disease, through Resistance

Flexibility I have experienced a dramatic improvement in my posture, gait, rigidity, facial expression, and vocal strength along with gaining a new sense of peace and well being. This has had a tremendous impact on my life. Recently I was with my mother whom I had not seen since prior to beginning RFST. She also had no knowledge of RFST or that I was involved in any type of training program. As soon as she saw me she said, 'Oh my gosh you look great! You look younger…and taller. Wait…how can you be taller?? I don't know what you have been doing; all I know is that I want to do it too!' "
Susie Nocia Santa Barbara CA

"A greater foundation for me has occurred in terms of understanding my physiological health from doing this work. It connects dots for me in a beautifully natural but sophisticated way. The way I can access the health of my organ by doing a specific group of stretches is paramount information for every person to know and use. When I get intense thymus stretches I feel unbreakable internally. There's this heat that shows up for me and I feel it's the light or fire of protection that fuels me and keeps me safe."
Chris Pearsall@TheGeniusofFlexibility.com Resistance Flexibility Intern

"After 26 years I had become accustomed to sleeping on my right side. Back in 1987, I injured my left hip when I fell cross-country skiing. I hadn't been able to sleep on that side since. I tried everything, physical therapy, chiropractic, massage, acupuncture, and nothing worked. I was convinced that emotions had been trapped in my hip. I searched for help in releasing this. In 2013, I was introduced to Resistance Flexibility and it was the beginning of some very significant changes for me. In my first session the emotion that was trapped in my hip was released. After several sessions I was able to lie on my left side for a short amount of time. And now, I wake up in the morning smiling when I realize I am on my left side!"
Ruth Wishengrad, M.Ed., Songs To Change Your Tune™ (www.SongsToChangeYourTune.com)

"Resistance Stretching has certainly given me significant increases in my ease of movement. Of course it has removed chronic knee, back, and neck pain from my body…but what I didn't expect is the new movement I now have and relish. I am very aware that there is so much more to go. Experiencing the ease and explosiveness that comes from muscles being able to shorten and fire is something I had never identified in my body before Resistance Flexibility. One evening I was running home in the rain and after a few minutes my legs and arms started to move as a whole…the movement felt so secure and powerful that I found myself gaining access to deeper levels of breathing and my lung power to propel my body forward with ease. Now that I have discovered Resistance Flexibility, I can only imagine my movements will keep getting better."
BerylHagenburg@TheGeniusofFlexibility.com Resistance Flexibility Intern

2. PSYCHOLOGICAL BENEFITS FROM RESISTANCE FLEXIBILITY

High/Low Personality Traits, Mastery, Free-Attentional Focus, GPT traits,

There is a concomitance between each of the 16 different muscle groups or *types* of Resistance Flexibility stretches and personality trait development according to the theory of Genetic Personality Types (GPT)™. For example, the muscles that twist you are concomitant with your ability to be trusting, other muscles that untwist you are concomitant with your ability to be intimate, the muscles that that use to throw are concomitant with empowerment, etc. There are sixteen of these high personality traits that can be developed while simultaneously dismantling their opposite low traits.

According to Genetic Personality Type (GPT) Theory, each *type* of stretch can help to develop the high traits of one of the 16 genetic personality *types* while dismantling the opposite low traits. Anyone can develop their sobriety, creativity, trust, etc. while dismantling the opposite low traits. For example, by Resistance Flexibility training the muscles on the outside of your lower body associated with the Gall Bladder (GB), you can increase your ability to make decisions and be more devotional while dismantling dependency problems. Other Resistance Flexibility *types* of stretches can increase our sobriety, creativity, honesty, trust, etc.

Each of the different personality types has predicable relationships with the other *types*. The nature of those relationships mirrors the high/low traits of each type. One of those is called the balancing *types* who are good matches for long-term intimate relationships.

The hallmark of Resistance Flexibility is the ability to advance one's psychological health in predictable ways from different *types* of stretches. There are four groups of *types* that have equivalent qualities. What is so important about the equivalency principle is that it allows everyone to better understand how other people have equivalent things happening for them that match what they are having. For example, if you see someone that is being emotional compared to yourself, you are being viewed as not being as emotional as them, and instead maybe more physical. This allows everyone to not be so triggered by other things people find irritating.

There are four groups of *types*: Physical, Thinking, Emotional, and Spiritual each having equivalent viewpoints, time references, awareness, instincts, etc.

The following is a chart comparing the four groups of *types* and how they are equivalent.

FOUR GROUPS OF GENETIC PERSONALITY TYPES EQUIVALANCEY CHART

	PHYSICAL	THINKING	EMOTIONAL	SPIRITUAL
VIEWPOINT	*Instinct*	*Knowledge*	*Being*	*Perspective*
TIME	*Present*	*Future*	*Past*	*Relative*
AWARENESS	*Awake* *Asleep*	*Clear* *Confused*	*Conscious* *Unconscious*	*Alive* *Suffering*
INSTINCT	*Love* *Anger*	*Fearless* *Fear*	*Excited* *Anxious*	*Calm* *Frightened*
PROCESS	*Active*	*Proactive*	*Retroactive*	*Reactive*
INTERFACE	*Relate* *Defensive*	*Detach* *Clueless*	*Attach* *Uncaring*	*Connect* *Unconnected*
BODY	*Arms*	*Legs*	*Face*	*Trunk*
LONGING	*Dream*	*Aspiration*	*Fantasize*	*Imagine*
PERCEPTION	*Discernment*	*Insight*	*Shrewdness*	*Judgment*
STRETCHING	*Position*	*Identification*	*Breathing*	*Resistance*

CATEGORIES: Viewpoint; Time Reference; Awareness; Instinct; Process; Interface; Body; Impression; Perception; Stretching

Viewpoint—the group *type's* essential or natural way of identifying, recognizing, and displaying to others the *type* of information they collect about the world. Each group develops one of the four viewpoints initially before learning how to develop the others.

Time—the group *type's* natural time reference and preference; each group uses one of the four time references initially disproportionately to the others before learning how to develop the others.

Awareness—the group *type's* state of sentience. Being awake or asleep refers to being aware of information from the five senses or not. Being clear or confused refers to being aware of mental clarity on an idea or not. Being conscious or unconscious refers to being aware of one own and others desires or not. Being alive or suffering refers to being aware of one's perspective on one's own or others lives or not.

Instinct—the group *type's* innate impulse to the world. Love and anger refers to a person feeling accord or conflict with others. Fearless and fearful refers to a person feeling knowledgeable or not about ideas. Excitement and anxiety refers to a person feeling satisfied or not about what they desire. Calm and indifferent refers to a person feeling alive and connected to their life and others or not.

Process—the group *type's* way of processing their life's events. Active refers to a person taking action in response to a situation. Proactive refers to a person taking action in preparation before a situation. Retroactive refers to a person processing a situation after the event. Reactive refers to a person having a perspective reaction to a situation.

Interface—the group *type's* interchange with the world. Relating or defensive refers to a person's response as protective of themselves or others or not. Detach or clueless refers to a person's response as associating with themselves or others or not. Attach or uncaring refers to a person's response to themselves or others as intimate or not. Connected or unconnected refers to a person's response to themselves or others as linked or not.

Body—the group *type's* most often experienced body part. Either the arms, legs, face or torso.

Longing—the group *type's* style of yearning for ultimate gratification. Either by having a dream, aspiration, fantasy, or imagination.

Perception—the group *type's* form of assessing the world. Discernment refers to a person having the ability to discriminate and perceive the present difference between things. Insight refers to a person having the ability to internally differentiate subtleties between things. Shrewdness refers to a person having strategic and careful approach to things. Judgment refers to a person having objective perspective between things.

Flexibility—the group *type's* contribution in Resistance Flexibility. The four aspects of stretching are the movement and position of the body, the identification of what is happening during the stretch, the natural way to breathe during the stretch and how to resist during the stretch.

Diaries

"Each major muscle group that I Resistance Flexibility train brings different sensations to my awareness. Some are more familiar than others. I've found that my success in getting a stretch in any particular muscle group depends on my ability to 'be' with this new sensation, which translates into a new way of being in my life. I love how this turns stretching, which I would normally consider a boring physical exercise, into an activity that allows me to explore all aspects of myself, including my behavior, and develop my personality in all ways."
LutherCowden@TheGeniusofFlexibility.com Elite Resistance Flexibility Trainer

"I have been taken, and taken myself, into distinctly different somatic and perceptive states many times, as well as observed others doing that, by focusing on different stretches. And these particular states are predictable and repeatable. I continue to be astonished by the fact that simply by targeting stretches on certain parts of my body I can enter into markedly distinct and pleasurable new ways of being."
KajHoffman@TheGeniusofFlexibility.com Elite Resistance Flexibility Intern

"I decided to spend time in heart pose because it is one of my least favorites. I did the pose for an hour- interspersing the stretch with the balancing and opposing muscle groups so I could get deeper into it. The very next morning I found myself in a typical situation for my life at the time. However, my behavior was radically different. I spontaneously acted unconditionally loving in a situation that I normally would have been defensive and irritated in."
BerylHgenburg@TheGeniusofFlexibility.com Resistance Flexibility Intern

"Its all in the body...working a specific muscle group that will help you reveal and experience that certain personality trait is profound at best. Experiencing these different traits means a better understanding of how other people on this planet are doing it different than you."
BonnieCrotzer@TheGeniusofFlexibility.com Elite Resistance Flexibility Trainer

"The personality information has made me realize how many different ways people are seeing and experiencing the world and each other. I used to assume if everyone were 'healthy' they would be having similar perceptions and experiences of the world, and similar thoughts about it. Now I am aware how very different the experience of different types can be."
KajHoffman@TheGeniusofFlexibility.com Elite Resistance Flexibility Trainer

"The equivalency chart puts words to the varieties of behaviors I see in people. It makes it so much easier to understand that different people really think and behave using different processes and tools. When I interact with people now I am more open to learning about what they do, rather than being frustrated with their differing approach. Stretching muscle groups intensely in the other worldviews also gives me a direct perception of these equivalent but different behaviors..., which in turn gives me a clearer view of what I am innately doing. This perspective makes the road to growth and development so much clearer."
BerylHagenburg@ThegeniusofFlexibility.com Resistance Flexibility Intern

"When I first learned about the four worlds (physical, thinking, emotional and spiritual) it was very humbling. By practicing the stretches associated with each worldview, I experienced how dramatically different these worldviews are from each other. I realized that I had spent my life operating from a limited viewpoint and that I had low odds of success because of this. I felt both validated for my strengths and challenged to work on my weaknesses. Understanding the four worlds allows me to learn enormously from other people who are developed in ways that I am working on. Now, everyone is endlessly interesting."
NickWare@ThegenusofFlexibility.com Elite Resistance Flexibility Trainer

"I was leaving my house and a neighbor was walking her dog. I hadn't seen her before so I said 'Good morning.' Before I said good morning, I was able to naturally process the following internal dialogue that used to overtake me for several hours: 'She probably doesn't like me because I am a renter in a guesthouse invading her "neighborhood" environment.' So in the past, I would have said 'hi' to her while still unable to get through this feeling that assumed her criticism of me. But yesterday, that negative feeling burned off and I felt a nice connection with her before I spoke. She responded, 'Hi, do you live here?' and stopped walking. We had a brief conversation. She told me which house she lived in, etc. Then, as if scripted, she smiled and said to me (quote), "Well, thank you for being so friendly." I was so shocked that I almost passed out and I said, 'Have a great day.' 'You too,' she said, and we walked away.

"It's not an easy thing to handle how differently people are interacting with me and how I relate to others. I have to change everything. It's as if one day, out of nowhere, everyone started looking at you differently than they have for your entire life. When this happens, I am conscious of burning my self-criticism and criticisms of others—it turns into the something else that I am learning about each day. It frees me to diversify my ways of being with others, allows them to do the same with me, and it gives me a lot more variety and surprises in my life."
NickWare@TheGeniusofFlexibility.com Elite Resistance Flexibility Trainer

"I could not believe the first time I learned that this information all translated to the physical body. This work truly has the ability to take you wherever it is you want to go. It is at its core a healing modality, but truly when you get past that, this modality can develop you into a more complete person. You learn through experiences in your physical body, as well as through perspective from others that know just what you want to know. Whatever skill it is you want to develop, go to the body first. Resistance Flexibility definitely levels the field to give everyone an equal chance at achieving their goals."
EthanDupuis@TheGeniusofFlexibility.com Resistance Flexibility Intern

3. EMOTIONAL BENEFITS FROM RESISTANCE FLEXIBILITY

Relaxation, Tension, Breathing, Looks, Emotional Maturation, Intelligences

RELAXATION AND TENSION

Deferring to your body when you stretch allows you to learn how your body produces tension in order to relax. As your muscles tense when being stretched, you feel there is an endless well of possible tension that is available. Using the right amount brings satisfaction to the stretch. Doing the emotional *type* stretches allows you to learn when you are tense how to relax, by allowing your attention to be outside yourself while feeling tense.

BREATHING

There are an unlimited number of ways to breathe, and each stretch show you how to allow yourself to breathe differently. This transfers over into your life so you can allow yourself to breathe differently in different situations with different people. Many disciplines instruct a person to breath in different ways, but I have always found this forced. I prefer to allow my body to show me how to breathe.

GOOD LOOKS

Everyone wants to feel good looking. Unbeknownst to most people, is that being good looking comes from acknowledging what is special in another person. Also the development of your self-affirmation, self-esteem, self-worth, and self-liking is what is reflected in your looks. There are many different *types* of good looks. Some examples include: sensual, pleasing, pretty, ravishing, remarkable, bedazzling, lovely, beautiful, alluring, precious, magnificent, delightful, reflective, absorbing, glowing, etc.

EMOTIONAL MATURATION

It is commonly known to most people that in order to advance their understanding about something, they have to talk out their ideas with others, and as a result of that exchange, a better understanding of the results. But it is less commonly known, that the same principle is true in order to mature emotionally. When you like someone, it is necessary to engage with that person, and then his or her engagement with your attraction to him or her is what emotionally matures you. How the other person respond to your engagement results in a hormonal maturation. So if you ever tried to mature your own emotional feelings by considering them only from inside yourself and failing, then you might try engaging with others by putting your feeling out there so the other person can respond.

16 *TYPES* OF INTELLIGENCE/STUPIDITY

There are four general *types* of intelligence—a physical *type* of intelligence, a thinking *type* of intelligence, an emotional *type* of intelligence, and a spiritual *type* of intelligence, and within each of those groups are four differentiable *types* of intelligences, thus sixteen *types* of intelligences. The provenance of each type of intelligence is found in each *type*. A different *type* of intelligence and foolishness lives within each *type*. Each *type* woos the world with their characteristic perspicacious nature and intelligence, and boggles everyone's mind with their

16 GENETIC *TYPES* OF INTELLIGENCES

Gall Bladder	Decision Making
Liver	Strategy
Lung	Leadership
Large Intestine	Actualization
Stomach	Speculation
Pancreas	Communication
Heart	Mediation
Small Intestine	Creative
Brain	Problem Solving
Sexual	Conceptualization
Pericardium	Judgment
Skin	Venture
Bladder	Diversity
Kidney	Understanding
Appendix	Changing
Thymus	Healing

Diaries

"When I first observed Bob working with the trainers and asking them to look in the mirrors in the studio and talk about what they saw in themselves, I didn't think I'd be able to do that…let alone want to! But watching them change and grow exponentially, persuaded me to join in. It's truly amazing to see my own face change, and looks improve, after doing certain stretches, and feel comfortable looking in the mirror as I develop emotionally. I'm so grateful for this work!"
MimiAmrit@TheGeniusofFlexibility.com Resistance Flexibility Intern

"As a person who is naturally analytical, I've always wanted to gain more access to my emotions. Practicing the emotional exercises (Small Intestine, Bladder, Sexual, Liver) gives me access. My desires and attractions arise more easily and deeply. I am also more able to see the needs and desires of others. Each time I get stretched, I learn something new about how to tense, relax and be free."
NickWare@TheGeniusofFlexibility.com Elite Resistance Flexibility Trainer

"All the sudden I was attracted to everyone! I almost couldn't believe the contrast of what I was doing before and what I saw now. Time slowed down and the density of the air seemed to increase between people, it was like information was being exchanged through breathing. I can see what is so special about each individual then allow myself to process the next feeling that comes up, jealously, envy, love, excitement and so on. When I let this process run its course I get to have more of that particular high trait and in return realize what is so special about myself. Imagine if every single person on the planet had the support to experience this."
SamuelCamburn@TheGeniusofFlexibility.com Resistance Flexibility Intern

"I think that adults have a false, or somewhat illusory sense of what emotional maturity actually means, much less how they can track it within themselves as we age…at least that shoe fits on me. Feedback has given me great room to explore myself in the realm of how I am connecting with the outside world through my emotional body. I always thought of myself as emotional, but being told as a child that you're sensitive or moody, doesn't grant you a free pass to emotional relating in the world as we grow and change over the years. I can now see how I have been very much like a child, or a teenager in some of my ways of being that simply don't serve me as I am intending, and now have a more relaxed sense of how to perceive emotion in myself and others. I just feel more free and at ease with awkward moments of processing my experience, instead of pretending things aren't really effecting me and sweeping them under the carpet, because let's face it, nobody likes to go back and clean under that carpet. It's such a much more satisfying thing to be able to handle life when you aren't lying to yourself for self-protection or out fear of not knowing."
JohnBagasarian@TheGeniusofFlexibility.com Resistance Flexibility Intern

"Funny that everyone talks about projecting, that is, if I am upset at someone for being jealous, then 'pop psychology' says that I must be the jealous one. More than likely I have a problem equal (or worse than) jealousy like paranoia or lust or bias, etc. The concept of equivalency creates much more space when interfacing with the rough parts of a person, and with our own. It softens the edges a bit, and provides a way to resolve an issue. If I feel impatient then I can ask someone who does have patience how they do it."
BonnieCrotzer@TheGeniusofFlexibility.com Elite Resistance Flexibility Trainer

"For my entire life I have always spent much of my time noticing what is attractive, likeable, good-looking, beautiful, desirable and appealing in other people and also in objects. The more I do this, the more I get clarification on what I like and am attracted to. I hadn't realized it until Bob put it to words, but I am also aware of absorbing those qualities into myself that I find so desirable on the outside. So it would have to follow that I am projecting out all that I am able to absorb."
BerylHagenburg@TheGeniusofFlexibility.com Resistance Flexibility Intern

"When I am assisted in RF stretching, I often come out of it with a higher awareness of my emotional self. For many reasons, in my development as a young person this part of me was somewhat suppressed or that I falsely matured emotionally. So it's a big deal after getting stretched to feel a higher degree of personal satisfaction, attachment to others, and to like my looks, all concepts that are related to emotionality. The process to get there may or may not have that intention; really we just have to work the areas of the body that has a behavioral association with emotionality. As I am getting stretched, I become aware of all my effort building like a storm cloud, that tension I am using to get a result, and most important for me, that for those that are helping me, are getting satisfaction as they help me. Whoa, that's a big one to learn, being cared for and helped by others, most amazing feeling. Just like Mother Theresa, she must have liked helping folks and got a lot out of it, how else could she have kept going? When I come out of the stretch, I feel exhilarated, wanting to be so much closer to those around me, I see aspects of them that make me like them more, and a desire to help all humans feel the same kind of satisfaction in simply 'being.' As that sense of being or being in the becoming, pours out of me, I actually feel it in return. What a gift. And I feel soft enough to receive it."
BonnieCrotzer@TheGeniusofFlexibility.com Elite Resistance Flexibility Trainer

"It is totally surprising to me that my anxiety states can be turned into very positive emotional states. I have found that I can be in social situations in relaxed ways where before I was not really functioning well. I found I can accept other people's desires, what they like and dislike, while also having consciousness of what I like and dislike. Being able to handle my own and other emotions has freed me, and paved the way for me to be more spiritual."
BobCooley@TheGeniusofFlexibility.com

"When you ask a type about their high traits or their 'intelligence,' they can connect you to that way of being instantly. It feels like a download- it is that powerful. It might be one of the fastest ways to change and develop. People are just waiting to give and share what they have in abundance. We just don't know what or how to ask! Learning about the types and their intelligence gives the question and allows you to receive the answer. I never cease to be amazed at how much I have misunderstood qualities associated with types other than my own. Everything becomes so much easier when you know the innately human way to do what you are trying to do. Did you know that a decision is made with the knowledge and anticipation that the decision will have to change as soon as you get more information on the topic? I never knew that- but now that I do I am so much more free to make a 'wrong' decision"
BerylHagenburg@TheGeniusofFlexibility.com Resistance Flexibility Intern

4. SPIRITUAL BENEFITS FROM RESISTANCE FLEXIBILITY

Values, perspective, energy, practicality, life

It is perhaps unbelievable that you can develop your spirituality by increasing the flexibility in specific parts of your body. Spiritual development includes values, energy, practicality, perspective, and life awareness. It is important to know that the four different *types* of spiritual stretches specifically develop different *types* of spirituality: goodness, principles, integrity, and judicious. Spirituality is all about how to live well, and that depends on your ability to yield and resist and to process your reactions to events, people, etc.

The concomitance between each of the different muscle groups or *types* of Resistance Flexibility stretches and your spiritual development are extraordinary. For example, the deep muscles in your chest are concomitant with having better judgment, while muscles on the inside back of your legs connect you to being peaceful, while muscles on the sides of your body connect you with your integrity, etc. Your ability to know how and when to resist or yield, how to process your reaction to negative traits in others, all occur from developing different muscle groups.

Resistance Flexibility allows you to develop your spirituality from your body as a source. Is it possible, that the 16 types highest personality traits form the basis for all the different types of religions? Perhaps each spiritual tradition is a magnificent pillar that supports spirituality, each providing their high traits as paths to spiritual enlightening. All of these different pathways must be equal in value, none better than any other, yet each offering a different way to the top.

16 Types of Enlightenment—

Joy, Delight, Health, Empowerment,

Sobriety, Devotion, Trust, Understanding,

Romance, Bliss, Ecstasy, Freedom, and

Peace, Harmony, Integrity, and Pity.

After knowing types for a while, an unusual insight occurs…

Anytime someone behaves in an extraordinary positive manner, you find yourself absorbing their high traits, learning how to be like them, and then exhibiting these unexpectedly when you are doing something with just the right person, at the right time, and in the right place. And when you or someone behaves in a horrible manner in any way whatsoever, you simply realize that person, who is sometimes you, is simply malfunctioning internally, and that when their internal functionings are repaired, just like when you fix a broken part inside a car, you and everyone else can run more humanly, sometimes for the first time, in a particular way, in a very long time!

You probably have always hated the negative parts of yourself and others and either wanted to know how to defend yourself from these things or wanted these horrific behaviors to simply go away. But by knowing *types,* you will develop a new and infinitely better understanding of why these negative aspects of yourself and others exist. You will realize that these negative things, the vices in you and others, are exactly the 'stuff' in everyone that are transmuted into virtues.

Knowing types results in you developing the virtues of:

Humility, empowerment, temperance, love,

chastity, pity, moderation, and integrity.

while your mistakes of

pride, suppression, gluttony, sloth,

lust, anger, greed, and envy metamorphose.

You grow vegetables out of compost, they don't grow out of the flower, and such is the same for all the virtues, as they all grow out of the dark side of people. The negative aspects of people are the essential ingredients that are converted into the greatest behaviors of humanity. Learn how to transform the negative side of yourself into gold.

It is no longer good against bad precept,

goodness only comes out of the transmutation of what is bad.

It is only through having an awareness of the dark side of yourself and others that you then can create the opposite light side of yourself and others. In the process of converting your undesirable shortcomings, you learn how to turn the worst parts of yourself and others into the most righteous and admirable advantages for everyone—alchemizing that which you hate the most into gold.

Knowing types will break down

the fear and bias you have about people forever,

and elevate your predation instinct

into its higher trait of being uplifting

towards yourself or others that are

in need of personal development.

Diaries

"The more perspective I have on myself and those around me and on life in general, the more I find I am able to accept the changes that happen to me during a stretch. I let go of things like time, self and other judgment. This speeds up my recovery and integration of the stretch. Time stops and allows me to absorb."
BerylHagenburg@TheGeniusofFlexibility.com Resistance Flexibility Intern

"Last night was the first time that the feelings I had inside matched how people were looking at me and experiencing me. I've been waiting for this to happen, because when the inside view of myself comes to me, I can integrate what I am demonstrating in that moment. It felt very harmonious to experience a balance between how I felt about myself and how people were looking at me- a completion of the circle of energy exchange.

"I am certain that my weak link usually creates a gap in how I feel and how others feel about me. In the past, I have spent a lot of energy to figure out how people feel about me, because I didn't have this inside connection that I am developing."
NickWare@TheGeniusofFlexibility.com Elite Resistance Flexibility Trainer

"The organ concomitance is a miraculous discovery! The appendix is associated with removing toxicity from the face and brain. I had a toxic exposure when I was young and later in my adult life found myself seeking out activities that require the use of the muscles in the upper body associated with the appendix organ. I was very drawn to skateboarding! This might seem normal, but given my life situation at the time, it was the opposite! I remember craving the movement that you make on the skateboard and really wanting to learn and experience it. The Lattissimus Dorsi muscle associated with the appendix is dominant during skateboarding. When I found myself afraid of falling on the skateboard and also slow to learn it... I moved onto gardening. Again, gardening is associated with the appendix meridian muscle group and I craved it. As I remove the toxicity from my body, I still love to garden, but it doesn't consume me in the way that it use to. The stretch I did when I first started resistance stretching was pigeon for the gall bladder meridian muscle group. I would spend 15-30 minutes a night in the pose. My digestion radically changed in a matter of a week or so. I began digesting fats! I had no idea before this that I wasn't. I just thought that is the way it is."
BerylHagenburg@TheGeniusofFlexibility.com Resistance Flexibility Intern

"I've had emotional moments of release and being humbled come up for me doing this work and just being around it. I get moved by people. I had a moment during my level 4 training where I was taken to a place during an intense medial hamstring stretch that overwhelmed me in such a way that I started to deeply cry. I felt like I was crying for the worlds sadness, not just my own. I had never been taken to that place of healing with 5 sets of hands on me. I'm grateful this work has the power to help take people at times so gracefully, to a place they've never been before."
ChrisPearsall@TheGeniusofFlexibility.com Resistance Flexibility Trainer

"Having experienced the equivalencies of the different groups of types, has allow me to transfer this comparative perspective into my life. When I am being with another person, I can see how they are not

'doing' their life mostly like I am, they are 'doing' life a different ways. I love learning more and more different ways to be living."
BobCooley@TheGeniusofFlexibility.com

"My original thought that was that to further allow a muscle to stretch you would just have to continue stretching it and it would slowly become more flexible. Working with Resistance Flexibility quickly changed that view for me. After starting my work at the studio, it was brought to my attention that my body cannot digest sugars properly and that it results in my body over producing an almost disgusting amount of mucous. This immediately made sense to me, but was not something that I had ever thought of before. I had not changed my diet after hearing this (bad move on my part but turned into a learning experience in the end thankfully), and continued with my stretching as I had before. I decided to start focusing more and more on my Spleen-Pancreas meridian, hoping that this would help stimulate my body to produce more digestive enzymes that would break down the sugars so that I would not have as much mucous pooling throughout my body. After about 2 weeks, I had little to no change in my true range of my medial hamstrings. I talked to some of the Elite Trainers and Bob about it, and they all came up with the idea that I should actually change my diet so that I am not taking in as many of the foods that require the spleen and pancreas to fully operate. I decided to try it out, not fully understanding at the time how that it would be linked to getting more flexibility in my medial hamstrings. Alas, it worked. After just 4 days of changing my diet, and continuing the same stretching routine that I had been previously doing, I had a significant amount of more flexibility in my spleen-pancreas meridian. The crazy part? I also started to lose POUNDS of mucous from my body. I no longer have to spit out mucous every 5-10 minutes, and my tissue is much less 'puffy' than it used to be. In the end, it turned out that changing my diet and eating nutrient rich food that supported the inabilities of my body immediately changed my flexibility in those problem areas."
AlexNolte@TheGeniusofFlexibility.com Elite Resistance Flexibility Intern

"The next profound realization was that who I am is a particular kind of person, oriented by birth in a certain way. As I develop that, and move through greater awareness of my gifts and challenges, I realize that I can have the life And love I have always longed for. The WAY I stretch determines the result. The ways I listen and learn add tension or surrender, subtle or strong. The journey is deep and endless and cannot be done alone. The world is full of infinite possibilities instead of limitations. For all this and more, I am grateful and challenged!"
KateRabinowitz@TheGeniusofFlexibility.com Resistance Flexibility Intern

"For me I have always struggled to make my life happen, now as I am learning about being in the becoming and building on contentment, life is just taking me, taking me places I always knew I had the potential to go, places where I have always wanted to be."
BonnieCrotzer@TheGeniusofFlexibility.com Elite Resistance Flexibility Trainer

"I see how they are doing the thing that brings them into their authentic self. I am beginning to see what is so special about everyone, when I do this I allow the next reaction of jealousy, envy, anger, excitement, love and so on to process, I try and be with it with out judgment. The more I out myself to the world the more they know how to heal me and me them. Of course there is a flip side to that and a healthy layer

of defense is natural. I learned about transmuting predatorily behavior into the higher trait, this really spoke to me, and put a database to the internal dialogue that I feel between people. My body healed more and more. I continue to be revived by the development of the individuals in my flexibility community. Now I am seeing more of the life of a person; this comes across as being more naturally able to pick up on what people and myself want, as well as being able to bridge into others from a pure interest that connects us to a solution together. Wow! People love to be seen, understood, and felt, all the things that people don't like about one another are just reactions from confusion, at least that's what I know right now."

SamuelCamburn@TheGeniusofFlexibility.com Resistance Flexibility Intern

"I could not believe the first time I learned that this information all translated to the physical body. This work truly has the ability to take you wherever it is you want to go. It is at its core a healing modality, but truly when you get past that, this modality can develop you into a more complete person. You learn through experiences in your physical body, as well as through perspective from others that know just what you want to know. Whatever skill it is you want to develop, go to the body first. Resistance Flexibility definitely levels the field to give everyone an equal chance at achieving their goals.With the help and support of the RF community, and through your own journey in stretching, you will learn more than you could have ever imagined about the interaction of people and why we do what we do. You gain a perspective that tells you that people aren't necessarily thinking the same way, or doing what you're doing. From my experience I have discovered that not everyone is as future minded as I am. I was even unaware that this was what I was doing, or that there was anything else to do. I spend a lot of my time now staying present minded and out of my head, which allows me to connect with more people and have many more satisfying experiences with people."

EthanDupuis@TheGeniusofFlexibility.com Resistance Flexibility Intern

"The psychological component of the RF stretch is the most intriguing part of the stretch for me. It's what drew me in, keeps me coming back and hanging in there when I want to bolt. I know somewhere during my stretch a jewel of an insight will be revealed. I've been interested in, motivated by, propelled forward by personal growth since I can remember. It's the psychological revelations and insights that keep me coming back/ motivated to continue RF stretching. For example: I had NO idea how much I was resisting everything in my life. I was basically saying NO to my life. My resistance was disconnecting me from others and my life. I was enduring my life rather than living my life. Feeling dead or shutting me down to certain aspects of my life. As I have learned to yield, I've opened up more fully to my life. I am more myself. Living more fully in my body and more ALIVE in my life."

KatConnor-Longo@TheGeniusofFlexibility.com Resistance Flexibility Intern

"Sharing perspective was new for me. It basically scared me to death. The first time I was asked to share I just stood there like a deer in head lights. I really wasn't aware of what I was being asked. I was use to being on my yoga mat in a quiet space with an internal focus. I've now since learned the perspective we gain from each other is quite invaluable. We see things about others that they don't see for themselves and vice versa they see things about me I don't or can't see for myself. Just this week a huge insight was revealed to me through shared perspective regarding controlling my external environment. I hadn't realized that I was controlling my external environment because I was feeling uncontrollable internally.

Once I allowed myself to actually feel uncontrollable internally I was no longer terrified by it. There was an easy and a softening that flowed through me internally and through the room. I want to say an acceptance. I realized I had been fighting and trying to avoid feeling uncontrollable for years. Once I allowed the internal feeling of being uncontrollable it dissipated."

KatConnor-Longo@TheGeniusofFlexibility.com Resistance Flexibility Intern

CHAPTER 7

HEALTH CHECK USING RESISTANCE FLEXIBILITY

Proactive and preventative health strategies

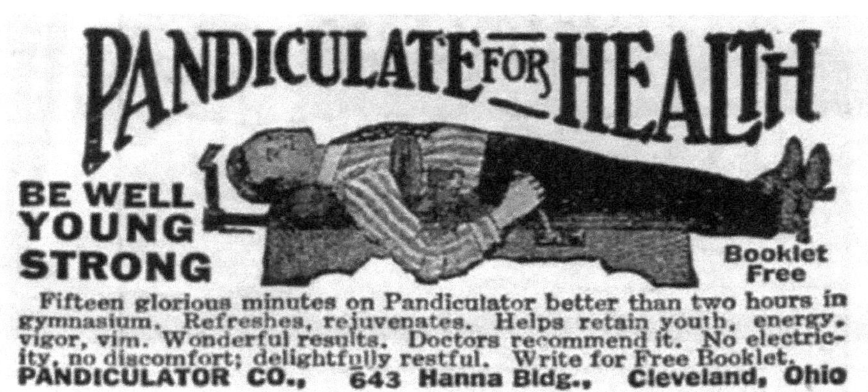

WHERE AND HOW TO START

I discovered Resistance Flexibility because I found it completely unacceptable that I could not move well nor be healthy after my pedestrian automobile accident. However, decades later I identified that there was a much bigger reason: I had been disconnected from my life because of my accident, and I wanted my life back. When I began to teach other people what I discovered that worked to bring me back to health, more often than not, everyone begins like myself with a problem they wish to solve. So lets begin there.

You can use Resistance Flexibility to help solve physical and physiological, psychological, emotional, or life concerns. What follows are simple questions to help you to begin to solve your concerns.

BEING AND STAYING HEALTHY IS A PROACTIVE THING

Everybody wants to know what their state or level of health is, and not wait until they get sick, can't move well, are too unsatisfied, or their life is not happening as they always imagined it could. So there is a way to learn something about the physical and physiological health of all of your sixteen *types* of your muscle groups, organs, tissues, as well as your psychological, emotional and spiritual wellness. You can use the results you gain from these two simple tests to monitor your level of wellness, and be proactive about your health?

People that first try Resistance Flexibility often come to The Genius of Flexibility Centers because they have lack a of physical functioning in their back, knee, shoulder, elbows, wrists etc. or because of physiological concerns. Others come for psychological snags, needed emotional maturation, or life concerns. And they usually find that many of their concerns are much easier to remedy than they imagined, but also requires more help from others than they imagined. As they begin to solve their problems, everyone begins to realize how much more it takes than they would ever have imagined. Yet their constant progress and the support of others cheer them on.

Then a lot of people find themselves returning for sessions or classes not because of chronic pain but because they want specific physiological upgrades that they learned were possible. Perhaps more unexpectedly, they also noticed advancements that were possible in personality trait developments, and better looks and more mature emotionality, and finally in new ways to develop spiritually. Now they come for classes or private sessions for all four reasons—physical/physiological, psychological, emotional, and spiritual.

SIMPLE QUESTIONS ABOUT WELLNESS

Why is there a simply way to help you know more about your health? Because in TCM, each of the different muscles groups are uniquely associated with different organ and tissue health and movements. For example if you don't already know, in TCM the muscles on the outside of your leg are associated with the Gall Bladder and ligaments. So if that is true, and that has been my experience, then if you RF test those muscles for flexibility and strength it may tell you something about the health of that organ. You can Resistance Flexibility train those muscles for a while and then see if the health of those organs has occurred through your personal experience or by medical tests.

POSTURE

1. Question: Do you have lower back pain?

If yes, then I would recommend to do Stretch #13 (Bladder)

2. Question: Do you lack rotation at your hip joints?

If yes, then I would recommend to do Stretch #6 (Pancreas)

3. Question: Do your knees bend too much backwards?

If yes, then I would recommend to do Stretch #9 (Brain)

4. Question: Does your spine curve too much backwards in your middle or upper back?

If yes, then I would recommend to do Stretch #15 (Appendix) and #16 (Thymus)

5. Question: Do you slouch when you sit?
If yes, then I would recommend to do Stretch # 8 (Small Intestine).

6. Question: Do you stand with your legs too wide?
If yes, then I would recommend to do Stretch #1 (Gall Bladder) and Stretch #2 (Liver)

7. Question: Do you have concerns with your ankles and feet
If yes, then I would recommend to do Stretch #13 (Bladder) and #14 (Kidney).

8. Question: Are your shoulders too narrow and tilted forward?
If yes, then I would recommend to do Stretch #12 (Skin) and Stretch #16 (Thymus)

9. Question: Do you have shoulder joint pain or lack of movement there?
If yes, then I would recommend to do Stretch #7 (Heart) and Stretch #8 (Small Intestine).

10. Question: Do your elbows hurt when you play tennis or golf?
If yes, then I would recommend to do Stretch #11 (Pericardium) and Stretch #12 (Skin)

11. Question: Do you have discomfort in your wrists and hands?
If yes, then I would recommend to do Stretch #15 (Appendix) and Stretch #16 (Thymus)

MOVEMENTS—16 KINETIC PATTERNS.

Which of the following movements do you want to have more of?

<u>Lower body:</u>

Turning outward (#1 GB)

Turning inward (#2 LV)

Advancing (#5 ST)

Retreat (#6 PA)

Twisting (#9 BR)

Untwisting (#10 SE)

Jumping (#13 BL)

Squatting (#14 KI)

Upper body:

Throw (#3 LU)

Catch (#4 LI)

Punch (#7 HE)

Elbow stroke (#8 SI)

Open (#11 PE)

Close (#12 SK)

Lift (#15 AP)

Lower (#16 TH)

JOINTS

Which of the following joints do you need to be freer?

Hip Girdle—#1Gall Bladder and #2 Liver

Hip Joint—#5 Stomach and #6Pancreas

Knee—#9 Brain and #10 Sexual

Ankle and Foot—#13 Bladder and #14 Kidneys

Shoulder girdle—#3Large Intestine and #4 Lung

Shoulder joint—#7 Heart and #8 Small Intestine

Elbow—#11Pericardium and #12 Skin

Wrist and Hand—#15 Appendix and #16 Thymus

TCM Check

Another more thorough way to learn more about your health is to test the flexibilities and strengths of each of the sixteen different *types* of Resistance Flexibility™ exercises that are concomitant with their respective organ and physiological systems, and personality traits. Based on the flexibility and strength of different muscle groups you can quickly determine which health concerns you need to prioritize.

Use the following sixteen *types* of Resistance Flexibility stretches to evaluate each area of your body and its TCM concomitance with organ wellness.

<u>HIP GIRDLE - GB AND LV</u>

GB BACK LYING LEG CLOSERS

LV BACK LYING LEG OPENERS

<u>SHOUDLER GIRDLE - LU AND LI</u>

LU HAND STAND

LI KNEELING TWIST

<u>HIP JOINT ST AND PA</u>

ST QUAD WALL

PA TURTLE

<u>SHOULDER JOINT SI AND HE</u>

HE HEART STRETCH

SI PRAYER ARMS IN FRONT

<u>KNEES BRAIN AND SEXUAL</u>

BR BACK LYING BENT LEG HAMSTRING

SE HIP FLEXOR ON FLOOR

<u>ELBOWS SK AND PE</u>

PE INCLINE PLANE

SK COBRA

ANKLE AND BL AND KI

BL BACK LYING LEG CROSS OVER

KI LOTUS SEATED

WRIST AND HAND AP AND TH

AP LOCUST WALKING UP WALL

TH ROLLDOWN

ORGANS/TISSUE/PHYSIOLOGICAL SYSTEMS

Which of the following organs, tissues, or physiological systems do you want to help?

ORGAN—TISSUE—SYSTEM

GB—Ligaments—Digestive System (Fat Metabolism)

LV—Tendons—Detoxification

LU—Oxygenation—Air Elimination System

LI—Venous Blood Flow—Waste Elimination System

ST—Muscles—Muscular System

PS—Fascia—Digestive System (Enzyme Catalysts)

HE—Blood Volume—Arterial Circulation

SI—Cerebral Spinal Fluid—Cranial Sacral System

BR—Nerves—Nervous System

SE—Hormones—Endocrine and Reproduction System

PE—Arterial Blood Flow—Arterial Circulation

SK—Skin—External Immune System (Integument)

BL—Bones—Skeleton System

KI—Joints—Urinary System

AP—Cartilage—Elimination of Toxins

TH—Lymph Nodes—Internal Immune System

DESIGNING YOUR OWN PROGRAM

On The GeniusofFlexibiliy.com web page, there are over 200+ videos of all the different types of stretches at all levels of difficulty. You can create your own Resistance Flexibility program or take prerecorded classes, or train with an Elite Trainer On Line. Each stretch is explained how to do each stretch is in video format with text explanation as well as all four aspects for each stretch.

https://www.thegeniusofflexibility.com/training-archive/join.html

A SUMMARY OF RESISTANCE FLEXIBILITY HEALTH BENEFITS

Immediate, cumulative, and lasting increases in true flexibility through Resistance Flexibility through the removal of ADFST ultimately frees all the myofascial structures to move optimally.

Increases in muscle mass, circulation, and lymphatic drainage occur because of removal of ADFST.

Increase joint movement in three planes, increase in joint capsule lubrication and elasticity, repair of joint capsules and ligaments.

Increase tendon elasticity, springiness, and repair of tendons.

Increase in muscle strength, especially throughout the entire muscle range instead of just in one section of the muscle.

Increase in endurance, and oxygenation saturation in the blood.

Decrease in recovery time from exercise. Damaged tissue has characteristically dramatic reductions in circulation and lymphatic flow, which starves the myofascial structures and greatly prolongs recovery.

Elimination of overly dense accumulated fascia and scar tissue in the anterior torso, posterior neck, and shoulders causes significant improvements in looks and attractiveness and feelings of self-liking, self-worth, self-esteem, and self-affirmation occur.

Remarkable recovery from concussions is being reported by individuals who suffered debilitating concussions.

Remarkable recovery from viral infections and elimination of the toxins

Increase in accuracy, replicability, and consistency of skill level.

Elimination of pain and referred pain in areas sometimes far from the ADFST location (e.g. low back pain resulting from hamstrings ADFST).

Reduce BRI substitutions and compensations; return the body to true, natural, and pain-free movement. Characteristically, fascia damage located in one area always affects areas of the body far away from the original site. Compensatory Bone Rotational Substitutions are forced to occur because the ADFST prevent movement at one or more joints thus requesting that adjacent joints make the movements they cannot make. Bone Rotational Interrelatonships (BRI): optimize BRI to allow optimal and efficient movements.

PART II: RESISTANCE FLEXIBILITY EXERCISES

Introduction to 16 types of Resistance Flexibility exercises

CHAPTER 8

RESISTANCE FLEXIBILITY STRETCHES

Two Page Layout: Beginners, Intermediate, Advanced and Assisted

HOW TO USE THE TWO PAGE STRETCH LAYOUT

THE TRAINING ARCHIVE—200+ STRETCH VIDEOS

All of the Resistance Flexibility exercises in this book are in video format on our web page www.TheGeniusofFlexibility.com called The Training Archive with additional instructions and content. The first month is free and then only costs $15/month for 6 months. Check it out:

https://www.thegeniusofflexibility.com/training-archive/join.html

Diaries

"I learned about Resistance Flexibility through Oprah.com. I joined the Training Archive for free for my first month, and then subscribed for only $15/month for six months. For every stretch there is a video, how the stretch can affect my physiological and psychological health, looks, and spirituality. Any question I ever had about a stretch is presented in video, graphics and text on the Training Archive. Incredible."

"I subscribed to the Training Archive and learned that I could hire one of the Elite Resistance Flexibility Trainers for On-Line private sessions. I tried one with my personal trainer present also, and we both learned how to do the self stretches I needed, and how to have my trainer assist me."

"I have been taking Resistance Flexibility classes for the last year Bob's Sunday morning class. As a small group we learn and practice different types of stretches but always hamstrings because they need the most work. We always laugh a lot, and learn from each person on how the different stretches are affecting them. Everyone is honored as a knower, and we each give our perspective on how the stretches affect each other. A great way to learn."

"I have always been frustrated with stretching in general. I've tried many different brands of stretching and truthfully they don't work. I'm willing to put in the effort, I'm smart enough to understand what I need to do, but only Resistance Flexibility works. It is not that it works so well that is the most amazing, it is how fast it works. I did not believe that flexibility training would affect my personality, looks, or my values. But when I first started I watched as other people self stretched or got assisted and afterwards I saw and hear incredible things by everyone. You don't have to believe the claims; you get to experience them yourself. The results say it all."

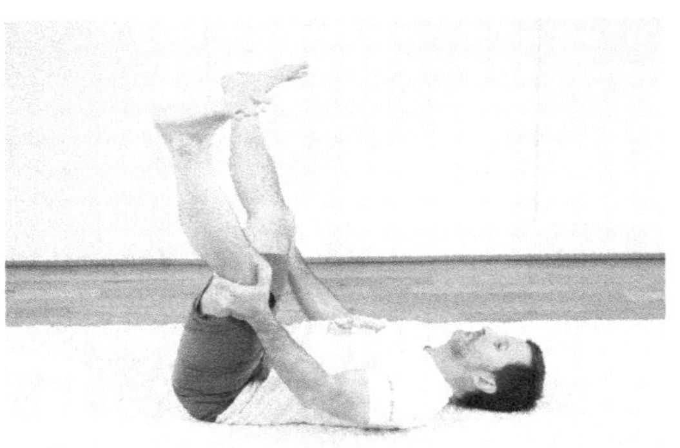

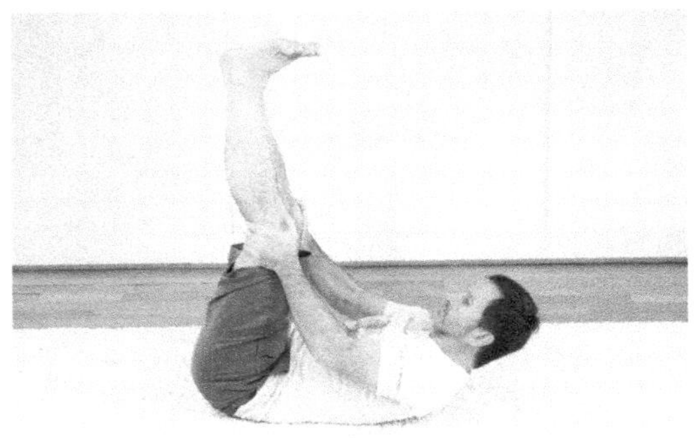

FOUR OPTIONS (LEVELS) FOR EACH OF THE 16 TYPES OF STRETCH = 64 TOTAL RESISTANCE FLEXIBILITY STRETCHES

There are four versions for each *type* of Resistance Flexibility exercise: Beginners, Intermediate, Advanced, and Assisted. For example, for Resistance Flexibility Stretch #1 there are four levels of practice. And of course there are a total of sixteen different *types* for your whole body—eight for your lower body and eight for your upper body. Choose whichever level for each *type* of stretch that works best for you. Each *type* of stretch is presented in that order so you can pick whichever level works best for you. Each of the same *type* of stretch is on a page that has the same color code on the bottom of the pages. The Two-page Layout includes:

1. THE NAME OF THE STRETCH

Includes the number of the stretch #1—#16, and a name. For example:

#1 BEGINNER (GALL BLADDER) - BACK LYING LEG CLOSING

#1 Beginner (Gall Bladder) is on the left page, and

Back Lying Leg Closing is on the right page.

Some people like remembering the stretch by the number and difficulty level, and other people like remembering the stretch by the name. Help yourself.

2. THE ORDER OF THE STRETCHES #1- #16

All the stretches are ordered based on the theory of Traditional Chinese Medicine (TCM) energy flow. What I discovered is that the muscles in my body are organized by depth, and that the Energy Cycle in TCM is identical to the depth of muscles, organizing them from lower and upper and lower continuously in a loop.

ENERGY FLOW TRELLIS

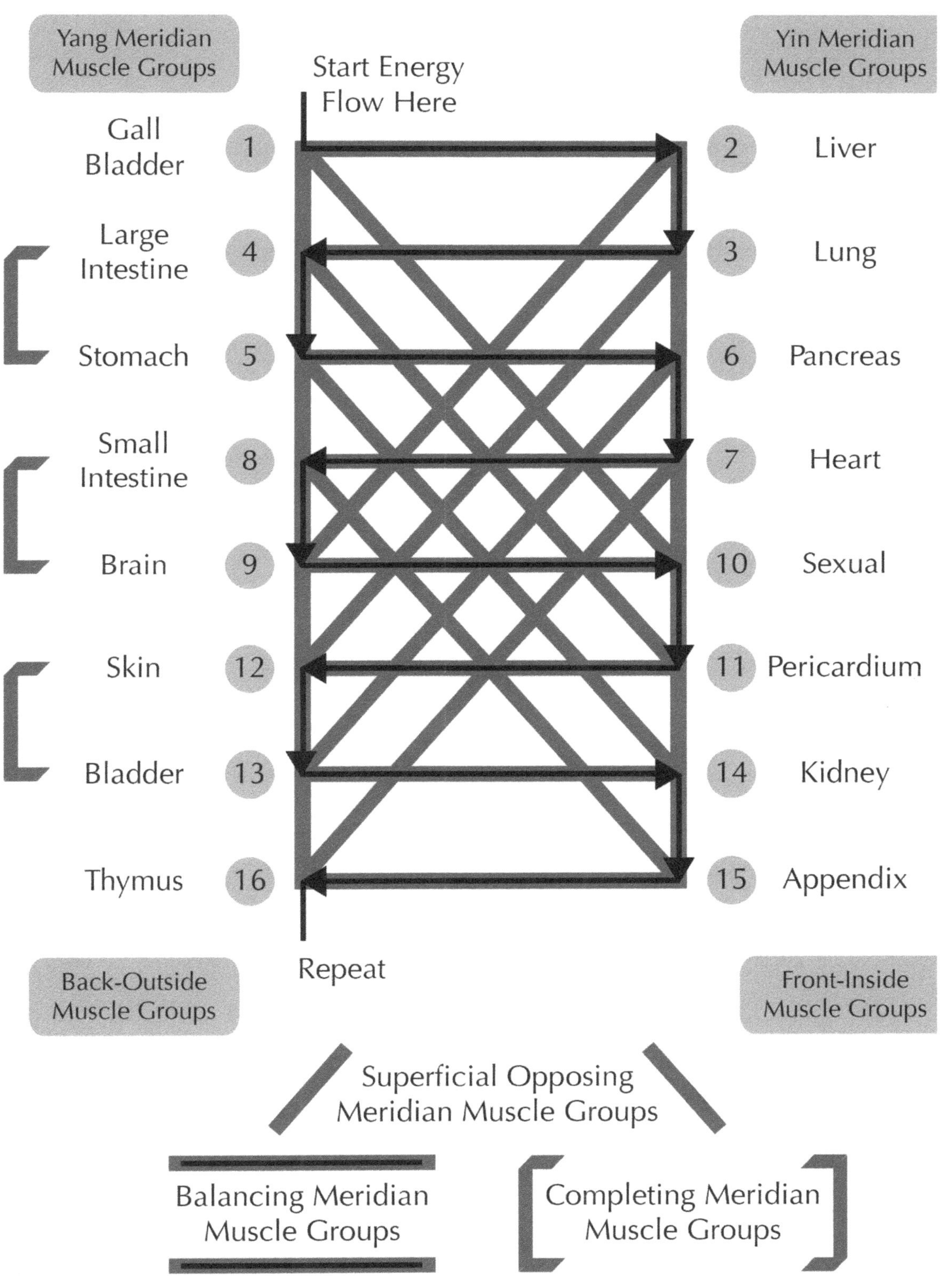
Yang Meridian Muscle Groups
Start Energy Flow Here
Yin Meridian Muscle Groups
Gall Bladder
1
2
Liver
Large Intestine
4
3
Lung
Stomach
5
6
Pancreas
Small Intestine
8
7
Heart
Brain
9
10
Sexual
Skin
12
11
Pericardium
Bladder
13
14
Kidney
Thymus
16
15
Appendix
Back-Outside Muscle Groups
Repeat
Front-Inside Muscle Groups
Superficial Opposing Meridian Muscle Groups
Balancing Meridian Muscle Groups
Completing Meridian Muscle Groups

3. THE STARTING POSITION AND RESISTANCE FLEXIBILITY PHOTOS AND INSTRUCTIONS

Example from #1 stretch:

#1. BACK LYING LEG CLOSING (GALL BLADDER)

STARTING POSITION: Lie on your back with both legs perpendicular to your torso and opened wide apart. Grasp the outside of your knees with your hands, palms facing in.	RESISTANCE FLEXIBILITY: Your legs push outwards to resist as your hands close your legs together. Return to the starting position and repeat 10 times.

Each stretch has two large photos with explanations centered in each page. On the left page is the starting position with an explanation of how to get into the starting position, and the right page how to Resistance Flexibility train during that stretch.

4. THE BENEFITS

There are six potential health benefits for each type of stretch including: your physiological health, the body part and joint that are targeted, the movement that can be improved by doing this type of stretch, the good looks that this type of stretch helps to create, and how this type of stretch can affect your life. For example for stretch #1 Beginner (Gall Bladder) Back Lying Leg Closing Stretch:

BENEFITS

Health: Fat Metabolism
Body Part: Hips
Joint: Hip Girdle
Movement: Turn Outward
Good Looks: Sensual
Life: Committed, Advocate

5. MUSCLES

Specific muscles are primarily stretched for each type of stretch. And when those muscles contract or stretch they produce a specific kinematic pattern. For example, for stretch #1 Beginner (Gall Bladder) Back Lying Leg Closing Stretch this is the list and a more complete list can be seen on The Training Archive on TheGeniusofFlexibility.com web page.

MUSCLES

Frontalis, Temporalis, Trapezius, Pectoralis Major, Oblique Abdominals, Gluteus Minimus and Medius, TFL, IT Band, Vastus Lateralis, Peroneals

Action: Flexion/Abduction/Inward

Stretch: Extension/Adduction/Outward

6. TRADITIONAL CHINESE MEDICINE

In Traditional Chinese Medicine (TCM) each group of contiguous muscles is uniquely associated (concomitant) with an organ, type of tissue, physiological system, type of receptors, and Yin or Yang element. When you practice each of the 16 different *types* of stretches, each *type* can positively affect these aspects of yourself. For example, for Stretch #1 Beginner (Gall Bladder) Back Lying Leg Closing Stretch:

(TCM)

Organ: Gall Bladder
Tissue: Ligaments
Body Part: Legs
System: Fat Metabolism
Sensory: Nervous System
Yin/Yang Element: Yang Wood

7. PERSONALITY *(GPT)*

Each of the sixteen different types of stretches is also concomitant with capable of developing specific personality traits. There are four groups of *types:* Physical, Thinking, Emotional, and Spiritual. Each of these groups is innately more time aware in the present, future, past, or has a relative sense of time. There are many high and low traits for each *type,* and five high traits, and two low traits are offered as a quick review. And each *type* innately has either a physical, thinking, emotional, or spiritual instinct. Please see Chapter 6 for a beginning explanation of these concepts, and in March of 2016 my second book *The Sixteen Geniuses—sixteen Genetic Personality Types 1.0* will be available with support from *The16Geniuses.com* web page. For example, the genetic personality *type* (GPT) information for Stretch #1 Beginner (Gall Bladder) Back Lying Leg Closing Stretch:

PERSONALITY (GPT)

Group: Thinking
Time and Attention: Future and Inside
High Traits: Decision Maker, Advocacy,
Devotional, Abundance, Certainty
Low Traits: Dependent, Guilt
Instinct: Fearless/Fearful

8. BALANCING STRETCH

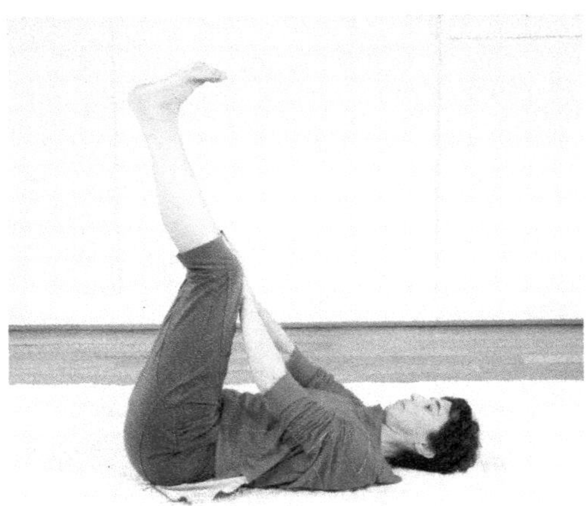

The ability to stretch any muscle is dependent on the muscles on the opposite side of the body to shorten. So when you try any stretch, your ability to get into that position is not just determined by the flexibility of the muscles that are targeted to be stretched in that position but instead mostly by the ability of their balancing muscles on the opposite side of the body capacity to shorten. Remember that the capacity of a muscle to shorten is dependent on its flexibility not just its strength, so if you want to get a great stretch for any muscle group, the limiting factor is NOT the muscles you are stretching but the flexibility of the muscles on the opposite side of the body. (See Chapter 1 and 2 for more information on the Balancing Muscles capacity to shorten. For example, for Stretch #1 Beginner (Gall Bladder) Back Lying Leg Closing Stretch the Balancing Stretch is its balancing stretch: #2 Beginners (Liver).

9. OPPOSING STRETCH

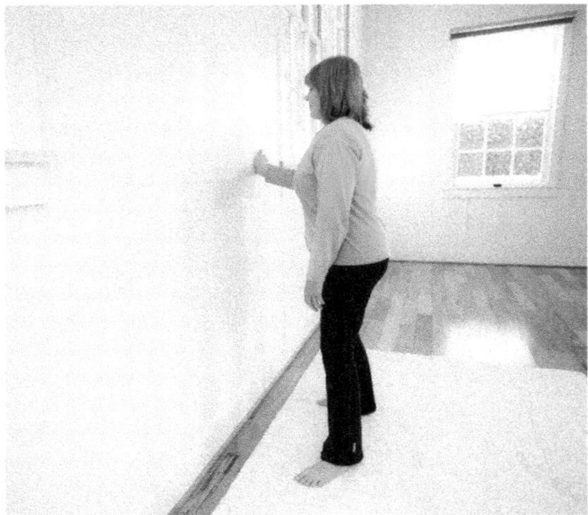

When any muscles stretches besides the balancing muscles needing to shorten, your bones need to rotate either inward or outward in order for the natural movement to happen. This is largely determined by muscles that are at a ninety-degree angle to the muscles you are stretching—called the Opposing Muscles. (See Chapter 2 for a more in depth explanation). For example, for Stretch #1 Beginner (Gall Bladder) Back Lying Leg Closing Stretch the Opposing Stretch is its balancing stretch: #7 Beginners (Heart).

10. HELPFUL REMINDERS

HELPFUL REMINDERS

1. Reverse movement for strengthening.
2. The Balancing Stretch muscles help you get into the stretch position.
3. The Opposing Stretch muscles help you get the necessary rotation.
4. Your stretch occurs only while you contract and resist.
5. Your breathing is different in every *type* of stretch.
6. Get perspective from others on how each stretch affects you.

For each of the stretches on every two-page layout on the bottom right, there are constant reminders of how to get the best stretch. This includes:

1. Reverse movement for strengthening.

When you are at the end of the stretch you can of course return to the starting position and then repeat the stretch, OR you can reverse what you did and strengthen those muscles. For example, when you stretch your hamstrings in #9 Beginner Stretch (Brain), after you have lifted you ankle and foot upward while resisting to cause a stretch in your hamstrings in the back of your leg, you can strengthen those muscles by continuing to lift your ankle and foot upward while you use your hands to pull them back towards your hips while those muscles contract for strength training.

2. Your Balancing Stretch muscles help you get into the stretch position.

Remember that the muscles on the opposite side of your body need to shorten in order to get you into the best position of leverage to stretch your target muscles, and those muscles on the opposite side of your body are called your Balancing muscles. So if you need better leverage to get a stretch, go stretch the balancing muscles first so they can contract and shorten and pull you into a great position so that you can then contract and resist the muscles you are stretching.

3. Your Opposing Stretch muscles help you get the necessary rotation.

Again, the opposing muscles that are at a 90-degree angle of the muscles you are stretching determine whether your bones are rotating correctly in order to get a stretch. So stretch those first so that you can get the best stretch possible.

4. Your stretch occurs only while you contract and resist.

The ground-breaking discovery of Resistance Flexibility is that all muscles naturally contract and the fascia resists when you stretch any muscle. Learn from your body how your muscles want to contract and how your fascia wants to resist when you stretch. Defer to your body to learn this.

5. Your breathing is different in every *type* of stretch.

Surprisingly and contrary to many instructions about breathing, your body wants to naturally breathe different for each *type* of stretch. So learn from your body how your body wants you to breathe for each *type* of stretch. When you defer to your bodies natural way to breathe, you will find that your body will use just the right amount of tension as well as relaxation for each *type* of stretch.

6. Get perspective from others on how each stretch affects you.

A hallmark of Resistance Flexibility is the community that is created. Most important to each community is the request for other people in the room to give their perspective on the results others received from a stretch. Each person watching has a unique perspective on what a person received from a stretch, and this greatly helps that person identify the most important benefits.

11. EASY 'TAB' COLOR CODE AT THE BOTTOM OF EACH STRETCH PAGE

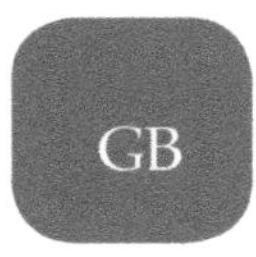

There are four versions of each type of stretch: Beginner, Intermediate, Advanced, and Assisted. To make it easy for you to access all four, there is color bar on the bottom of each type of stretch, so you can flip through the four versions and decide which works best for you, and return to that version more easily. Again, on web page TheGeniusofFlexibility.com there is a Training Archive of 200 + videos of stretches with explanation when you want more options.

RECOMMENDATIONS FOR THE FOUR LEVELS OF RESISTANCE FLEXIBILITY STRETCHES

BEGINNERS

First, it is perhaps less obvious that most anyone would know, that it matters most which level for any of the sixteen types of stretches to practice that give you the best stretch. Regardless of your imagined sense of your flexibility, sometimes different levels work best. So chose the beginner even if you are advanced sometimes. It's not about the range of motion you can get in, it's about what gives you the best stretch.

In the beginner Resistance Flexibility exercises, you want to try to begin to learn how to defer to your body, that is, to feel into your body and find out from your body how to get into, move, and get a stretch naturally. Avoid if you can, thinking your way into the stretch, your body knows best. There are four things to do when stretching position and move, pay attention to the area that is being stretched, breathe naturally, and resist.

Observe how to defer to the four parts of themselves, and build on the involuntary responses to build better.

Physical: Deference to the body

Thinking: Deference to your mind directing your attention

Emotional: Ability to generate tension from involuntary reflex

Spiritual: Ability to resist or yield from involuntary reflex

You most probably find that you like some stretches better than others, everyone does, so do those and if you can stand it, do the ones you don't like as much. Remember in different stretches you will most probably need to concentrate on one of the four aspects of the stretch more than others. In some *types* of stretches you will need to fiddle with the position or movements, others paying close attention to the area being stretched and knowing what is happening, or how to learn how to breath in great ways that facilitate the stretch or how much tension to use or not use, or in others to resist or yield. Ask other people what is happening for them, and that will give you perspective on many of the possible things you can learn from each stretch.

Like in all the stretches, stand up after a stretch and discover what happened to you. Ask others what happened to them, and each of you tells each other what you see.

INTERMEDIATE

After you have stretched for a while, perhaps some of the intermediate stretches will give you more results. By the time you do intermediate stretches, best to have learned to allow your attention to go to what is important for you at any moment, some times you need to reposition, or move differently, other times you'll pay attention to memories or ideas associated with the areas you are stretching, other times how your became better looking, more relaxed or learned to use more tension, and other times how to resist better and how your perspective has changed.

As you advance through the series from beginners to advanced, the stretches are not just more sophisticated but they give you greater and greater leverage to get a better stretch and to develop that type of stretch throughout the whole muscle group. The beginner stretches start you off where that type of stretch begins and then the next level help to complete the stretch pathway until you have the entire muscle group associated with that stretch.

There are five conscious choices when stretching: Starting/Stopping, Force, Speed, Direction, Range. These determine the parameters of the stretch movement. The more each of these match what you like and need, the better the stretch.

ADVANCED

The advanced stretches specifically give you leverage to use rotational resistance. By feeling how the position you are in has arranged your bones in specific relationships, you can resist in the complimentary rotation to get the most optimal stretch.

It is most important when doing advanced Resistance Flexibility exercises to have other people around who can advise and give you feedback on details about the stretch. Don't think you can do these yourself. It takes a community to heal. Enjoy.

ASSISTED

Here are some things that are essential to know about when you are being Assisted RFST, or when you RFST Assist someone else.

• Besides stretching yourself, one or more other people can assist you. Being assisted allows your flexibility to increases much faster in many cases than when you stretch by yourself. The not so obvious advantage of having someone outside you giving objective analysis of what is tight in you is that this information is something that you cannot do for yourself.

So as you assist someone, you are moving the person through the stretch while they resist. It is very helpful to the other person if you give them as much feedback about what you discover about them while you assist them. For example, tell him or her where they are tight; how one side of their body compares to the other; or how their strength compares to their flexibility for each muscle group or movement. Don't underestimate just how valuable the almost limitless observations you can make of them as a person and how the stretch is affecting them. You are outside them, and they are inside! For them to compare the feelings they are having about themselves with what you tell them is priceless information.

• When you are being assisted, it is important that you not allow the person that is assisting you, to take you farther than you want to go. Keep your sense of authority on your own body, and always communicate with the person assisting you. Tell them when you want to start and stop, and when the range, speed, force, and the direction of the stretch is perfect. They will have their own ideas, and it is important that you both come up to the same conclusions together. Besides that, have a ball and remember to show your appreciation.

• As you assist someone, it is important to only take the person into a range a motion where they can continue to resist sufficiently nor excessively, and that the balancing muscle can continue to shorten. Move their body along their path of greatest resistance. Regulate the speed that feels great to them and to start and stop when they are ready. Decide how many repeats and sets to do based on their strength and fatigue. Stay away from exhausting them. If you bring them into exhaustion, it takes the muscles three times as long to recover, than if you stayed within their limits.

• When assisting anyone, guard against yourself being injured. The person being stretched can generate enormous amounts of force. Their force will be able at times to over come your strength, in which case, you can possibly become injured. Sometimes it takes several people to assist someone; for example, when you stretch their hamstrings or other strong muscles. Make sure your leverage is optimal. You can have optimal leverage by carefully positioning yourself in a direct line with their movement and resistance. When you have good leverage it should be relatively easy to overcome their resistance. If they are still overpowering you, then either have them reduce their resistance or get more people to help.

• As a rule of thumb, when you are *stretching* a particular group of muscles in someone else, the *balancing group of muscles* in you are being *strengthened*. And when you are *strengthening* a particular group of muscles in someone else, the *balancing group of muscles* in you are being *stretched*. If they can over power you while trying to stretch them, then those same muscles in your body are being strained. Ere on the side of caution. The person assisting is in as bigger of a risk of being injured then the person being stretched.

• Because much more force is being used when you assist someone, I would highly recommend that you "smash" those muscle groups you stretched so that you can help speed up the removal of the waste products produced from intense stretching."Smashing" someone's hamstrings, gluteals, and calfs can easily take 1/2 hour or more. Keep "smashing" the muscles until they feel "peachy."

• The person being stretched is asked to make a general movement, and the assister then feels the vectors of resistance, and moves the stretcher along those vector lines to remove acute and chronic biomechanical insufficiencies. Within any moment these vectors change. The skill level of the assister determines how quickly they can keep up with the vector changes that are necessary.

• Removing not normal facial densities but accumulated dense fascia requires significant feel on the assister part. Removing scar tissue requires a much greater level of expertise. The assister needs to be able to identify the 4 types of tissue for each of the 16 MMG and be able to explain to the person being assisted what they are dealing with; the person being assisted needs perspective on what type of tissue they have which they cannot have without being told by the assister.

• Skillful assisting involves moving a person in a way that helps them to defer to how their body wants to breathe, and communicating with them in a way that facilitates their breathing.

RESISTANCE FLEXIBILITY STRETCHES: BEGINNERS INTERMEDIATE ADVANCED ASSISTED

PREVIEW

In Chapter 9, there are Two Page Layouts of all the Beginner Stretches, Intermediate Stretches, Advanced Stretches, and Assisted Stretches so you can do all sixteen types of stretches in order. Again, when you do all 16 *types* of Resistance Flexibility exercises in that order, it has been coined The Energy Series of Stretches. Enjoy.

#1 BEGINNER (GALLBLADDER)

BENEFITS

Health: Fat Metabolism
Body Part: Hips
Joint: Hip Girdle
Movement: Turn Outward
Good Looks: Sensual
Life: Committed, Advocate

MUSCLES

Frontalis, Temporalis, Trapezius, Pectoralis Major, Oblique Abdominals, Gluteus Minimus and Medius, TFL, IT Band, Vastus Lateralis, Peroneals

Action: Flexion / Abduction / Inward
Stretch: Extension / Adduction / Outward

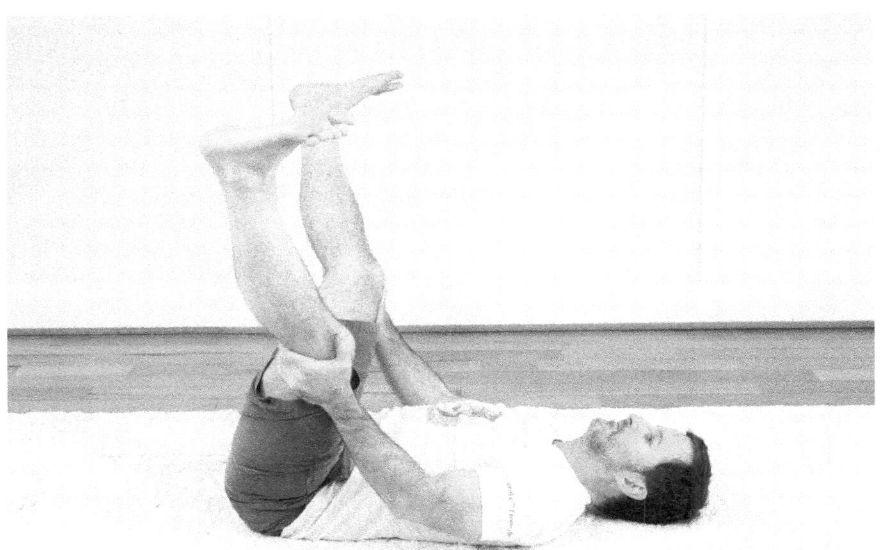

STARTING POSITION: Lie on your back with both legs perpendicular to your torso and opened wide apart. Grasp the outside of your knees with your hands, palms facing in.

BALANCING STRETCH

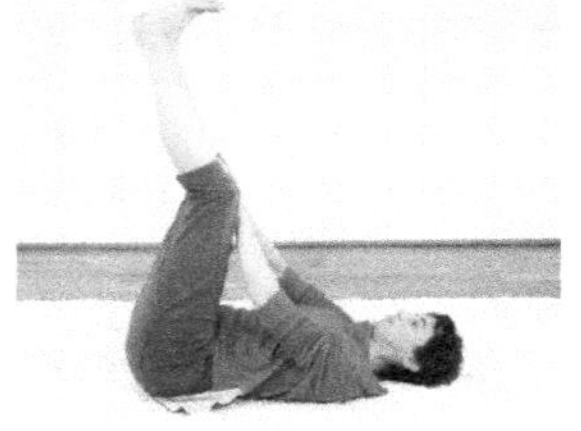

#2 Beginner (Liver)

OPPOSING STRETCH

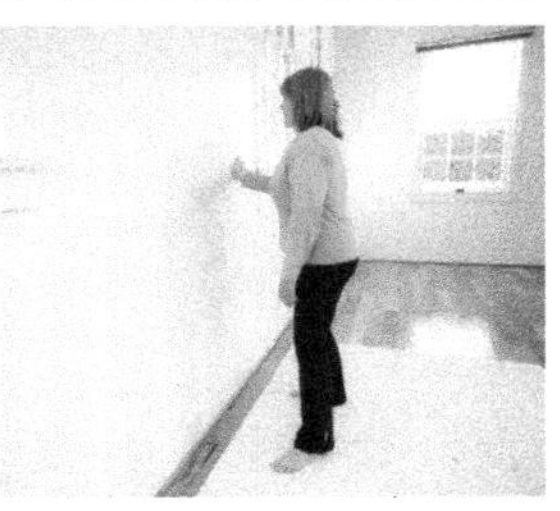

#7 Beginner (Heart)

BACK LYING LEG CLOSING STRETCH

CHINESE MEDICINE

Organ: Gallbladder
Tissue: Ligaments
Body Part: Legs
System: Fat Metabolism
Sensory: Nervous System
Yin/Yang Element: Yang Wood

PERSONALITY (GPT)

Group: Thinking
Time & Attention: Future and Inside
High Traits: Decision Maker, Advocacy, Devotional, Abundance, Certainty
Low Traits: Dependent, Guilt
Instinct: Fearless/Fearful

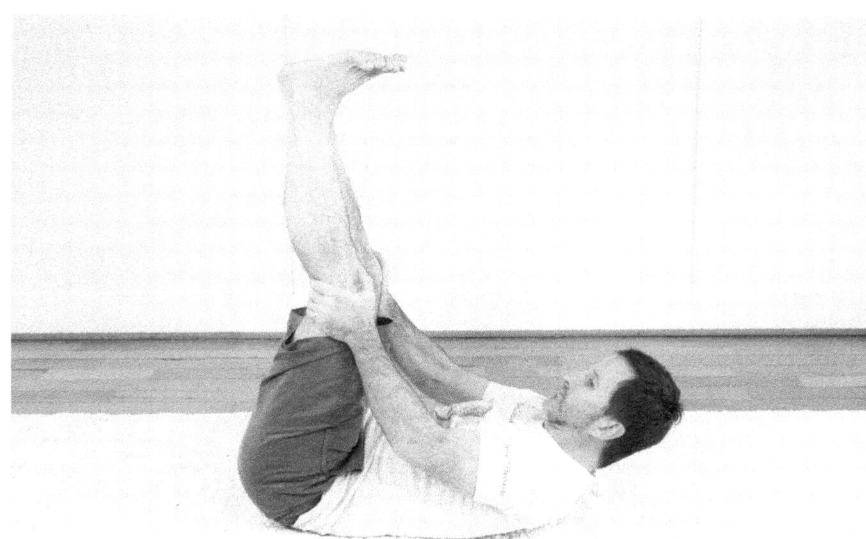

RESISTANCE FLEXIBILITY: Your legs push outwards to resist as your hands close your legs together. Return to the starting position and repeat 10 times.

HELPFUL REMINDERS

1. Reverse movement for strengthening.
2. The Balancing Stretch muscles help you get into the stretch position.
3. The Opposing Stretch muscles help you get the necessary rotation.
4. Your stretch occurs only while you contract and resist.
5. Your breathing is different in every *type* of stretch.
6. Get perspective from others on how each stretch affects you.

#1 INTERMEDIATE (GALLBLADDER)

BENEFITS

Health: Fat Metabolism
Body Part: Hips
Joint: Hip Girdle
Movement: Turn Outward
Good Looks: Sensual
Life: Committed, Advocate

MUSCLES

Frontalis, Temporalis, Trapezius, Pectoralis Major, Oblique Abdominals, Gluteus Minimus and Medius, TFL, IT Band, Vastus Lateralis, Peroneals

Action: Flexion / Abduction / Inward
Stretch: Extension / Adduction / Outward

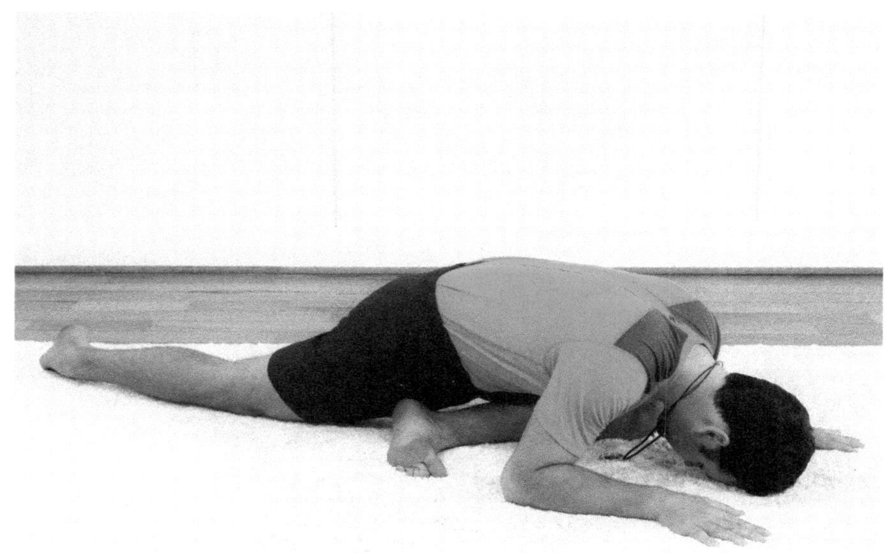

STARTING POSITION: Start on your hands and knees. Slide your right knee forwards as you bend it into a 35-degree angle, rotating your right thigh outwards. Straighten your left leg as you bring it behind you.

BALANCING STRETCH

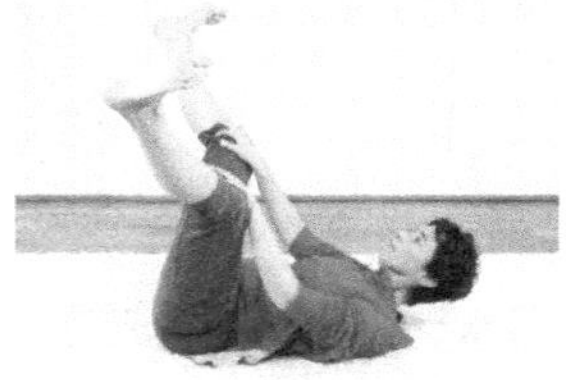

#2 Beginner (Liver)

OPPOSING STRETCH

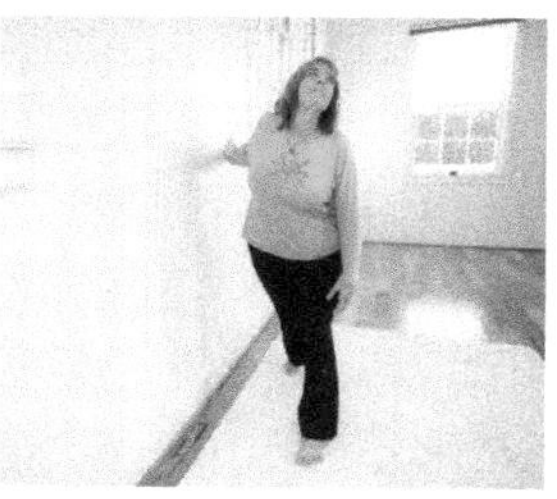

#7 Beginner (Heart)

EASY PIGEON

CHINESE MEDICINE

Organ: Gallbladder
Tissue: Ligaments
Body Part: Legs
System: Fat Metabolism
Sensory: Nervous System
Yin/Yang Element: Yang Wood

PERSONALITY (GPT)

Group: Thinking
Time & Attention: Future and Inside
High Traits: Decision Maker, Advocacy, Devotional, Abundance, Certainty
Low Traits: Dependent, Guilt
Instinct: Fearless/Fearful

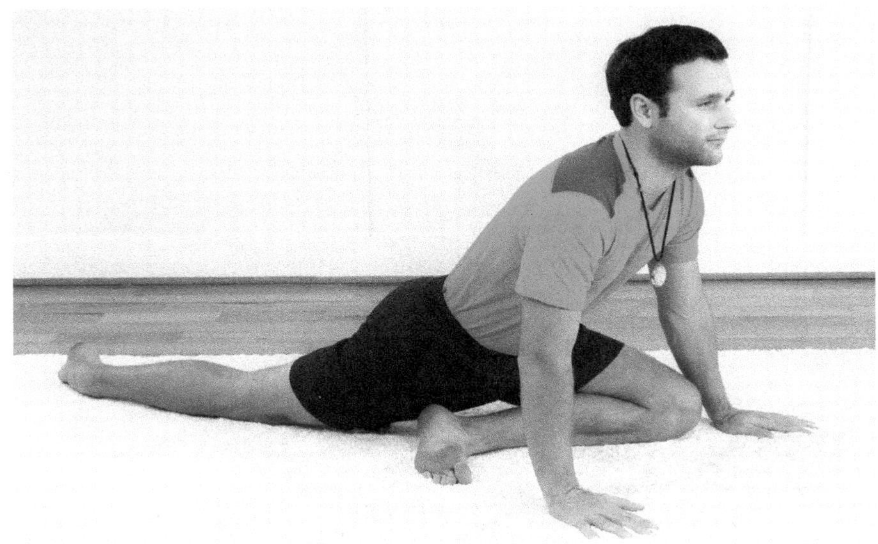

RESISTANCE FLEXIBILITY: Press both legs down against the floor and rotate your right thigh inwards to resist as your raise and lower your trunk. Return to the starting position and repeat 10 times on each side.

HELPFUL REMINDERS

1. Reverse movement for strengthening.
2. The Balancing Stretch muscles help you get into the stretch position.
3. The Opposing Stretch muscles help you get the necessary rotation.
4. Your stretch occurs only while you contract and resist.
5. Your breathing is different in every *type* of stretch.
6. Get perspective from others on how each stretch affects you.

#1 ADVANCED (GALLBLADDER)

BENEFITS

Health: Fat Metabolism
Body Part: Hips
Joint: Hip Girdle
Movement: Turn Outward
Good Looks: Sensual
Life: Committed, Advocate

MUSCLES

Frontalis, Temporalis, Trapezius, Pectoralis Major, Oblique Abdominals, Gluteus Minimus and Medius, TFL, IT Band, Vastus Lateralis, Peroneals

Action: Flexion / Abduction / Inward
Stretch: Extension / Adduction / Outward

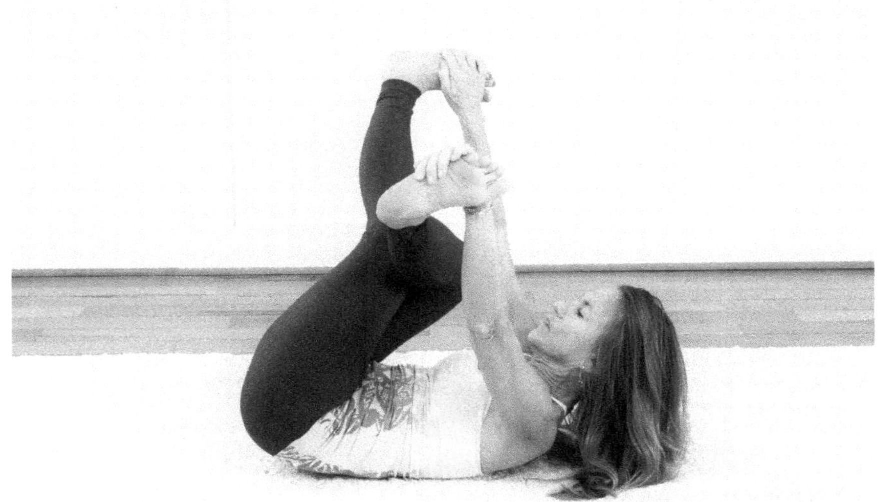

STARTING POSITION: Lie on your back. Cross your legs, bend your knees and grasp the outsides of your ankles with your hands.

BALANCING STRETCH

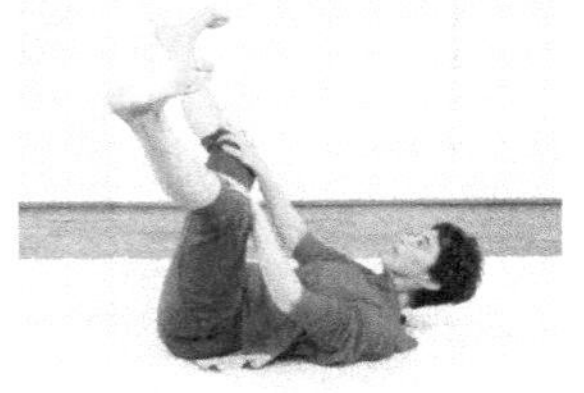

#2 Beginner (Liver)

OPPOSING STRETCH

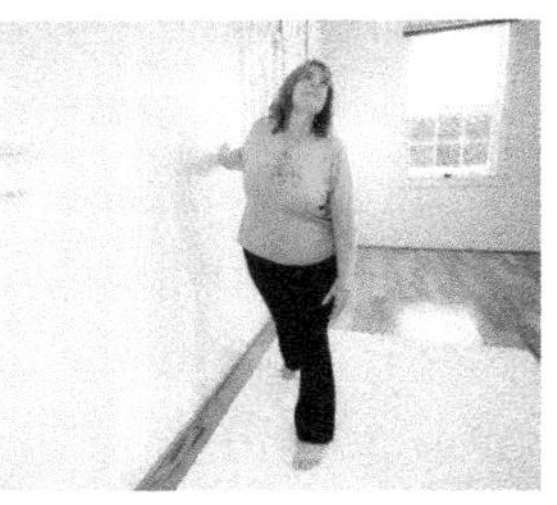

#7 Beginner (Heart)

BACK LYING LEG TURNS

CHINESE MEDICINE

Organ: Gallbladder
Tissue: Ligaments
Body Part: Legs
System: Fat Metabolism
Sensory: Nervous System
Yin/Yang Element: Yang Wood

PERSONALITY (GPT)

Group: Thinking
Time & Attention: Future and Inside
High Traits: Decision Maker, Advocacy, Devotional, Abundance, Certainty
Low Traits: Dependent, Guilt
Instinct: Fearless/Fearful

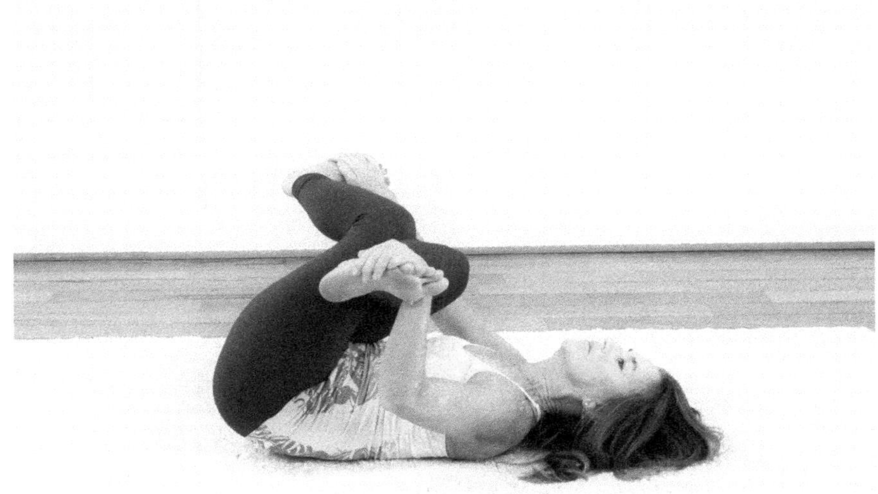

RESISTANCE FLEXIBILITY: Push your feet out and pull your legs apart to resist as your hands pull your feet down towards your shoulders. Keep your lower back and hips on the floor. Return to the starting position and repeat 10 times with legs crossed both ways

HELPFUL REMINDERS

1. Reverse movement for strengthening.
2. The Balancing Stretch muscles help you get into the stretch position.
3. The Opposing Stretch muscles help you get the necessary rotation.
4. Your stretch occurs only while you contract and resist.
5. Your breathing is different in every *type* of stretch.
6. Get perspective from others on how each stretch affects you.

#1 ASSISTED (GALLBLADDER)

BENEFITS

Health: Fat Metabolism
Body Part: Hips
Joint: Hip Girdle
Movement: Turn Outward
Good Looks: Sensual
Life: Committed, Advocate

MUSCLES

Frontalis, Temporalis, Trapezius, Pectoralis Major, Oblique Abdominals, Gluteus Minimus and Medius, TFL, IT Band, Vastus Lateralis, Peroneals

Action: Flexion/Abduction/Inward
Stretch: Extension/Adduction/Outward

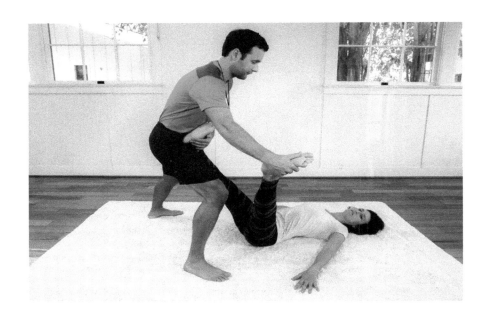

STARTING POSITION: Lie on your back with your knees straight and legs raised. Place your right ankle against the inside of your assister's right hip and open your left leg out away from their body. The assister grasps your left ankle with their right hand

BALANCING STRETCH

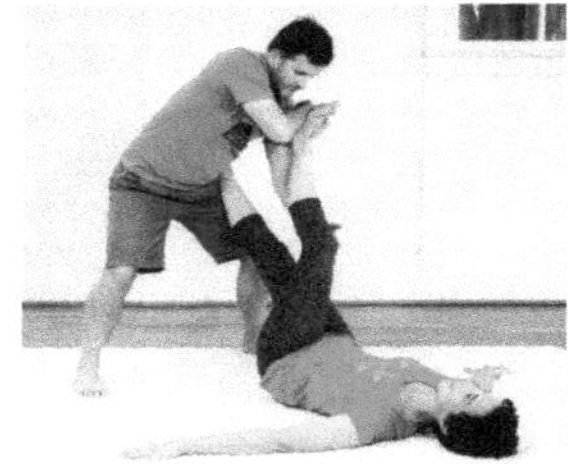

#2 Beginner (Liver)

OPPOSING STRETCH

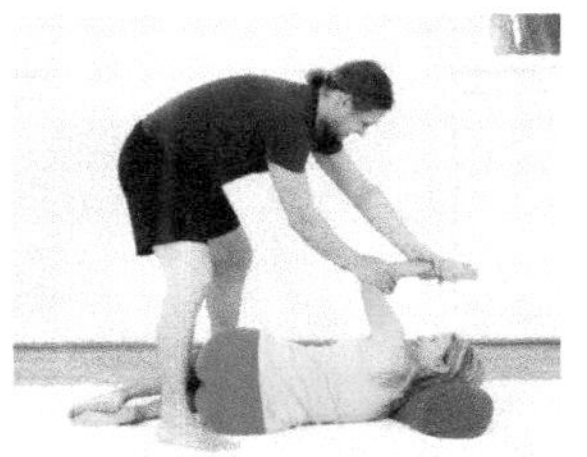

#7 Beginner (Heart)

ASSISTED LEG CLOSING

CHINESE MEDICINE

Organ: Gallbladder
Tissue: Ligaments
Body Part: Legs
System: Fat Metabolism
Sensory: Nervous System
Yin/Yang Element: Yang Wood

PERSONALITY (GPT)

Group: Thinking
Time & Attention: Future and Inside
High Traits: Decision Maker, Advocacy, Devotional, Abundance, Certainty
Low Traits: Dependent, Guilt
Instinct: Fearless/Fearful

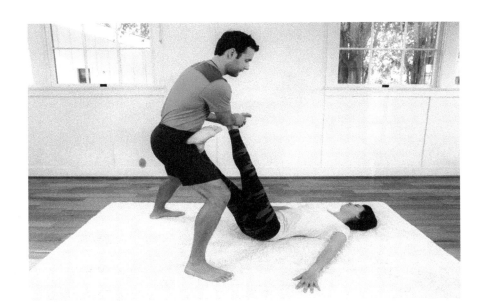

RESISTANCE FLEXIBILITY: Your left legs pushes out to the left to resist while the assister moves that leg across your body to your right. Return to the starting position and repeat 10 times on each leg.

HELPFUL REMINDERS

1. Reverse movement for strengthening.
2. The Balancing Stretch muscles help you get into the stretch position.
3. The Opposing Stretch muscles help you get the necessary rotation.
4. Your stretch occurs only while you contract and resist.
5. Your breathing is different in every *type* of stretch.
6. Get perspective from others on how each stretch affects you.

#2 BEGINNER (LIVER)

BENEFITS

Health: Detoxification
Body Part: Hips
Joint: Hip Girdle
Movement: Turn Inward
Good Looks: Pretty / Handsome
Life: Helpful, Free

MUSCLES

Extensor Hallucis Longus, Soleus, Gastrocnemius, Tibialis Posterior, Semimembranosus, Adductor Longus, Gracilis, Oblique Abdominals
Action: Extension / Adduction / Outward
Stretch: Flexion / Abduction / Inward

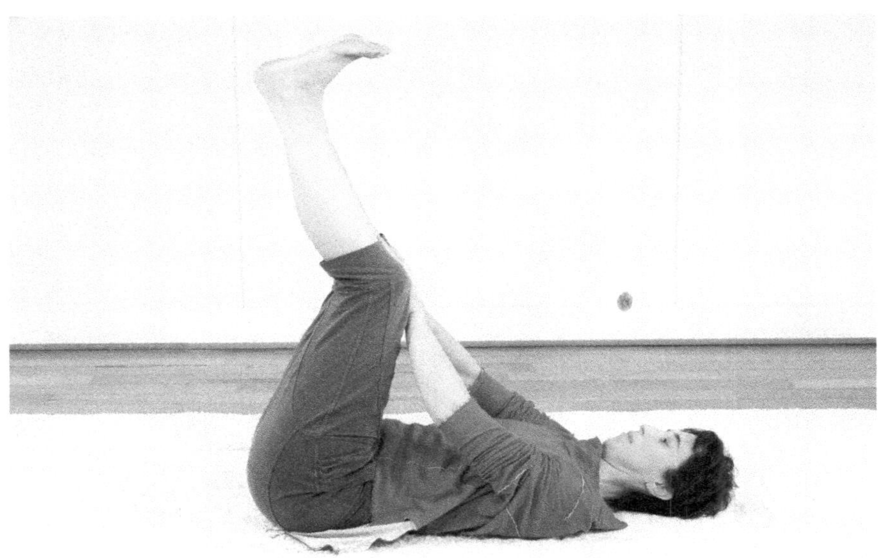

STARTING POSITION: Lie on your back with both legs perpendicular to your torso and together. Grasp the insides of your knees with your hands, palms facing out.

BALANCING STRETCH

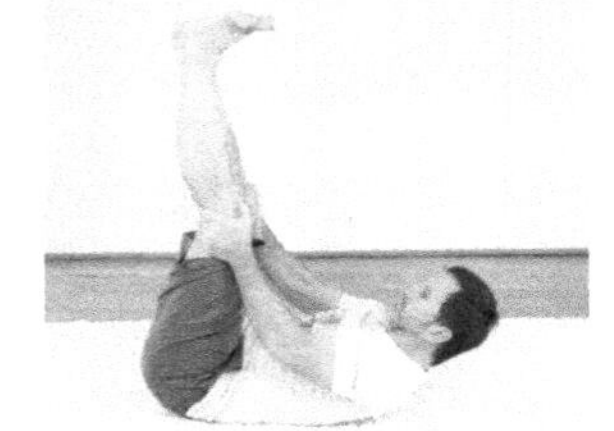

#1 Beginner (Gall Bladder)

OPPOSING STRETCH

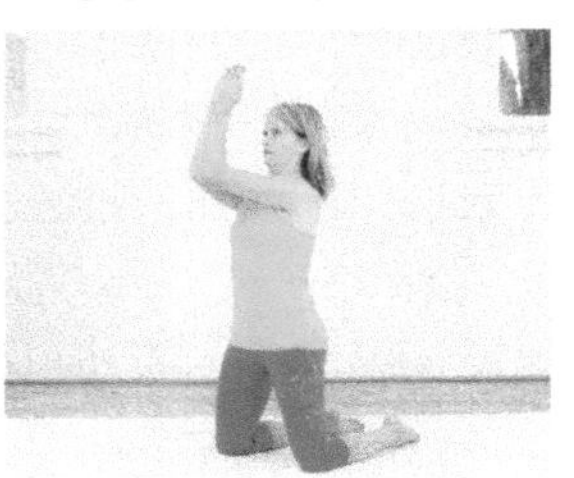

#8 Beginner (Small Intestine)

BACK LYING OPENERS STRETCH

(TCM)

Organ: Liver
Tissue: Tendons
Body Part: Face
System: Detoxification
Sensory: Hormonal Receptors
Yin / Yang Element: Yin Wood

PERSONALALITY (GPT)

Group: Emotional
Time and Attention: Past and Outside
High Traits: Strategist, Zeitgeist, Helper, Humble, Freedom
Low Traits: Codependent, Irritated
Instinct: Excited / Anxious

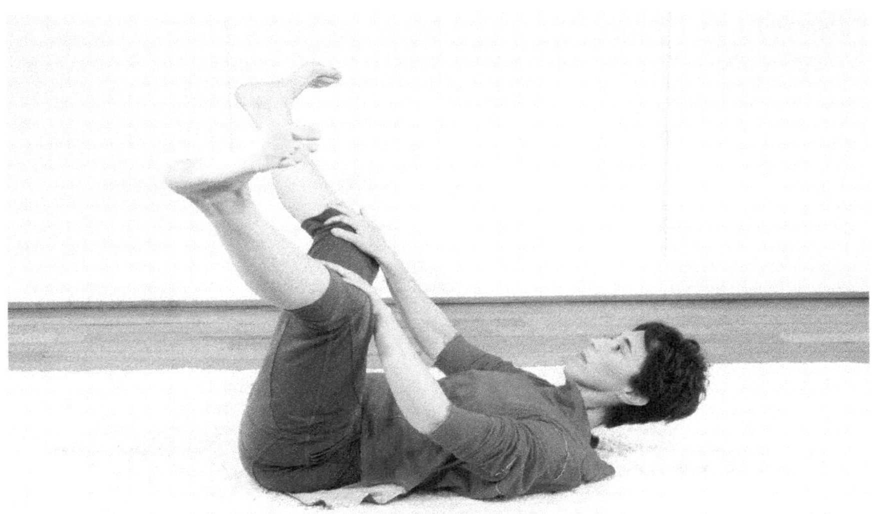

RESISTANCE FLEXIBILITY: Your legs squeeze together to resist as your hands pull your legs apart and open. Return to the starting position and repeat 10 times.

HELPFUL REMINDERS

1. Reverse movement for strengthening.
2. The Balancing Stretch muscles help you get into the stretch position.
3. The Opposing Stretch muscles help you get the necessary rotation.
4. Your stretch occurs only while you contract and resist.
5. Your breathing is different in every *type* of stretch.
6. Get perspective from others on how each stretch affects you.

#2 INTERMEDIATE (LIVER)

BENEFITS

Health: Detoxification
Body Part: Hips
Joint: Hip Girdle
Movement: Turn Inward
Good Looks: Pretty / Handsome
Life: Helpful, Free

MUSCLES

Extensor Hallucis Longus, Soleus, Gastrocnemius, Tibialis Posterior, Semimembranosus, Adductor Longus, Gracilis, Oblique Abdominals
Action: Extension / Adduction / Outward
Stretch: Flexion / Abduction / Inward

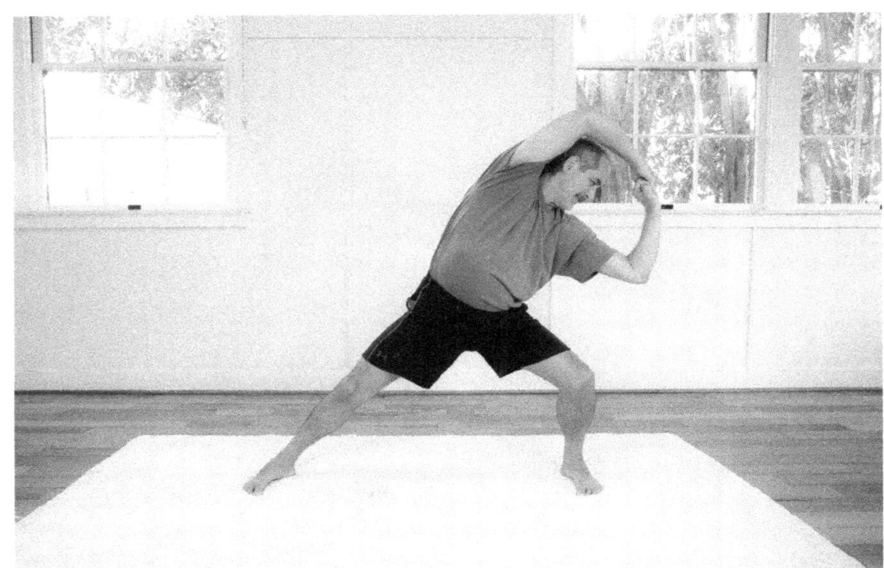

STARTING POSITION: Stand with your legs apart, wider than your hips. Bend forward, put your hands on the ground, and shift your body to one side.

BALANCING STRETCH

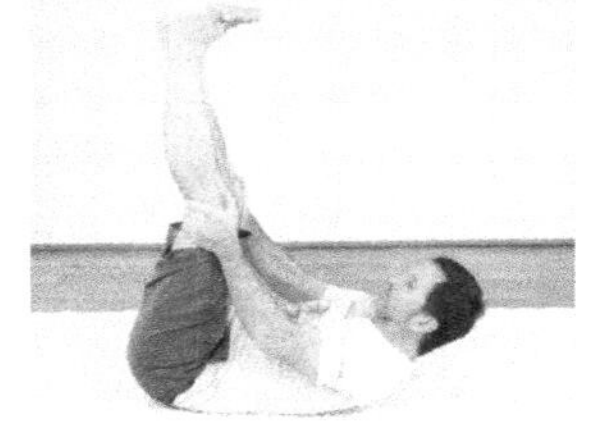

#1 Beginner (Gall Bladder)

OPPOSING STRETCH

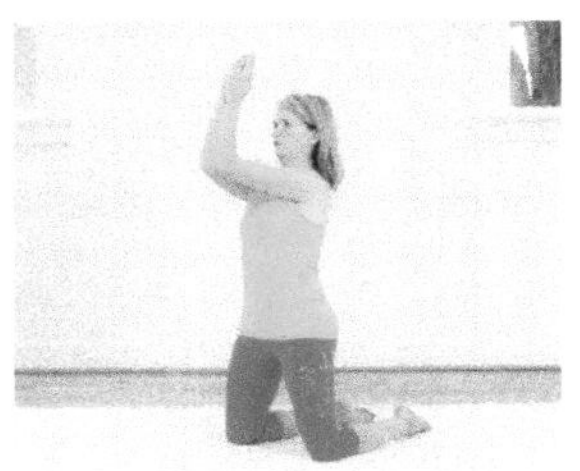

#8 Beginner (Small Intestine)

LATERAL SHIFT LUNGES

(TCM)

Organ: Liver
Tissue: Tendons
Body Part: Face
System: Detoxification
Sensory: Hormonal Receptors
Yin/Yang Element: Yin Wood

PERSONALALITY (GPT)

Group: Emotional
Time and Attention: Past and Outside
High Traits: Strategist, Zeitgeist, Helper, Humble, Freedom
Low Traits: Codependent, Irritated
Instinct: Excited/Anxious

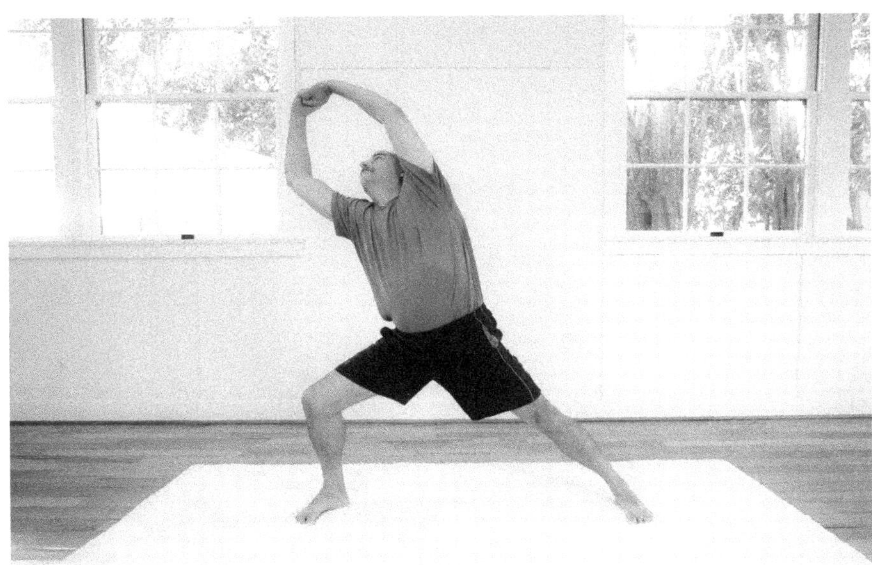

RESISTANCE FLEXIBILITY: Your legs squeeze together to resist while you shift your body to the other side. Repeat by shifting your body side to side 10 times.

HELPFUL REMINDERS

1. Reverse movement for strengthening.
2. The Balancing Stretch muscles help you get into the stretch position.
3. The Opposing Stretch muscles help you get the necessary rotation.
4. Your stretch occurs only while you contract and resist.
5. Your breathing is different in every *type* of stretch.
6. Get perspective from others on how each stretch affects you.

#2 ADVANCED (LIVER)

BENEFITS

Health: Detoxification
Body Part: Hips
Joint: Hip Girdle
Movement: Turn Inward
Good Looks: Pretty / Handsome
Life: Helpful, Free

MUSCLES

Extensor Hallucis Longus, Soleus, Gastrocnemius, Tibialis Posterior, Semimembranosus, Adductor Longus, Gracilis, Oblique Abdominals
Action: Extension / Adduction / Outward
Stretch: Flexion / Abduction / Inward

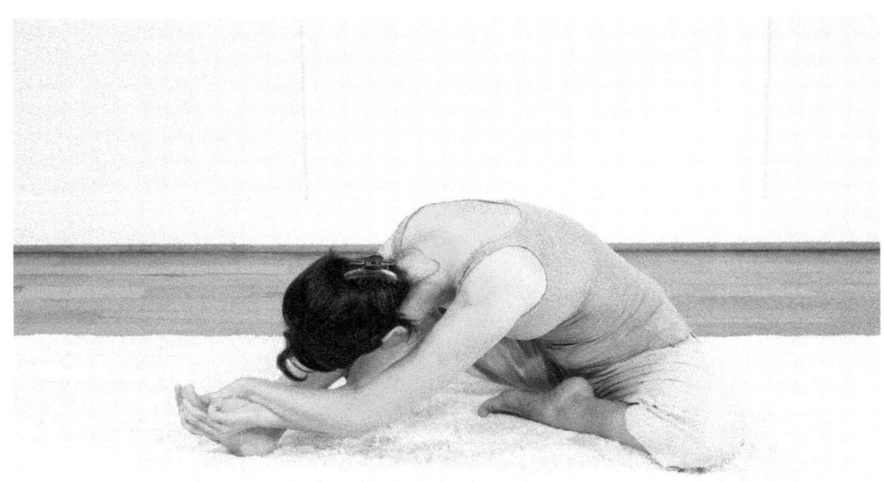

STARTING POSITION: Sit on the floor with your legs wide and knees bent. Bring your right knee wider and down to the floor, bending it further to bring your right foot towards your groin. With your left knee bent and left foot flexed, grasp the left foot with your right hand. Now bring your left arm inside your left leg and grasp the left foot with your left hand.

BALANCING STRETCH

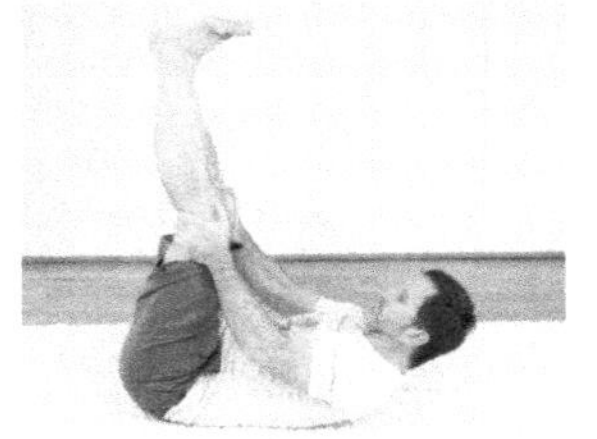

#1 Beginner (Gall Bladder)

OPPOSING STRETCH

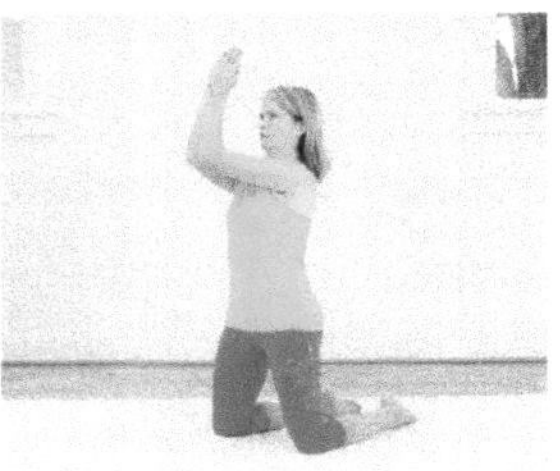

#8 Beginner (Small Intestine)

SEATED LATERAL BEND

(TCM)

Organ: Liver
Tissue: Tendons
Body Part: Face
System: Detoxification
Sensory: Hormonal Receptors
Yin/Yang Element: Yin Wood

PERSONALALITY (GPT)

Group: Emotional
Time and Attention: Past and Outside
High Traits: Strategist, Zeitgeist, Helper, Humble, Freedom
Low Traits: Codependent, Irritated
Instinct: Excited/Anxious

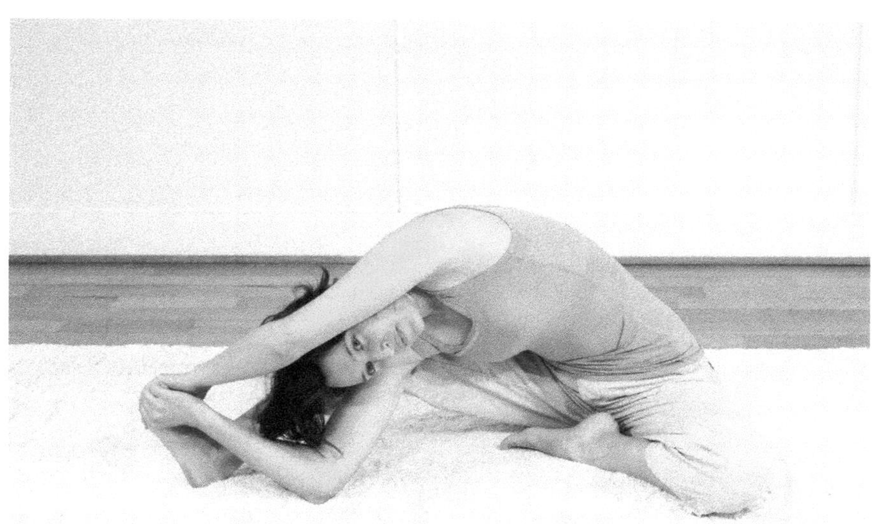

RESISTANCE FLEXIBILITY: Squeeze your legs together and pull your body upwards to resist as your arms pull your body down towards the floor. Also rotate your torso upwards and downwards while resisting that rotation in the opposite rotation. Return to the starting position and repeat 10 times on each side.

HELPFUL REMINDERS

1. Reverse movement for strengthening.
2. The Balancing Stretch muscles help you get into the stretch position.
3. The Opposing Stretch muscles help you get the necessary rotation.
4. Your stretch occurs only while you contract and resist.
5. Your breathing is different in every *type* of stretch.
6. Get perspective from others on how each stretch affects you.

#2 ASSISTED (LIVER)

BENEFITS

Health: Detoxification
Body Part: Hips
Joint: Hip Girdle
Movement: Turn Inward
Good Looks: Pretty / Handsome
Life: Helpful, Free

MUSCLES

Extensor Hallucis Longus, Soleus, Gastrocnemius, Tibialis Posterior, Semimembranosus, Adductor Longus, Gracilis, Oblique Abdominals

Action: Extension / Adduction / Outward
Stretch: Flexion / Abduction / Inward

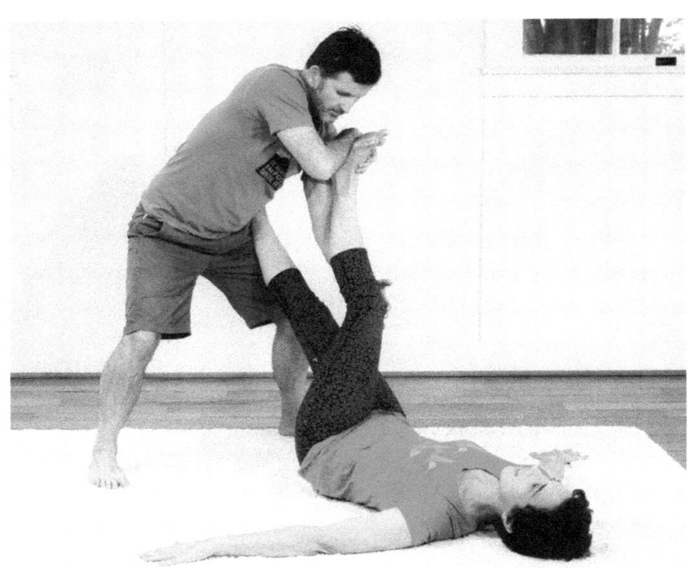

STARTING POSITION: Lie on your back with your knees straight and legs raised. Place your right ankle against the outside of your assister's left hip and cross your left leg over and to your right. The assister grasps your left ankle and knee with their hands.

BALANCING STRETCH

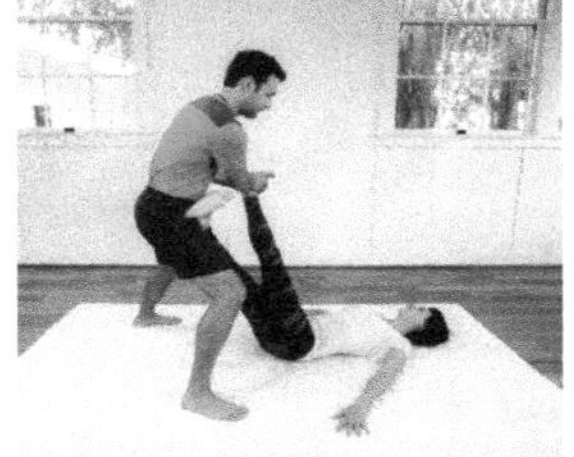

#1 Assisted (Gallbladder)

OPPOSING STRETCH

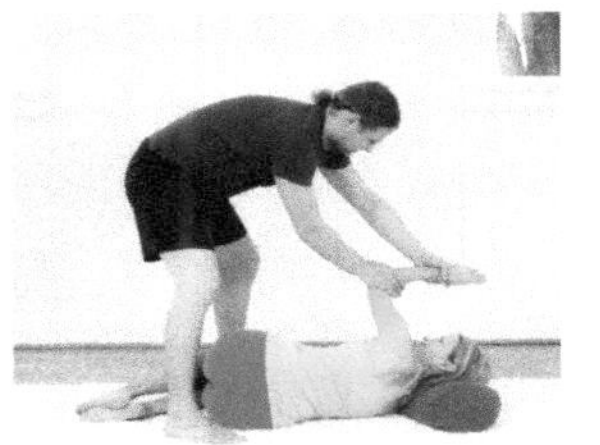

#8 Assisted (Small Intestine)

ASSISTED LEG OPENERS

(TCM)

Organ: Liver
Tissue: Tendons
Body Part: Face
System: Detoxification
Sensory: Hormonal Receptors
Yin / Yang Element: Yin Wood

PERSONALALITY (GPT)

Group: Emotional
Time and Attention: Past and Outside
High Traits: Strategist, Zeitgeist, Helper, Humble, Freedom
Low Traits: Codependent, Irritated
Instinct: Excited / Anxious

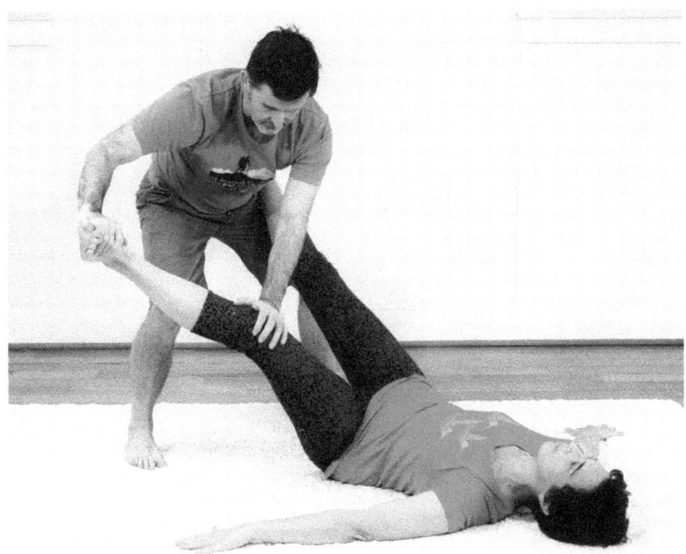

RESISTANCE FLEXIBILITY: Your legs squeeze inward to resist while the assister opens your left leg out to your left. Return to the starting position and repeat 10 times on each leg.

HELPFUL REMINDERS

1. Reverse movement for strengthening.
2. The Balancing Stretch muscles help you get into the stretch position.
3. The Opposing Stretch muscles help you get the necessary rotation.
4. Your stretch occurs only while you contract and resist.
5. Your breathing is different in every *type* of stretch.
6. Get perspective from others on how each stretch affects you.

#3 BEGINNER (LUNGS)

BENEFITS

Health: Endurance/Strength
Body Part: Shoulders
Joint: Shoulder Girdle
Movement: Throw
Good Looks: Powerful, Remarkable

MUSCLES

Opponens Pollicis, Pronator Quadratus, Flexors Forearm, Brachioradialis, Brachialis, Biceps Brachii, Subclavius, Anterior Deltoid, Pectoralis Major
Action: Flexion/Adduction/Inward
Stretch: Extension/Abduction/ Outward

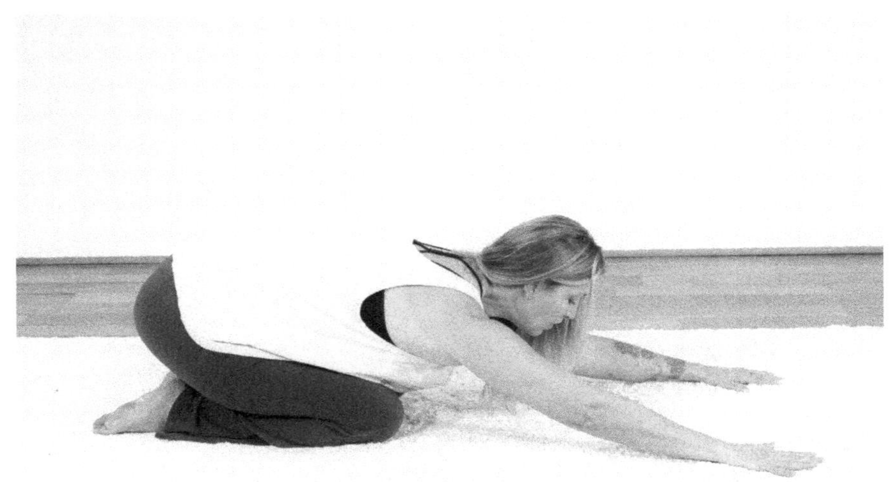

STARTING POSITION: Get on your hands and knees, bend your knees and reach your arms out straight, palms touching the floor.

BALANCING STRETCH

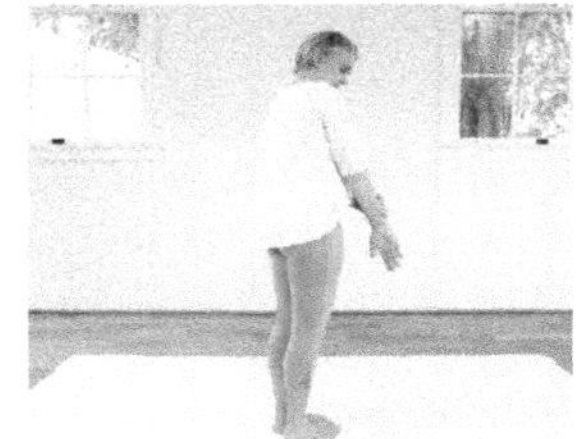

#4 Beginner (Large Intestine)

OPPOSING STRETCH

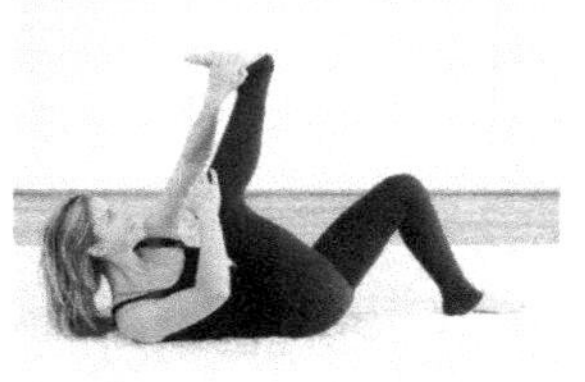

#13 Beginner (Bladder)

UPPER CHEST ADVANTAGE

(TCM)

Organ: Lungs
Tissue: Alveoli
Body Part: Arms
System: Respiratory
Sensory: Exteroceptive Receptors
Yin/Yang Element: Yin Metal

PERSONALITY (GPT)

Group: Physical
Time and Attention: Present and Inside
High Traits: Leadership, Strength, Power, Truth, Protector
Low Traits: Passive Aggressive, Apathetic
Instinct: Love/Anger

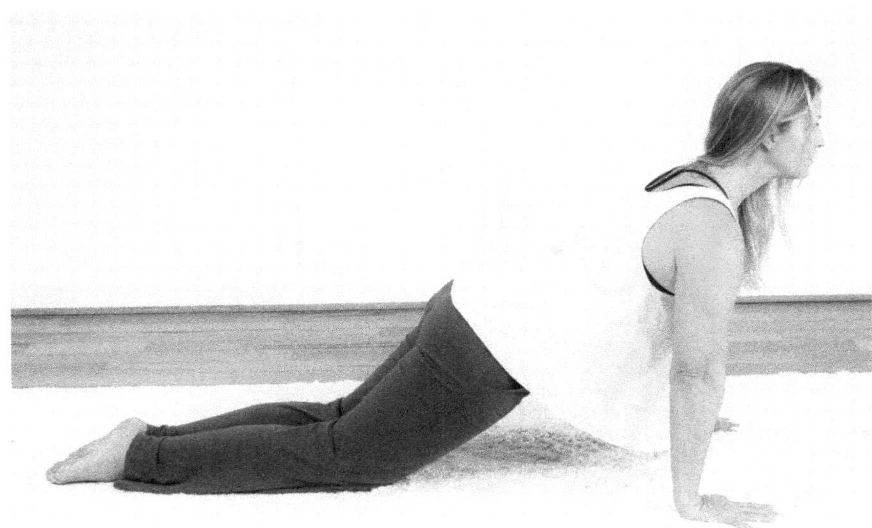

RESISTANCE FLEXIBILITY: Pull your knees toward your chest and pull your arms down toward your trunk to resist as you arch your head, neck and shoulders upwards and come up onto your arms. Return to the starting position and repeat 10 times.

HELPFUL REMINDERS

1. Reverse movement for strengthening.
2. The Balancing Stretch muscles help you get into the stretch position.
3. The Opposing Stretch muscles help you get the necessary rotation.
4. Your stretch occurs only while you contract and resist.
5. Your breathing is different in every *type* of stretch.
6. Get perspective from others on how each stretch affects you.

#3 INTERMEDIATE (LUNGS)

BENEFITS

Health: Endurance/Strength
Body Part: Shoulders
Joint: Shoulder Girdle
Movement: Throw
Good Looks: Powerful, Remarkable

MUSCLES

Opponens Pollicis, Pronator Quadratus, Flexors Forearm, Brachioradialis, Brachialis, Biceps Brachii, Subclavius, Anterior Deltoid, Pectoralis Major
Action: Flexion / Adduction / Inward
Stretch: Extension / Abduction / Outward

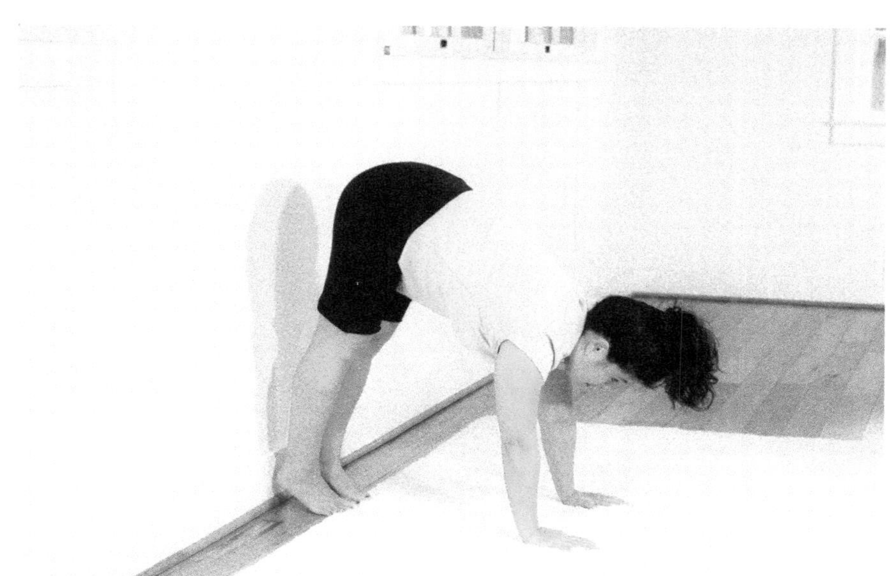

STARTING POSITION: Stand facing away from a wall. Bend down and put your hands on the floor, keeping your hips up off the ground.

BALANCING STRETCH

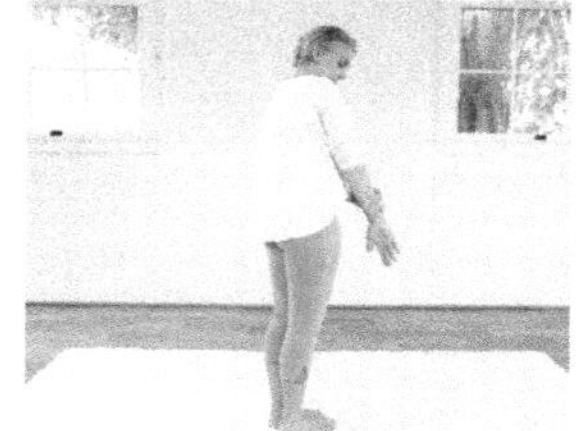

#4 Beginner (Large Intestine)

OPPOSING STRETCH

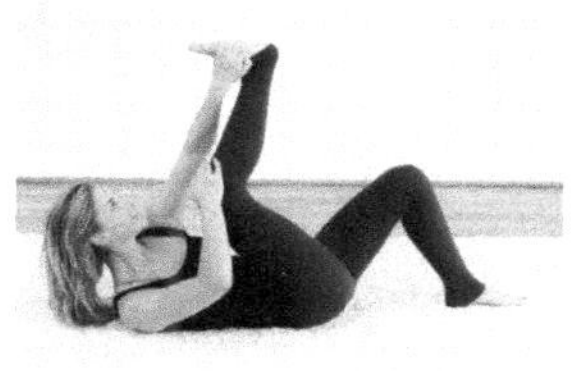

#13 Intermediate (Bladder)

HAND STAND WALL WALK UP

(TCM)

Organ: Lungs
Tissue: Alveoli
Body Part: Arms
System: Respiratory
Sensory: Exteroceptive Receptors
Yin/Yang Element: Yin Metal

PERSONALITY (GPT)

Group: Physical
Time and Attention: Present and Inside
High Traits: Leadership, Strength, Power, Truth, Protector
Low Traits: Passive Aggressive, Apathetic
Instinct: Love/Anger

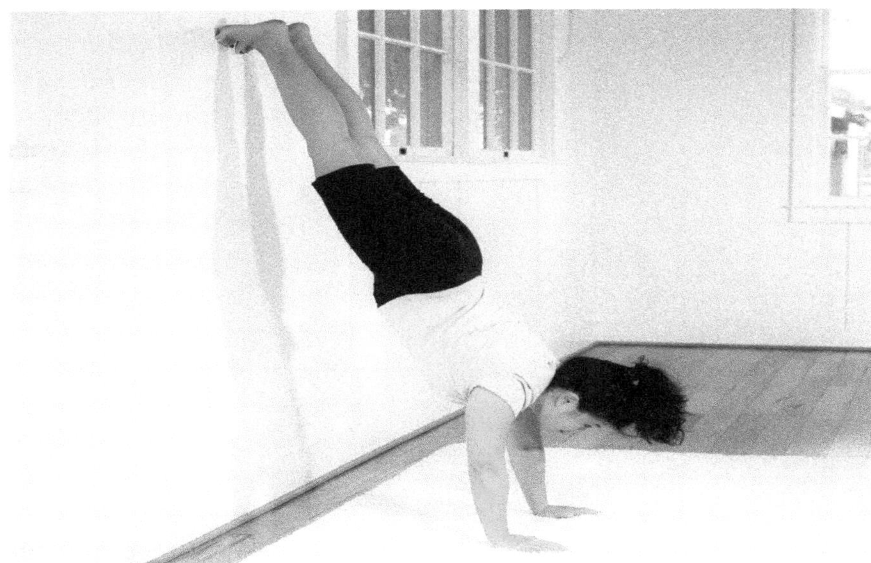

RESISTANCE FLEXIBILITY: Walk up the wall by taking a big step with one leg and then the other. Push your feet into the wall, pull your legs toward your chest and pull your arms down toward your trunk to resist as you arch your head, neck and shoulders upwards. Return to the starting position and repeat 10 times.

HELPFUL REMINDERS

1. Reverse movement for strengthening.
2. The Balancing Stretch muscles help you get into the stretch position.
3. The Opposing Stretch muscles help you get the necessary rotation.
4. Your stretch occurs only while you contract and resist.
5. Your breathing is different in every *type* of stretch.
6. Get perspective from others on how each stretch affects you.

#3 ADVANCED (LUNGS)

BENEFITS

Health: Endurance/Strength
Body Part: Shoulders
Joint: Shoulder Girdle
Movement: Throw
Good Looks: Powerful, Remarkable

MUSCLES

Opponens Pollicis, Pronator Quadratus, Flexors Forearm, Brachioradialis, Brachialis, Biceps Brachii, Subclavius, Anterior Deltoid, Pectoralis Major

Action: Flexion/Adduction/Inward
Stretch: Extension/Abduction/ Outward

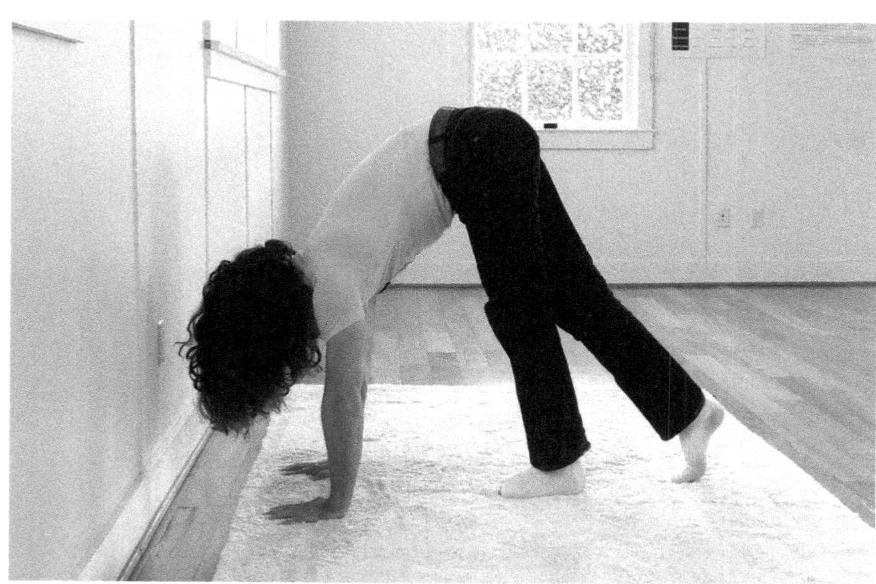

STARTING POSITION: Stand facing a wall and plant your hands shoulder distance apart on the floor, about a foot away from the wall. Kick your legs up onto the wall as you arch your head, neck and shoulders backwards.

BALANCING STRETCH

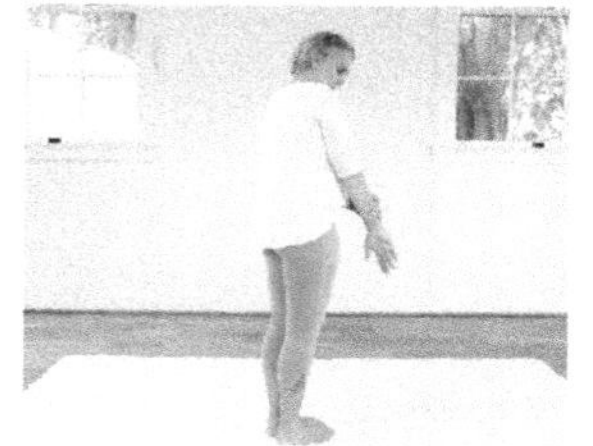

#4 Beginner (Large Intestine)

OPPOSING STRETCH

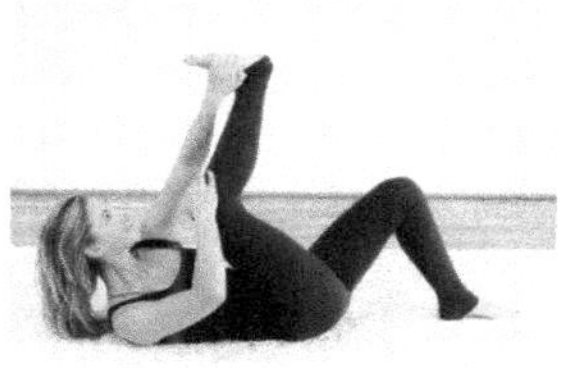

#13 Intermediate (Bladder)

HAND STAND FLIP UP

(TCM)

Organ: Lungs
Tissue: Alveoli
Body Part: Arms
System: Respiratory
Sensory: Exteroceptive Receptors
Yin/Yang Element: Yin Metal

PERSONALITY (GPT)

Group: Physical
Time and Attention: Present and Inside
High Traits: Leadership, Strength, Power, Truth, Protector
Low Traits: Passive Aggressive, Apathetic
Instinct: Love/Anger

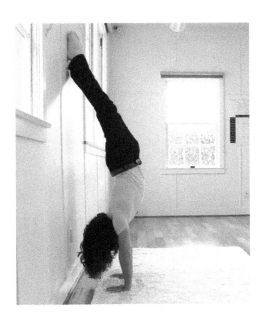

RESISTANCE FLEXIBILITY: Contract the muscles on the front of your body and pull your arms towards your chest to resist as you further arch up in your body, neck and head. Return to the starting position and repeat 10 times.

HELPFUL REMINDERS

1. Reverse movement for strengthening.
2. The Balancing Stretch muscles help you get into the stretch position.
3. The Opposing Stretch muscles help you get the necessary rotation.
4. Your stretch occurs only while you contract and resist.
5. Your breathing is different in every *type* of stretch.
6. Get perspective from others on how each stretch affects you.

#3 ASSISTED (LUNGS)

BENEFITS

Health: Endurance/Strength
Body Part: Shoulders
Joint: Shoulder Girdle
Movement: Throw
Good Looks: Powerful, Remarkable

MUSCLES

Flexors Forearm, Brachioradialis, Brachialis, Biceps Brachii, Subclavius, Anterior Deltoid, Pectoralis Major
Action: Flexion/Adduction/Inward
Stretch: Extension/Abduction/ Outward

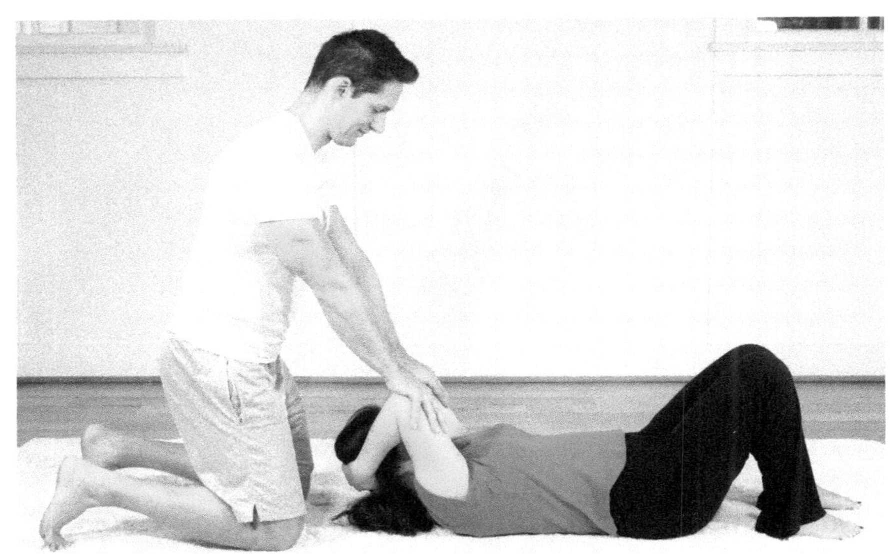

STARTING POSITION: Lie on your back with your hands clasped behind your head, your elbows bent and together, and knees bent. The assister grasps the inside of your elbows with their hands.

BALANCING STRETCH

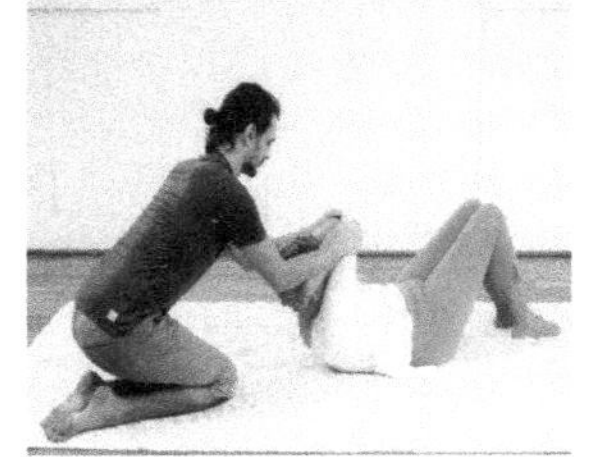

#4 Assisted (Large Intestine)

OPPOSING STRETCH

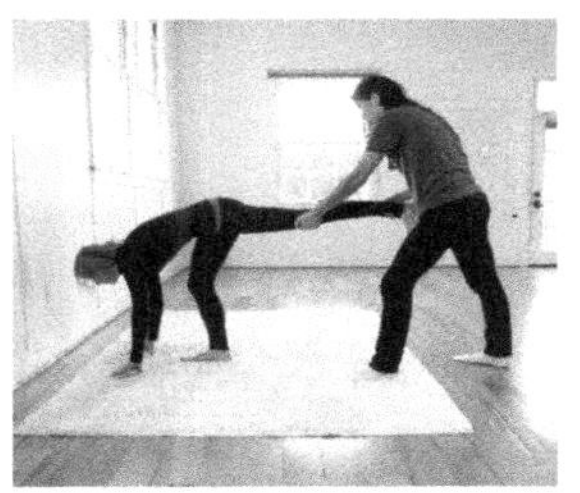

#13 Assisted (Bladder)

UPPER CHEST ADVANTAGE

(TCM)

Organ: Lungs
Tissue: Alveoli
Body Part: Arms
System: Respiratory
Sensory: Exteroceptive Receptors
Yin/Yang Element: Yin Metal

PERSONALITY (GPT)

Group: Physical
Time and Attention: Present and Inside
High Traits: Leadership, Strength,
Power, Truth, Protector
Low Traits: Passive Aggressive, Apathetic
Instinct: Love/Anger

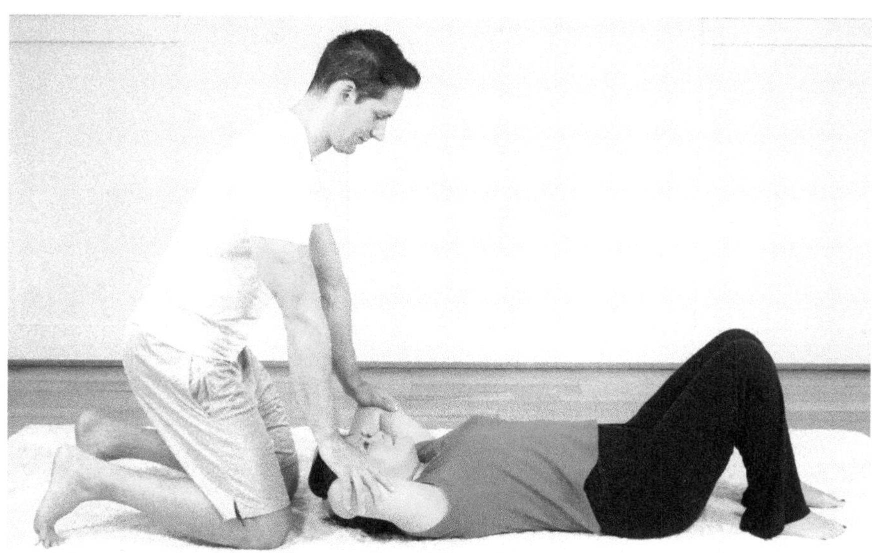

RESISTANCE FLEXIBILITY: Your arms squeeze inward to resist while the assister opens your arms apart. Return to the starting position and repeat 10 times.

HELPFUL REMINDERS

1. Reverse movement for strengthening.
2. The Balancing Stretch muscles help you get into the stretch position.
3. The Opposing Stretch muscles help you get the necessary rotation.
4. Your stretch occurs only while you contract and resist.
5. Your breathing is different in every *type* of stretch.
6. Get perspective from others on how each stretch affects you.

#4 BEGINNER (LARGE INTESTINE)

BENEFITS

Health: Blood Pressure
Body Part: Shoulders
Joint: Shoulder Girdle
Movement: Catch
Good Looks: Perfection, Charming
Life: Friendship, Actualize

MUSCLES

Levator Scapula, Trapezius, Posterior Deltoid, Supinator, Forearm Extensors, Adductor Pollicis, Dorsal Interosseous, Entensor Indicis

Action: Extension / Abduction / Outward
Stretch: Flexion / Adduction / Inward

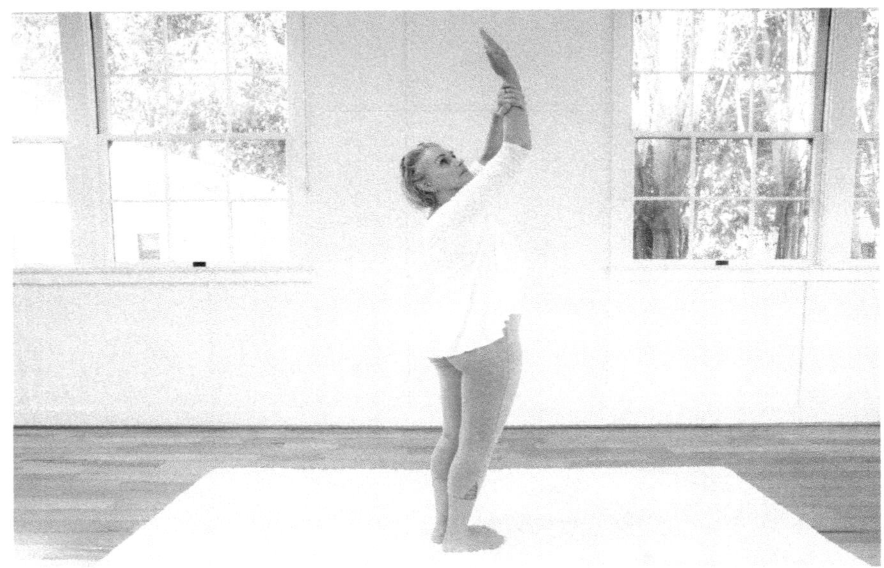

STARTING POSITION: Hold your right arm upward to your side and slightly forward. With your left hand, grasp the outside of your right arm or wrist.

BALANCING STRETCH

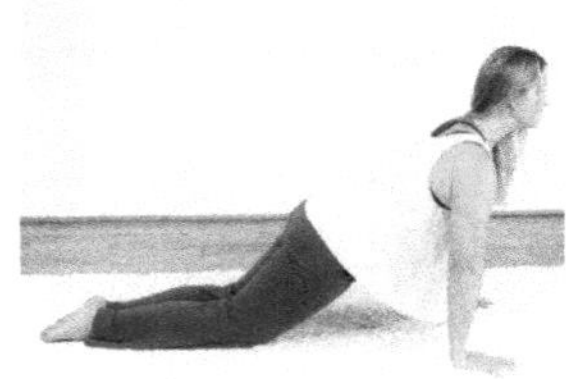

#3 Beginner (Lung)

OPPOSING STRETCH

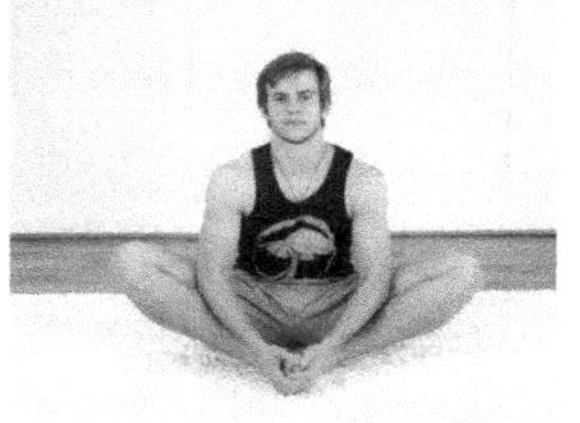

#14 Intermediate (Kidney)

BACK OF SHOULDER

(TCM)

Organ: Large Intestine
Tissue: Venous Blood
Body Part: Trunk
System: Elimination
Sensory: Energetic receptors
Yin/Yang Element: Yang Metal

PERSONALITY (GPT)

Group: Spiritual
Time and Attention: Relative and Outside
High Traits: Perfection, Ambition, Friendship, Fairness, Serene
Low Traits: Obsessive, Critical
Instinct: Calm/Frightened

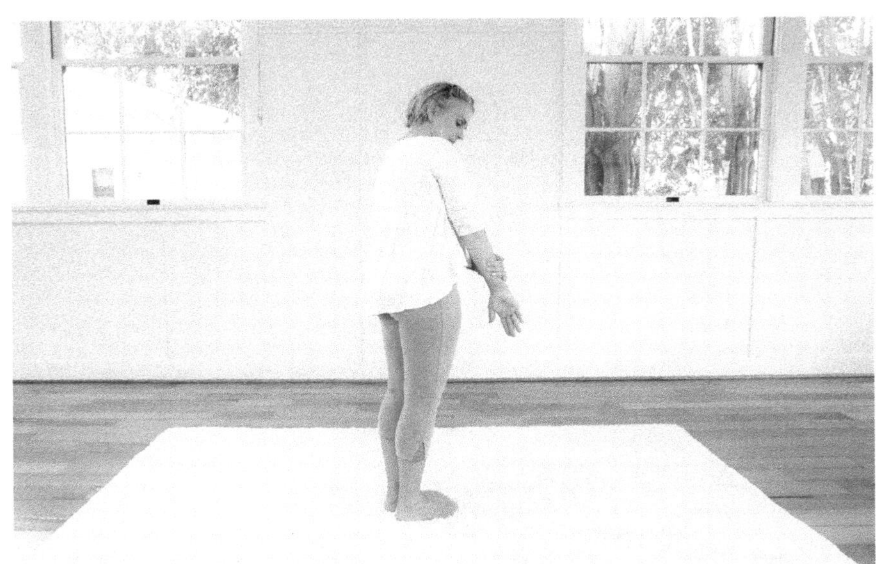

RESISTANCE FLEXIBILITY: Your right arm keeps lifting upward to resist as your left hand pulls the right arm downward and diagonally across your body towards your left hip. Return to the starting position and repeat 10 times on each arm.

HELPFUL REMINDERS

1. Reverse movement for strengthening.
2. The Balancing Stretch muscles help you get into the stretch position.
3. The Opposing Stretch muscles help you get the necessary rotation.
4. Your stretch occurs only while you contract and resist.
5. Your breathing is different in every *type* of stretch.
6. Get perspective from others on how each stretch affects you.

#4 INTERMEDIATE (LARGE INTESTINE)

BENEFITS

Health: Blood Pressure
Body Part: Shoulders
Joint: Shoulder Girdle
Movement: Catch
Good Looks: Perfection, Charming
Life: Friendship, Actualize

MUSCLES

Levator Scapula, Trapezius, Posterior Deltoid, Supinator, Forearm Extensors, Adductor Pollicis, Dorsal Interosseous, Entensor Indicis

Action: Extension / Abduction / Outward
Stretch: Flexion / Adduction / Inward

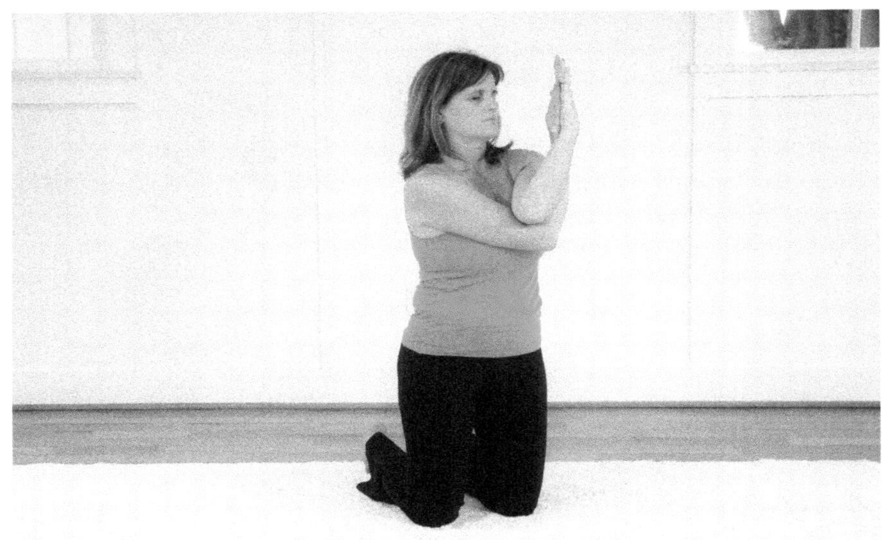

STARTING POSITION: While either standing or sitting, cross your arms at the elbows and twist your forearms around each other until your palms face each other and eventually clasp.

BALANCING STRETCH

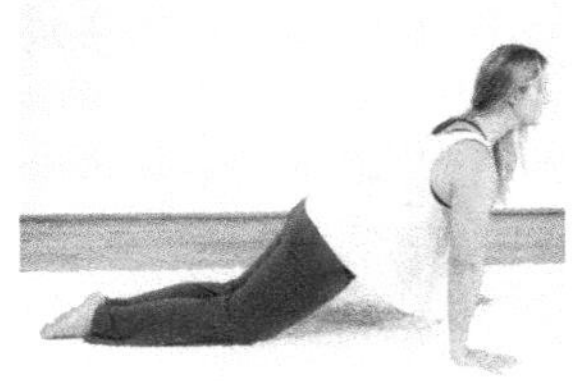

#3 Beginner (Lung)

OPPOSING STRETCH

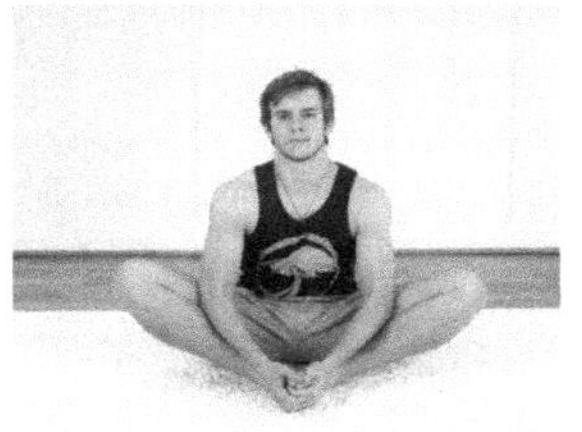

#14 Intermediate (Kidney)

TWISTING ARMS

(TCM)

Organ: Large Intestine
Tissue: Venous Blood
Body Part: Trunk
System: Elimination
Sensory: Energetic receptors
Yin/Yang Element: Yang Metal

PERSONALITY (GPT)

Group: Spiritual
Time and Attention: Relative and Outside
High Traits: Perfection, Ambition, Friendship, Fairness, Serene
Low Traits: Obsessive, Critical
Instinct: Calm/Frightened

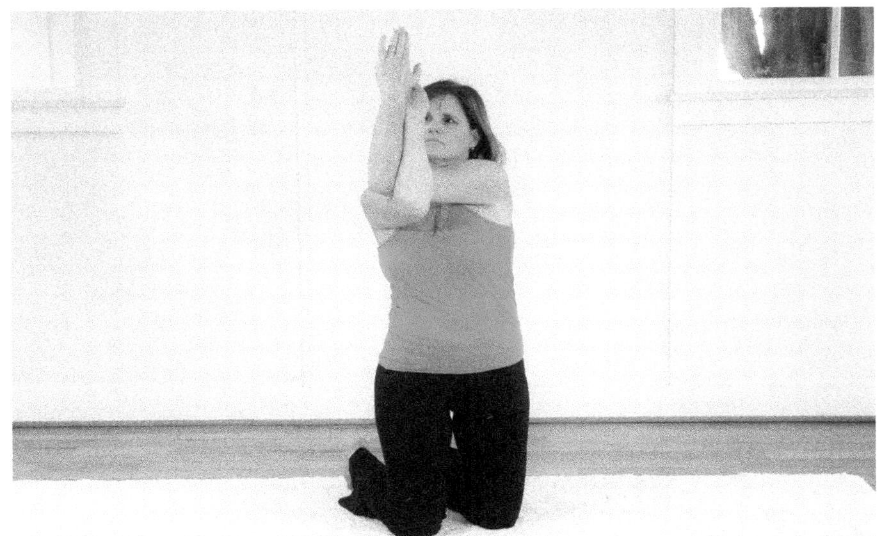

RESISTANCE FLEXIBILITY: Pull your arms apart so your elbows are squeezed together and attempt to untwist your arms to resist while your hands and forearms pull themselves back into their twisted starting position. Return to the starting position and repeat 10 times with your arms crossed in both possible directions.

HELPFUL REMINDERS

1. Reverse movement for strengthening.
2. The Balancing Stretch muscles help you get into the stretch position.
3. The Opposing Stretch muscles help you get the necessary rotation.
4. Your stretch occurs only while you contract and resist.
5. Your breathing is different in every *type* of stretch.
6. Get perspective from others on how each stretch affects you.

#4 ADVANCED (LARGE INTESTINE)

BENEFITS

Health: Blood Pressure
Body Part: Shoulders
Joint: Shoulder Girdle
Movement: Catch
Good Looks: Perfection, Charming
Life: Friendship, Actualize

MUSCLES

Levator Scapula, Trapezius, Posterior Deltoid, Supinator, Forearm Extensors, Adductor Pollicis, Dorsal Interosseous, Entensor Indicis

Action: Extension / Abduction / Outward
Stretch: Flexion / Adduction / Inward

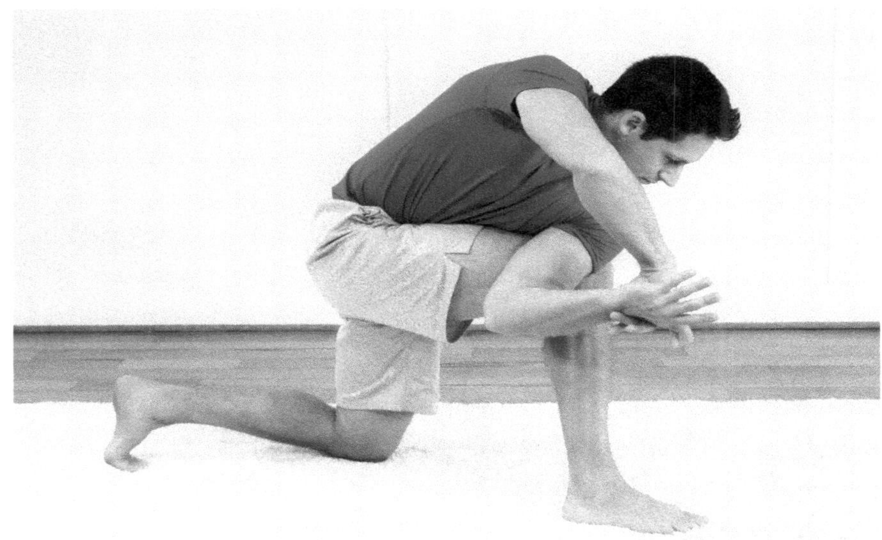

STARTING POSITION: Start on your hands and knees, then lift your left leg and assume a lunging position. Bring your right elbow across and against the outside of the left knee. Bend your right elbow and grasp the right wrist with your left hand.

BALANCING STRETCH

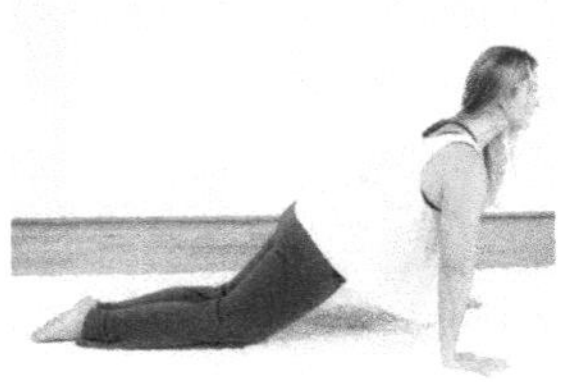

#3 Beginner (Lung)

OPPOSING STRETCH

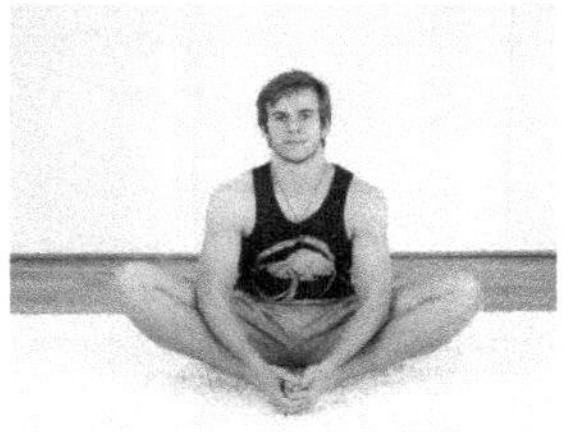

#14 Intermediate (Kidney)

KNEELING BACK OF SHOULDER

(TCM)

Organ: Large Intestine
Tissue: Venous Blood
Body Part: Trunk
System: Elimination
Sensory: Energetic receptors
Yin/Yang Element: Yang Metal

PERSONALITY (GPT)

Group: Spiritual
Time and Attention: Relative and Outside
High Traits: Perfection, Ambition, Friendship, Fairness, Serene
Low Traits: Obsessive, Critical
Instinct: Calm/Frightened

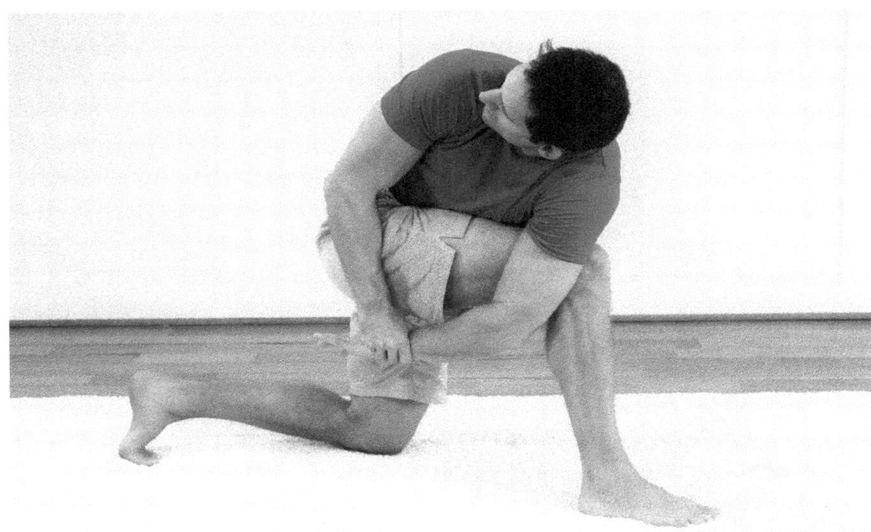

RESISTANCE FLEXIBILITY: Your right forearm pushes outward to resist as your left hand pulls the right wrist inward and under your left leg. Return to the starting position and repeat 10 times on each side.

HELPFUL REMINDERS

1. Reverse movement for strengthening.
2. The Balancing Stretch muscles help you get into the stretch position.
3. The Opposing Stretch muscles help you get the necessary rotation.
4. Your stretch occurs only while you contract and resist.
5. Your breathing is different in every *type* of stretch.
6. Get perspective from others on how each stretch affects you.

#4 ASSISTED (LARGE INTESTINE)

BENEFITS

Health: Blood Pressure
Body Part: Shoulders
Joint: Shoulder Girdle
Movement: Catch
Good Looks: Perfection, Charming
Life: Friendship, Actualize

MUSCLES

Levator Scapula, Trapezius, Posterior Deltoid, Supinator, Forearm Extensors, Adductor Pollicis, Dorsal Interosseous, Entensor Indicis

Action: Extension / Abduction / Outward
Stretch: Flexion / Adduction / Inward

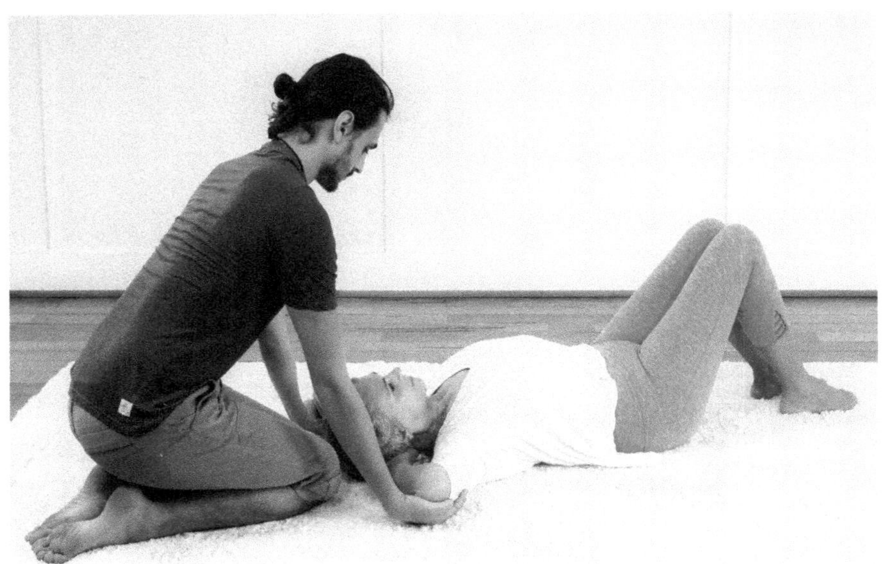

STARTING POSITION: Lie on your back with your hands clasped behind your head, your elbows bent and together, and knees bent. The assister grasps the outside of your elbows with their hands.

BALANCING STRETCH

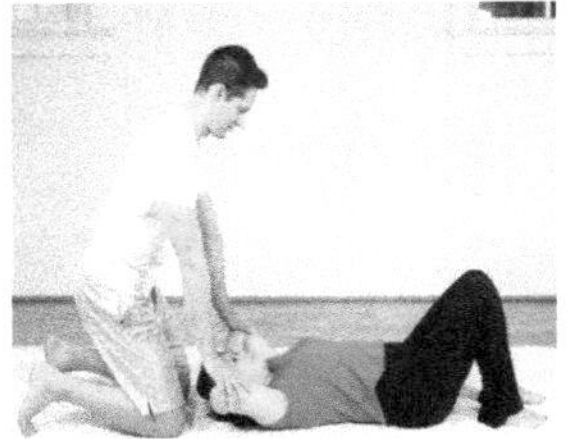

#3 Assisted (Lung)

OPPOSING STRETCH

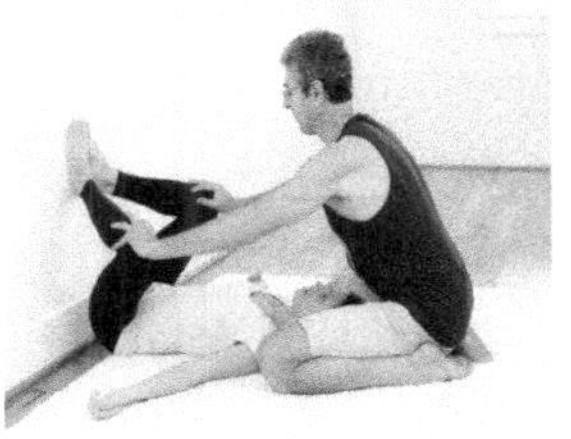

#14 Assisted (Kidney)

BACK OF SHOULDER

(TCM)

Organ: Large Intestine
Tissue: Venous Blood
Body Part: Trunk
System: Elimination
Sensory: Energetic receptors
Yin/Yang Element: Yang Metal

PERSONALITY (GPT)

Group: Spiritual
Time and Attention: Relative and Outside
High Traits: Perfection, Ambition, Friendship, Fairness, Serene
Low Traits: Obsessive, Critical
Instinct: Calm/Frightened

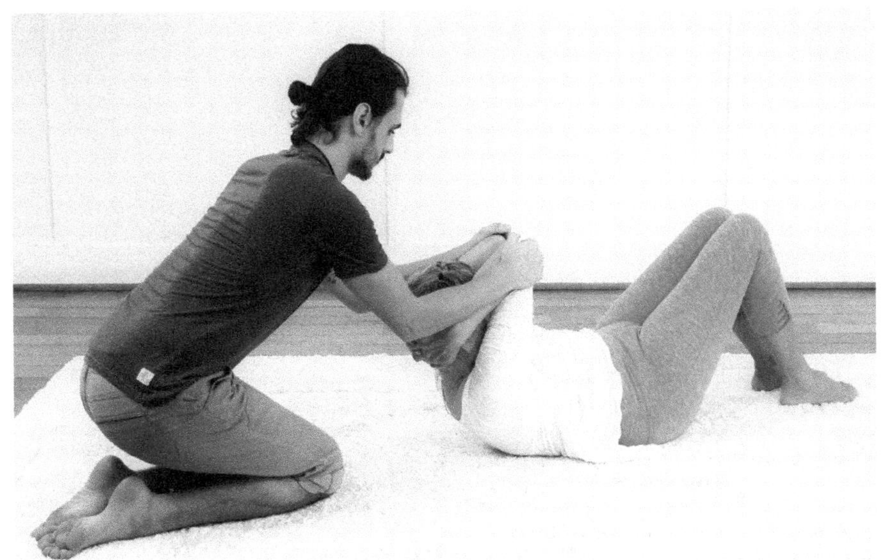

RESISTANCE FLEXIBILITY: Your arms push outward to resist while the assister squeezes your arms together. Return to the starting position and repeat 10 times.

HELPFUL REMINDERS

1. Reverse movement for strengthening.
2. The Balancing Stretch muscles help you get into the stretch position.
3. The Opposing Stretch muscles help you get the necessary rotation.
4. Your stretch occurs only while you contract and resist.
5. Your breathing is different in every *type* of stretch.
6. Get perspective from others on how each stretch affects you.

#5 BEGINNER (STOMACH)

BENEFITS

Health: Allergies / Asthma
Body Part: Thighs
Joint: Hip Joint
Movement: Step Forward
Good Looks: Cute, Unique
Life: Work, Singing and Dancing

MUSCLES

Orbicularis Oculi, Buccinator, Masseter, Vocal Cords, Platysma, Temoralis, Pectoralis Major, Oblique Abdominals, Vastus Lateralis, Tibialis Anterior,
Action: Flexion / Abduction / Outward
Stretch: Extension / Adduction / Inward

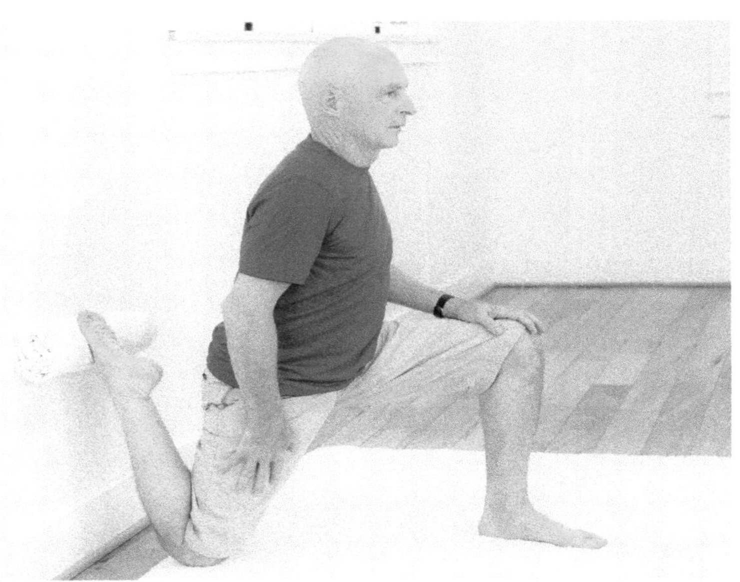

STARTING POSITION: Get on your hands and knees facing away from a wall. Bring your right knee close to the wall, bending it as you raise the right foot up against the wall. Step up onto your left foot, lunging forward with your torso arched upward. Put your right hand on the front outside of the right thigh in order to feel the upcoming stretch.

BALANCING STRETCH

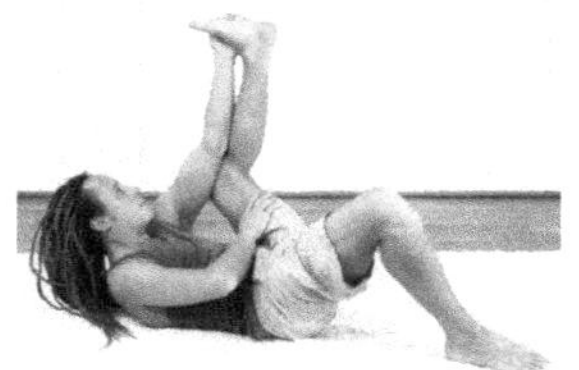

#6 Beginner (Pancreas)

OPPOSING STRETCH

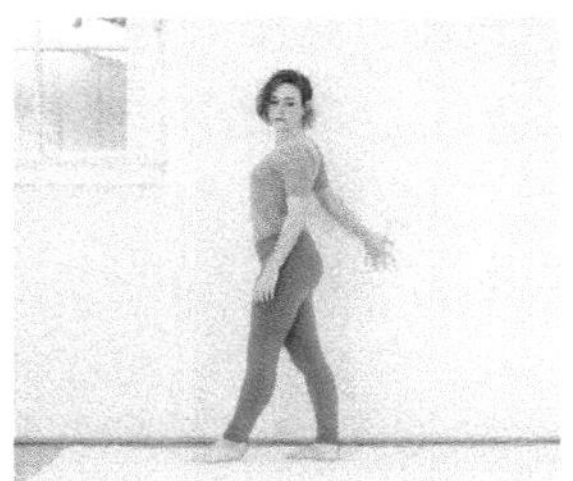

#11 Beginner (Pericardium)

QUAD WALL STRETCH

(TCM)

Organ: Stomach
Tissue: Muscles
Body Part: Legs
System: Digestion
Sensory: Nervous Receptors
Ying/Yang Element: Yang Earth

PERSONALITY (GPT)

Group: Thinking
Time and Attention: Future and Inside
High Traits: Sobriety, Quality, Work, Self Expression, Persevere
Low Traits: Addiction, Eccentric
Instinct: Fearless/Fear

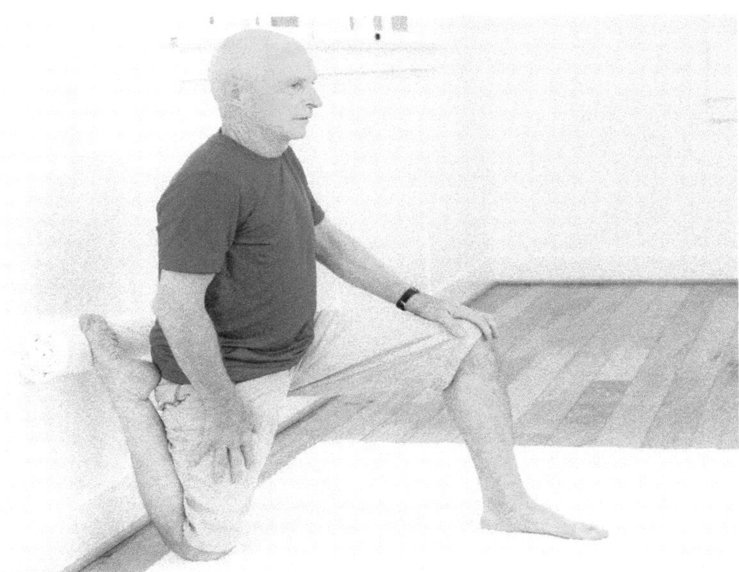

RESISTANCE FLEXIBILITY: Pull your right knee up towards your chest and push your right foot against the wall to resist while your left leg pushes your hips back towards the wall. Return to the starting position and repeat 10 times on each leg.

HELPFUL REMINDERS

1. Reverse movement for strengthening.
2. The Balancing Stretch muscles help you get into the stretch position.
3. The Opposing Stretch muscles help you get the necessary rotation.
4. Your stretch occurs only while you contract and resist.
5. Your breathing is different in every *type* of stretch.
6. Get perspective from others on how each stretch affects you.

#5 INTERMEDIATE (STOMACH)

BENEFITS

Health: Allergies/Asthma
Body Part: Thighs
Joint: Hip Joint
Movement: Step Forward
Good Looks: Cute, Unique
Life: Work, Singing and Dancing

MUSCLES

Orbicularis Oculi, Buccinator, Masseter, Vocal Cords, Platysma, Temoralis, Pectoralis Major, Oblique Abdominals, Vastus Lateralis, Tibialis Anterior,
Action: Flexion/Abduction/ Outward
Stretch: Extension/Adduction/Inward

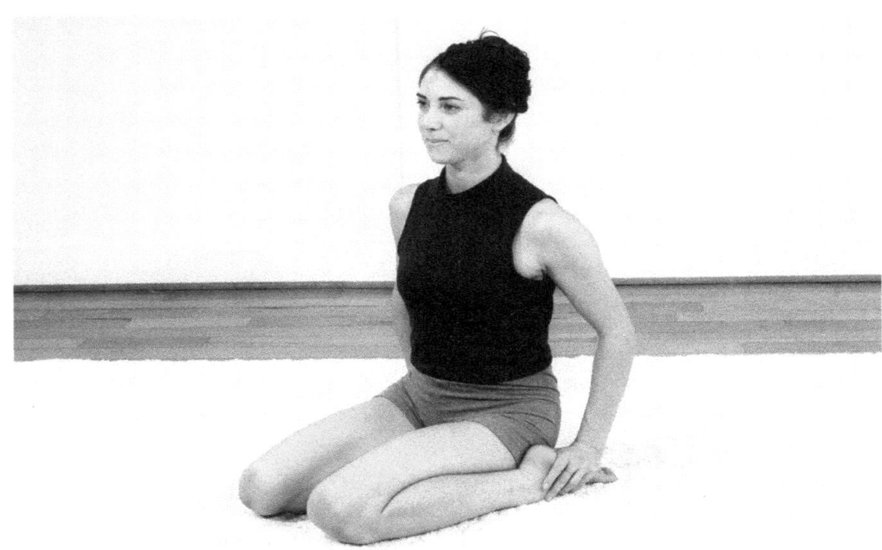

STARTING POSITION: Bend your knees and sit on both legs. Place your feet wide enough that they are next to your thighs.

BALANCING STRETCH

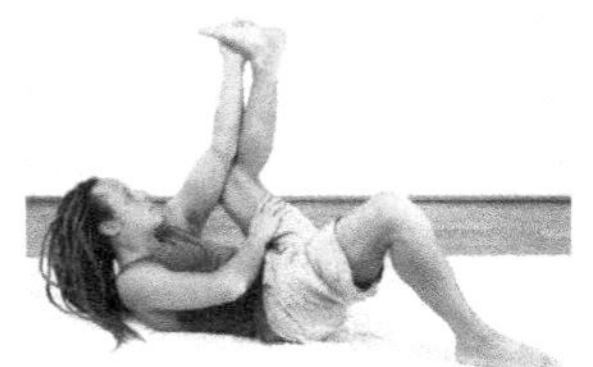

#6 Beginner (Pancreas)

OPPOSING STRETCH

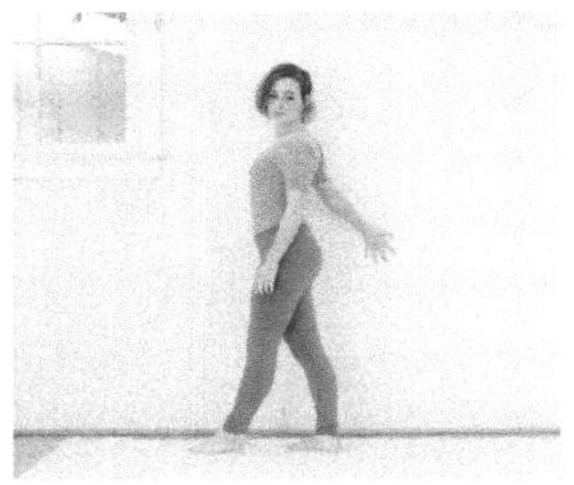

#11 Beginner (Pericardium)

BOTH QUAD STRECH ON FLOOR

(TCM)

Organ: Stomach
Tissue: Muscles
Body Part: Legs
System: Digestion
Sensory: Nervous Receptors
Ying/Yang Element: Yang Earth

PERSONALITY (GPT)

Group: Thinking
Time and Attention: Future and Inside
High Traits: Sobriety, Quality, Work, Self Expression, Persevere
Low Traits: Addiction, Eccentric
Instinct: Fearless/Fear

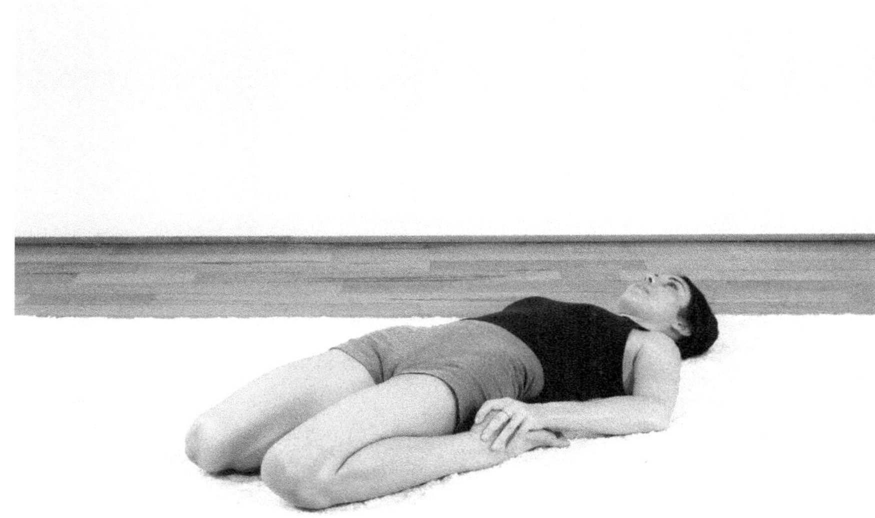

RESISTANCE FLEXIBILITY: Pull your knees up towards your chest and push your lower legs and feet into the ground to resist while you arch your body backwards. Return to the starting position and repeat 10 times.

HELPFUL REMINDERS

1. Reverse movement for strengthening.
2. The Balancing Stretch muscles help you get into the stretch position.
3. The Opposing Stretch muscles help you get the necessary rotation.
4. Your stretch occurs only while you contract and resist.
5. Your breathing is different in every *type* of stretch.
6. Get perspective from others on how each stretch affects you.

#5 ADVANCED (STOMACH)

BENEFITS

Health: Allergies / Asthma
Body Part: Thighs
Joint: Hip Joint
Movement: Step Forward
Good Looks: Cute, Unique
Life: Work, Singing and Dancing

MUSCLES

Orbicularis Oculi, Buccinator, Masseter, Vocal Cords, Platysma, Temoralis, Pectoralis Major, Oblique Abdominals, Vastus Lateralis, Tibialis Anterior,
Action: Flexion / Abduction / Outward
Stretch: Extension / Adduction / Inward

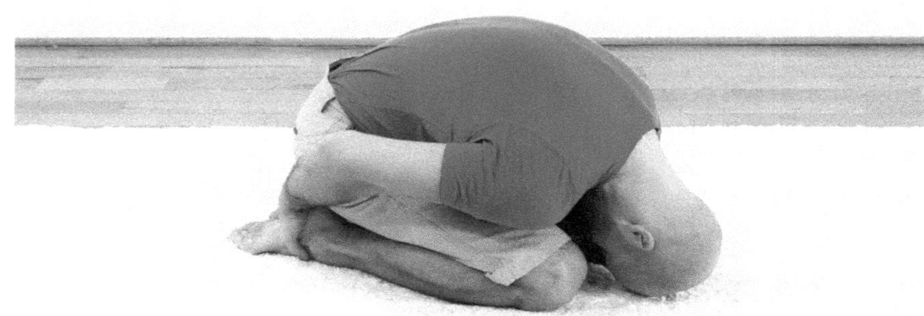

STARTING POSITION: Bend your knees and sit on both legs. Place your feet wide enough that they are next to your thighs. Grasp the insides of your ankles with your hands, palms facing out, and curl your body forward towards your knees.

BALANCING STRETCH

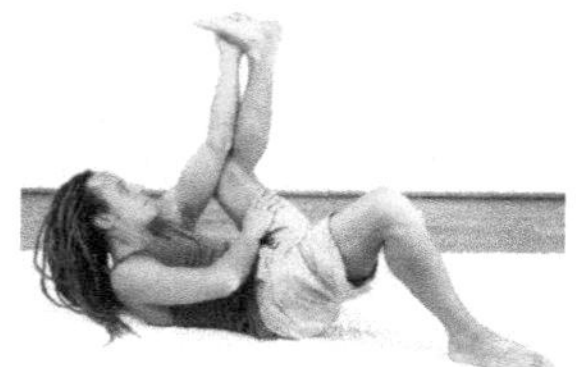

#6 Beginner (Pancreas)

OPPOSING STRETCH

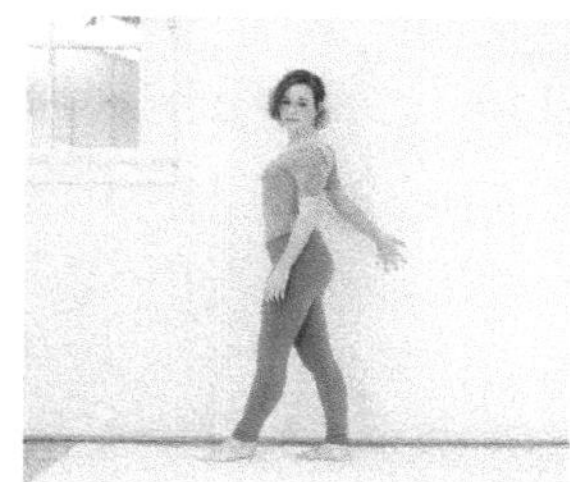

#11 Beginner (Pericardium)

KNEELING ARCH

(TCM)

Organ: Stomach
Tissue: Muscles
Body Part: Legs
System: Digestion
Sensory: Nervous Receptors
Ying/Yang Element: Yang Earth

PERSONALITY (GPT)

Group: Thinking
Time and Attention: Future and Inside
High Traits: Sobriety, Quality, Work, Self Expression, Persevere
Low Traits: Addiction, Eccentric
Instinct: Fearless/Fear

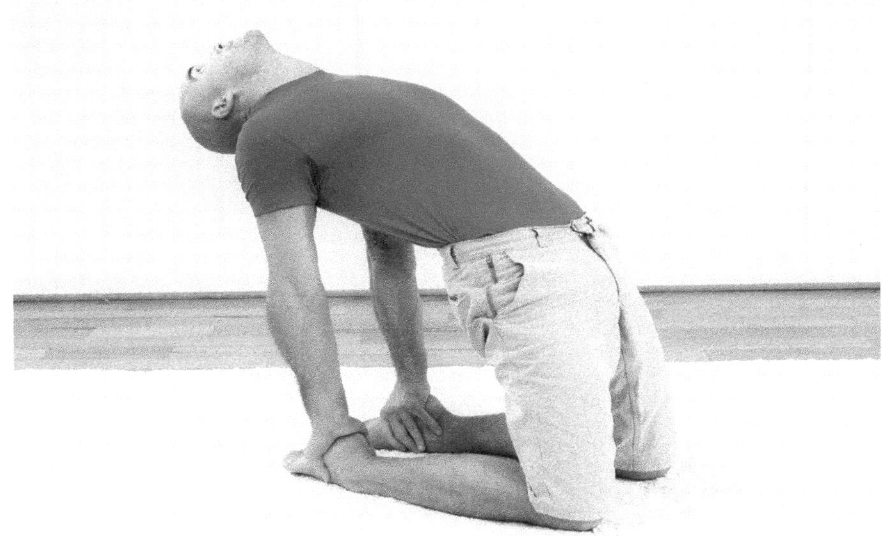

RESISTANCE FLEXIBILITY: Pull your knees up towards your chest, push your lower legs and feet into the ground, and contract your abdominals to resist while you arch your body up and backwards. Return to the starting position and repeat 10 times.

HELPFUL REMINDERS

1. Reverse movement for strengthening.
2. The Balancing Stretch muscles help you get into the stretch position.
3. The Opposing Stretch muscles help you get the necessary rotation.
4. Your stretch occurs only while you contract and resist.
5. Your breathing is different in every *type* of stretch.
6. Get perspective from others on how each stretch affects you.

#5 ASSISTED (STOMACH)

BENEFITS

Health: Allergies / Asthma
Body Part: Thighs
Joint: Hip Joint
Movement: Step Forward
Good Looks: Cute, Unique
Life: Work, Singing and Dancing

MUSCLES

Orbicularis Oculi, Buccinator, Masseter, Vocal Cords, Platysma, Temoralis, Pectoralis Major, Oblique Abdominals, Vastus Lateralis, Tibialis Anterior,

Action: Flexion / Abduction / Outward
Stretch: Extension / Adduction / Inward

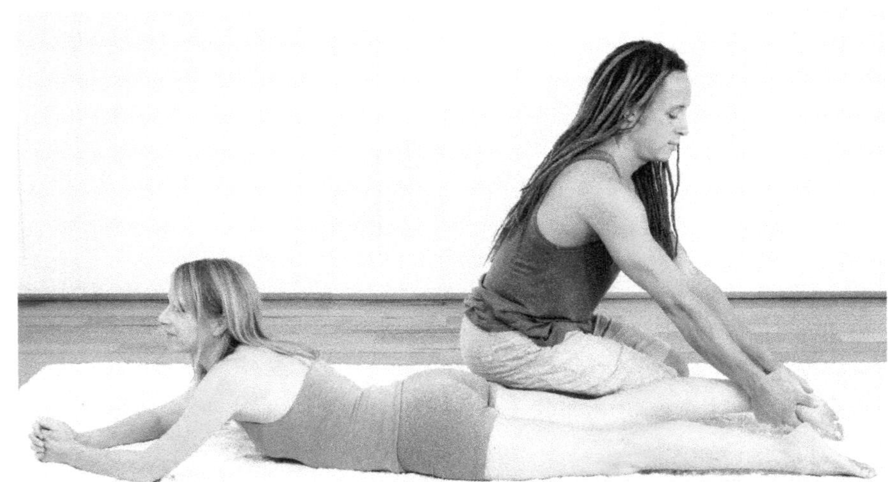

STARTING POSITION: Lie on your belly with your legs straight. The assister grasps your right ankle with their hands.

BALANCING STRETCH

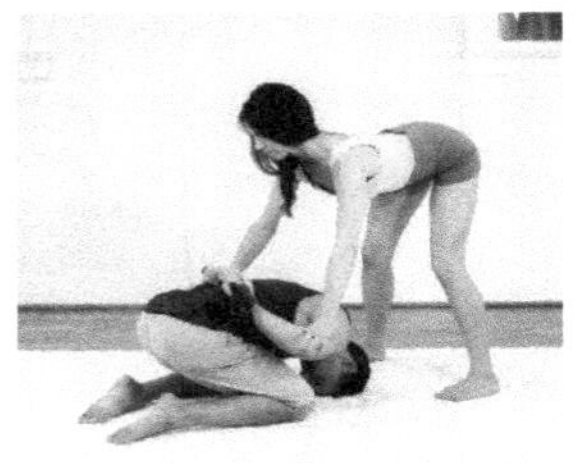

#6 Assisted (Pancreas)

OPPOSING STRETCH

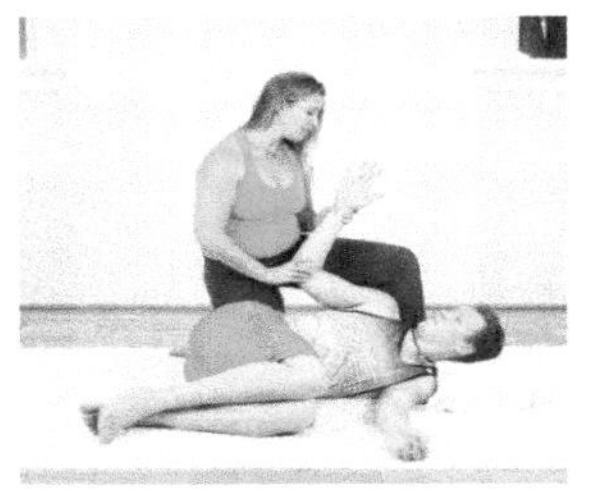

#11 Assisted (Pericardium)

FRONT LYING QUAD STRETCH

(TCM)

Organ: Stomach
Tissue: Muscles
Body Part: Legs
System: Digestion
Sensory: Nervous Receptors
Ying/Yang Element: Yang Earth

PERSONALITY (GPT)

Group: Thinking
Time and Attention: Future and Inside
High Traits: Sobriety, Quality, Work, Self Expression, Persevere
Low Traits: Addiction, Eccentric
Instinct: Fearless/Fear

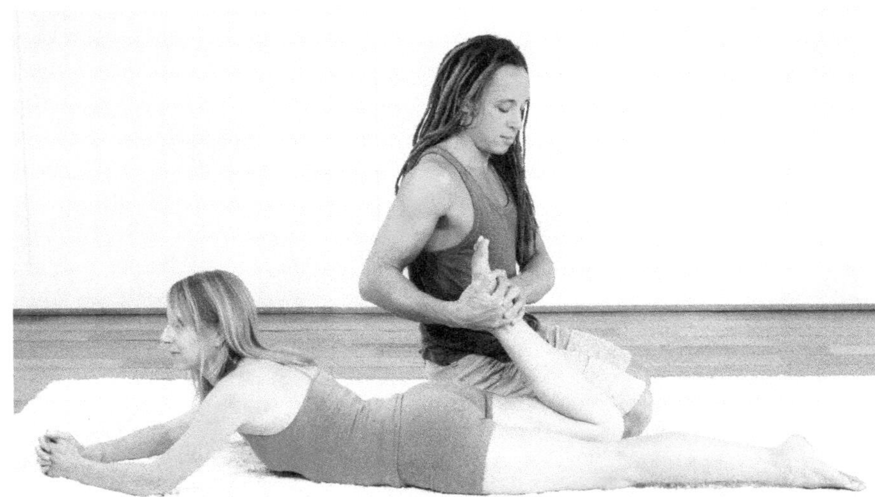

RESISTANCE FLEXIBILITY: Your right thigh presses into the floor and your right foot pushes back towards the floor to resist while the assister lifts your right ankle and bends your knee. Return to the starting position and repeat 10 times on each leg.

HELPFUL REMINDERS

1. Reverse movement for strengthening.
2. The Balancing Stretch muscles help you get into the stretch position.
3. The Opposing Stretch muscles help you get the necessary rotation.
4. Your stretch occurs only while you contract and resist.
5. Your breathing is different in every *type* of stretch.
6. Get perspective from others on how each stretch affects you.

#6 BEGINNER (PANCREAS)

BENEFITS

Health: Fascia
Body Part: Thighs
Joint: Hip Joint
Movement: Step Backwards
Good Looks: Bedazzling, Angelic
Life: Playful, Writing

MUSCLES

Palmar Flexor, Adductor Hallucis, Soleus, Flexor Digitorum Longus, Gastrocnemius, Semimembranosus, Vastus Medialis, Obliques, Serratus
Action: Extension/Adduction/Inward
Stretch: Flexion/Abduction/Outward

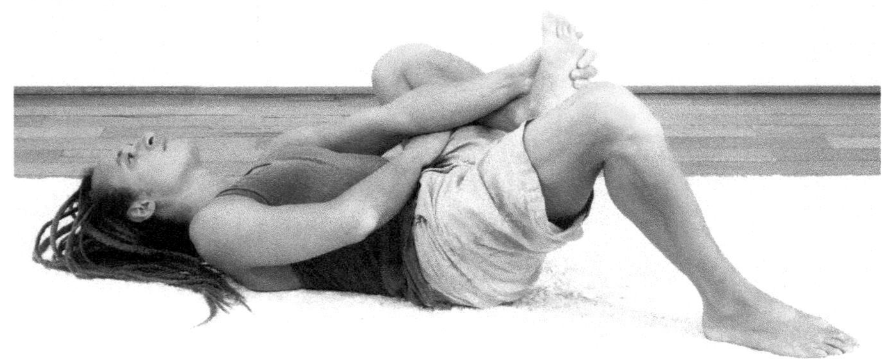

STARTING POSITION: Lie on your back with both knees bent. Bring your left knee up towards your chest and, with your left hand, grasp the outside of the left ankle. Put your right hand on the inside back of the left thigh in order to feel the upcoming stretch.

BALANCING STRETCH

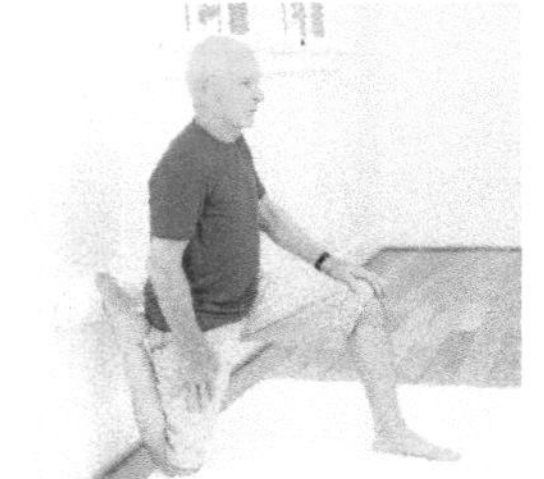

#5 Beginner (Stomach)

OPPOSING STRETCH

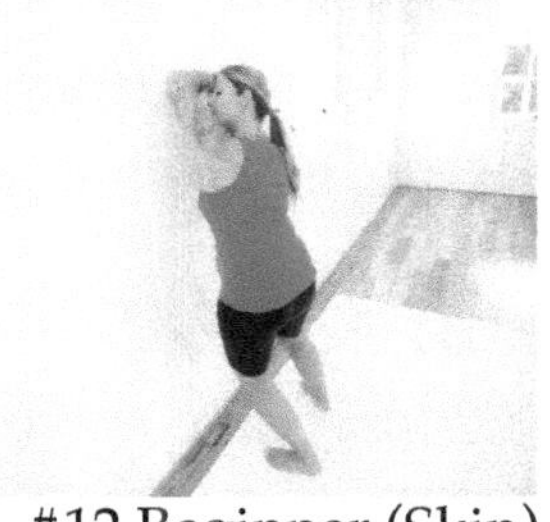

#12 Beginner (Skin)

BACK LYING MEDIAL HAMSTRING

(TCM)

Organ: Pancreas
Tissue: Fascia
Body Part: Legs
System: Enzymes
Sensory: Energetic receptors
Yin/Yang Element: Yang Earth

PERSONALITY (GPT)

Group: Spiritual
Time and Attention: Relative and Outside
High Traits: Balance, Communication, Empathy, Peace, Temperance
Low Traits: Martyrdom, Indifference
Instinct: Calm/Frightened

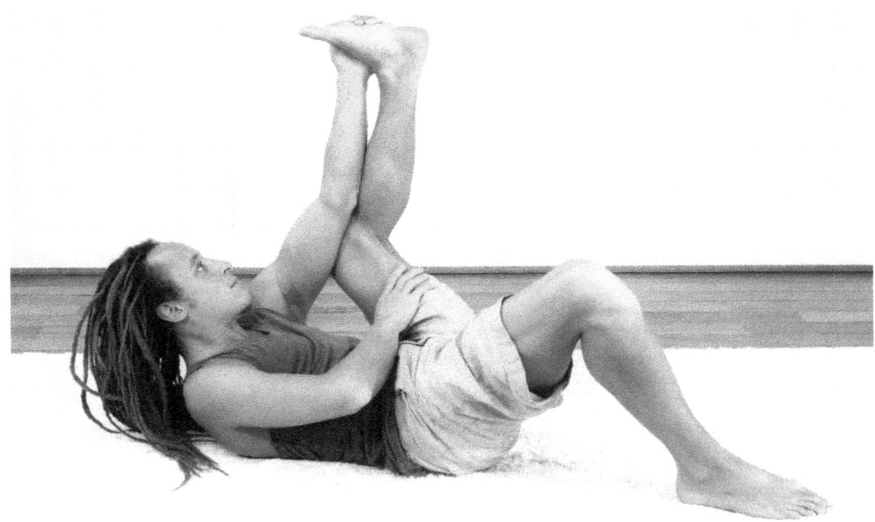

RESISTANCE FLEXIBILITY: Your left heel kicks down towards your butt to resist as your left hand lifts your leg upwards and to the left. Return to the starting position and repeat 10 times on each leg.

HELPFUL REMINDERS

1. Reverse movement for strengthening.
2. The Balancing Stretch muscles help you get into the stretch position.
3. The Opposing Stretch muscles help you get the necessary rotation.
4. Your stretch occurs only while you contract and resist.
5. Your breathing is different in every *type* of stretch.
6. Get perspective from others on how each stretch affects you.

#6 INTERMEDIATE (PANCREAS)

BENEFITS

Health: Fascia
Body Part: Thighs
Joint: Hip Joint
Movement: Step Backwards
Good Looks: Bedazzling, Angelic
Life: Playful, Writing

MUSCLES

Palmar Flexor, Adductor Hallucis, Soleus, Flexor Digitorum Longus, Gastrocnemius, Semimembranosus, Vastus Medialis, Obliques, Serratus
Action: Extension / Adduction / Inward
Stretch: Flexion / Abduction / Outward

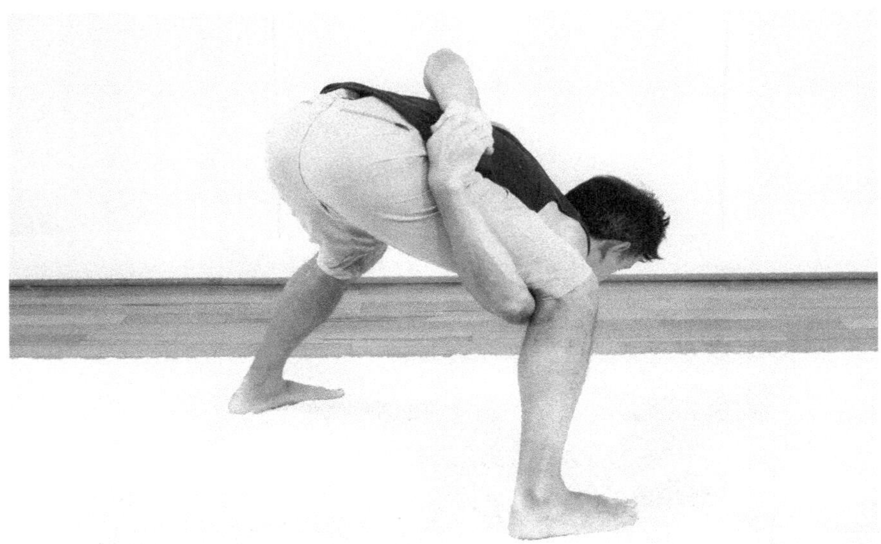

STARTING POSITION: Stand with your legs wide, then squat and bend over, placing your right elbow on the inside of your right knee. Bring your right hand under and behind your hips, and then reach your left hand behind your back to grasp your right hand. Arch your head and spine upwards.

BALANCING STRETCH

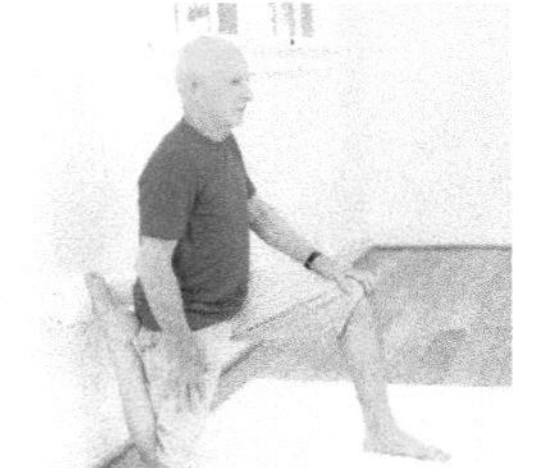

#5 Beginner (Stomach)

OPPOSING STRETCH

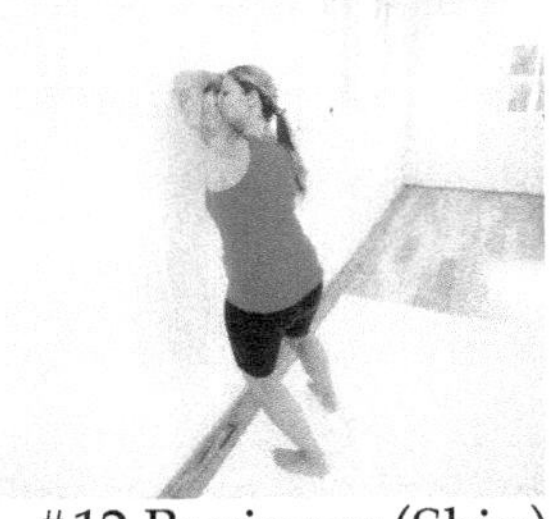

#12 Beginner (Skin)

TURTLE STANDING

(TCM)

Organ: Pancreas
Tissue: Fascia
Body Part: Legs
System: Enzymes
Sensory: Energetic receptors
Yin/Yang Element: Yang Earth

PERSONALITY (GPT)

Group: Spiritual
Time and Attention: Relative and Outside
High Traits: Balance, Communication, Empathy, Peace, Temperance
Low Traits: Martyrdom, Indifference
Instinct: Calm/Frightened

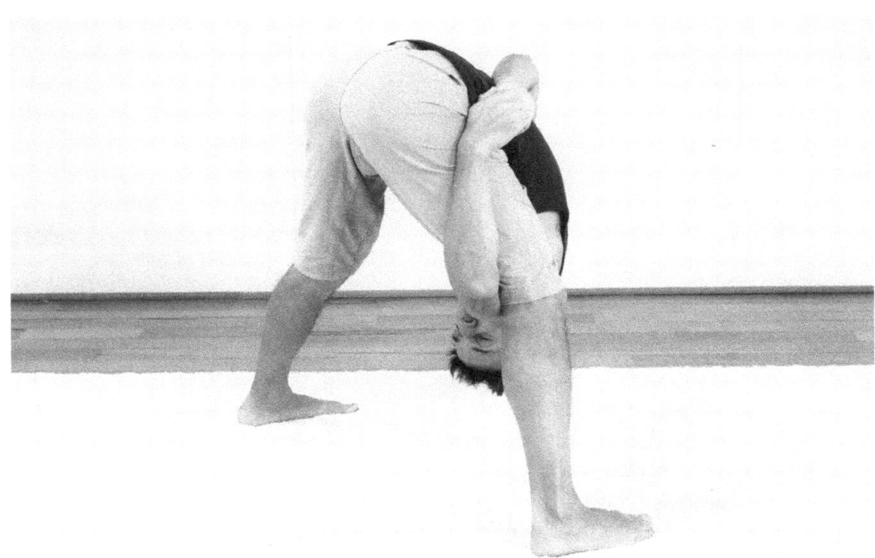

RESISTANCE FLEXIBILITY: Press the balls of your feet into the ground, pull your heels backwards towards your hips, pull your thighs backwards and squeeze your legs together to resist as you straighten your legs and drop your head down. Return to the starting position and repeat 10 times on the right and left sides.

HELPFUL REMINDERS

1. Reverse movement for strengthening.
2. The Balancing Stretch muscles help you get into the stretch position.
3. The Opposing Stretch muscles help you get the necessary rotation.
4. Your stretch occurs only while you contract and resist.
5. Your breathing is different in every *type* of stretch.
6. Get perspective from others on how each stretch affects you.

#6 ADVANCED (PANCREAS)

BENEFITS

Health: Fascia
Body Part: Thighs
Joint: Hip Joint
Movement: Step Backwards
Good Looks: Bedazzling, Angelic
Life: Playful, Writing

MUSCLES

Palmar Flexor, Adductor Hallucis, Soleus, Flexor Digitorum Longus, Gastrocnemius, Semimembranosus, Vastus Medialis, Obliques, Serratus

Action: Extension / Adduction / Inward
Stretch: Flexion / Abduction / Outward

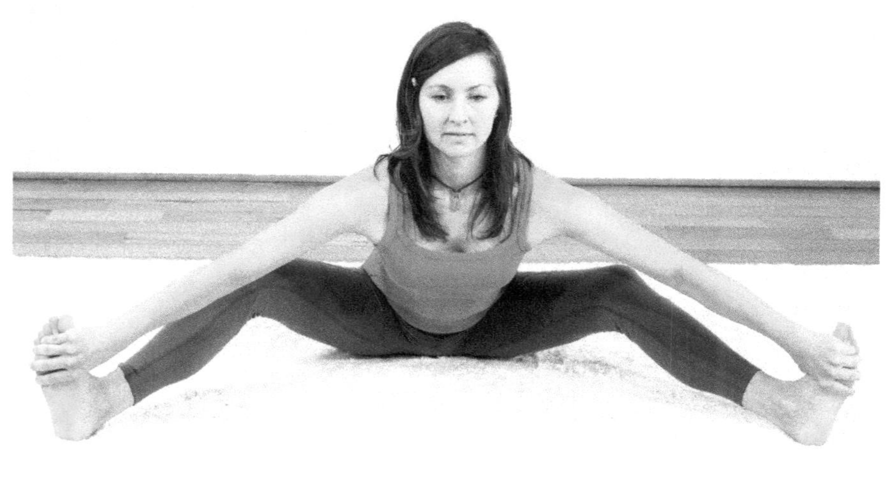

STARTING POSITION: Sit on the floor with your legs wide, knees bent, and feet flexed. Bend forward and grasp the insides of your ankles with your hands.

BALANCING STRETCH

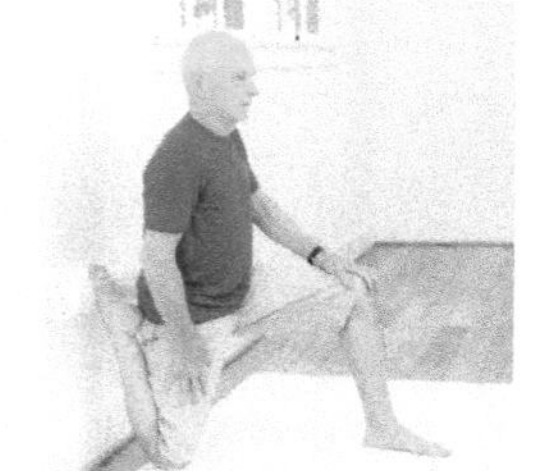

#5 Beginner (Stomach)

OPPOSING STRETCH

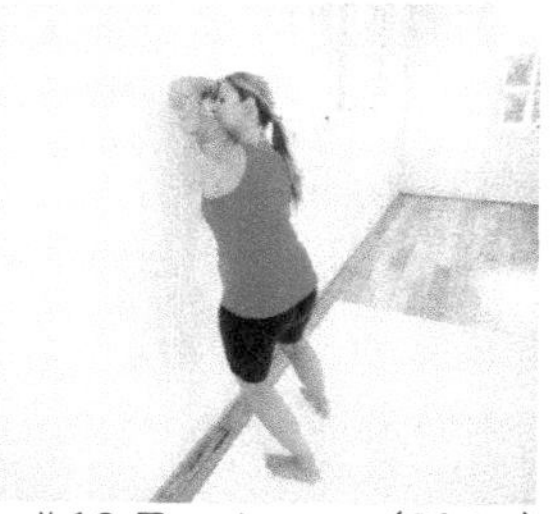

#12 Beginner (Skin)

SEATED WIDE LEG

(TCM)

Organ: Pancreas
Tissue: Fascia
Body Part: Legs
System: Enzymes
Sensory: Energetic receptors
Yin/Yang Element: Yang Earth

PERSONALITY (GPT)

Group: Spiritual
Time and Attention: Relative and Outside
High Traits: Balance, Communication, Empathy, Peace, Temperance
Low Traits: Martyrdom, Indifference
Instinct: Calm/Frightened

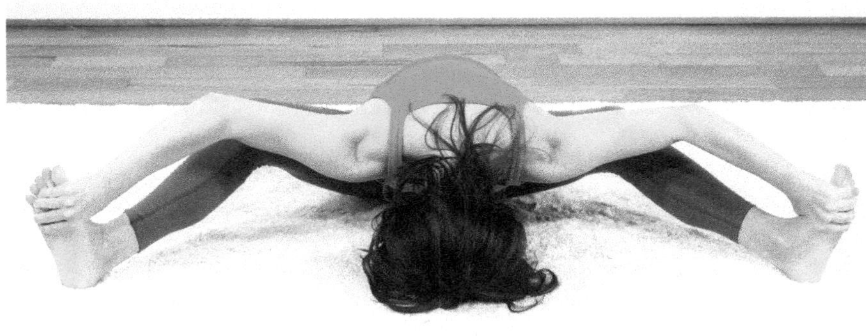

RESISTANCE FLEXIBILITY: Push your feet into your hands, kick your heels into the floor, push your thighs downward and squeeze them together to resist while your hands pull your feet and legs towards you and pull your body forwards. Return to the starting position and repeat 10 times.

HELPFUL REMINDERS

1. Reverse movement for strengthening.
2. The Balancing Stretch muscles help you get into the stretch position.
3. The Opposing Stretch muscles help you get the necessary rotation.
4. Your stretch occurs only while you contract and resist.
5. Your breathing is different in every *type* of stretch.
6. Get perspective from others on how each stretch affects you.

#6 ASSISTED (PANCREAS)

BENEFITS

Health: Fascia
Body Part: Thighs
Joint: Hip Joint
Movement: Step Backwards
Good Looks: Bedazzling, Angelic
Life: Playful, Writing

MUSCLES

Palmar Flexor, Adductor Hallucis, Soleus, Flexor Digitorum Longus, Gastrocnemius, Semimembranosus, Vastus Medialis, Obliques, Serratus
Action: Extension / Adduction / Inward
Stretch: Flexion / Abduction / Outward

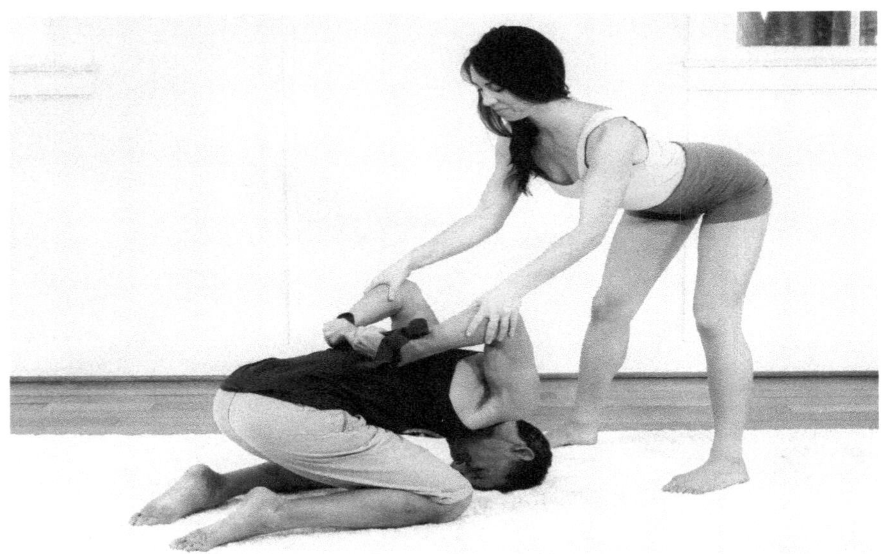

STARTING POSITION: Kneel on the floor and place your head on the floor. Bring your hands behind your back, holding a strap to connect them, and bring your elbows together. The assister grasps your elbows with their hands.

BALANCING STRETCH

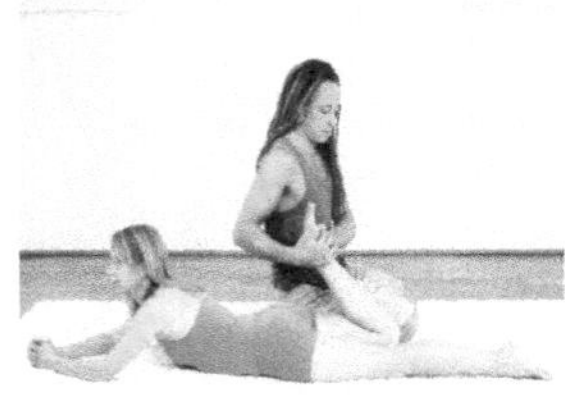

#5 Assisted (Stomach)

OPPOSING STRETCH

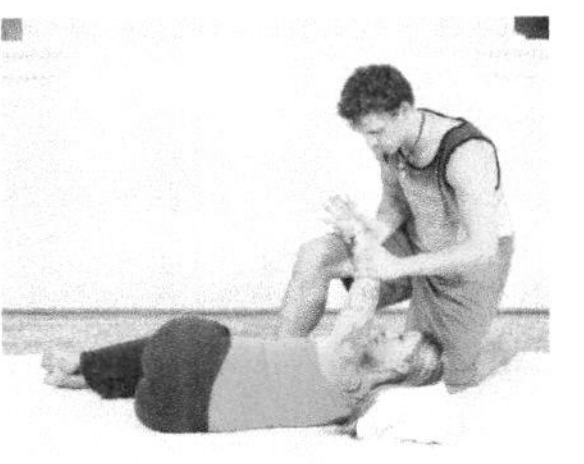

#12 Assisted (Skin)

BETWEEN SHOULDERS

(TCM)

Organ: Pancreas
Tissue: Fascia
Body Part: Legs
System: Enzymes
Sensory: Energetic receptors
Yin/Yang Element: Yang Earth

PERSONALITY (GPT)

Group: Spiritual
Time and Attention: Relative and Outside
High Traits: Balance, Communication, Empathy, Peace, Temperance
Low Traits: Martyrdom, Indifference
Instinct: Calm/Frightened

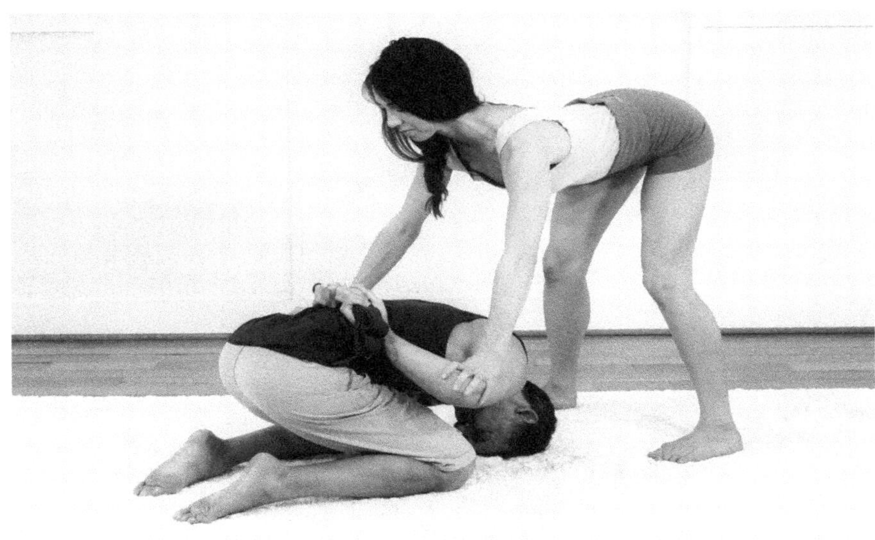

RESISTANCE FLEXIBILITY: Pull your arms backwards and together to resist while the assister pushes your elbows out and down. Return to the starting position and repeat 10 times.

HELPFUL REMINDERS

1. Reverse movement for strengthening.
2. The Balancing Stretch muscles help you get into the stretch position.
3. The Opposing Stretch muscles help you get the necessary rotation.
4. Your stretch occurs only while you contract and resist.
5. Your breathing is different in every *type* of stretch.
6. Get perspective from others on how each stretch affects you.

#7 BEGINNER (HEART)

BENEFITS

Health: Heart
Body Part: Upper Arm
Joint: Shoulder Joint
Movement: Push
Good Looks: Lovely, Joyful
Life: Political, Mediation

MUSCLES

Biceps, Pornator Teres, Brachialis, Forearm Flexors, Pronator Quadratus, Abductor Digit Minimi, Flexor Digiti Minimi Brevis, Lumbricals

Action: Flexion / Adduction / Inward
Stretch: Extension / Abduction / Outward

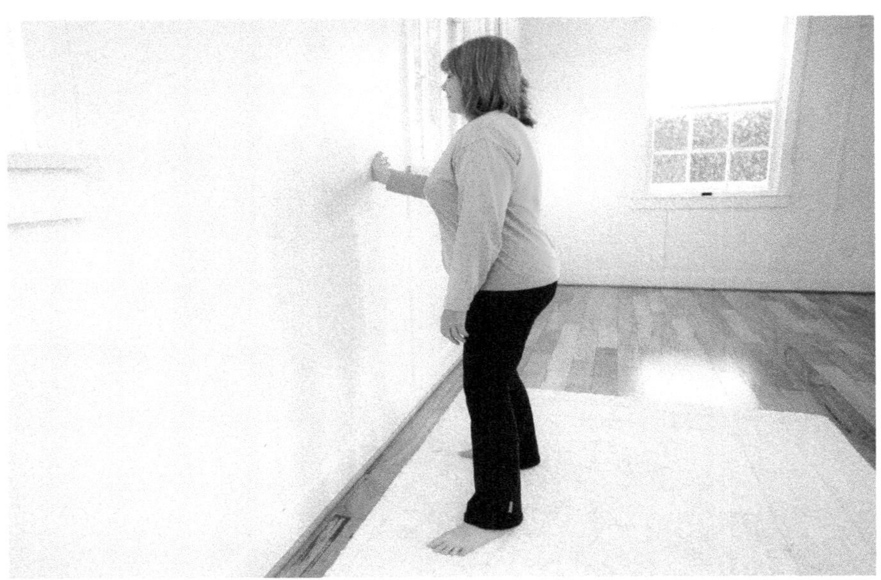

STARTING POSITION: Stand facing a wall. Open your right arm out to the right and place your palm against the wall.

BALANCING STRETCH

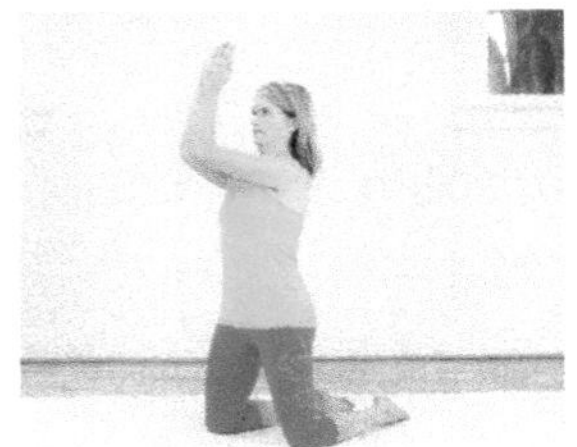

#8 Beginner (Small Intestine)

OPPOSING STRETCH

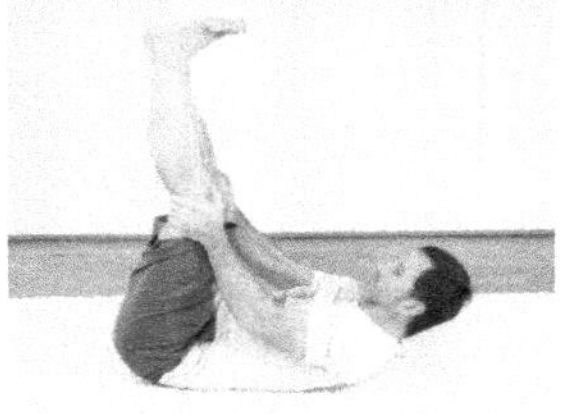

#1 Beginner (Gall Bladder)

HEART STRETCH AT WALL

(TCM)

Organ: Heart
Tissue: Arterial Blood Volume
Body Part: Arms
System: Circulation
Sensory: Exteroceptive receptors
Yin/Yang Element: Yin Fire

PERSONALITY (GPT)

Time and Attention: Present and Inside
High Traits: Right Action, Love
Mediation, Political, Joy
Low Traits: Avoidant, Sloth
Instinct: Love/Anger

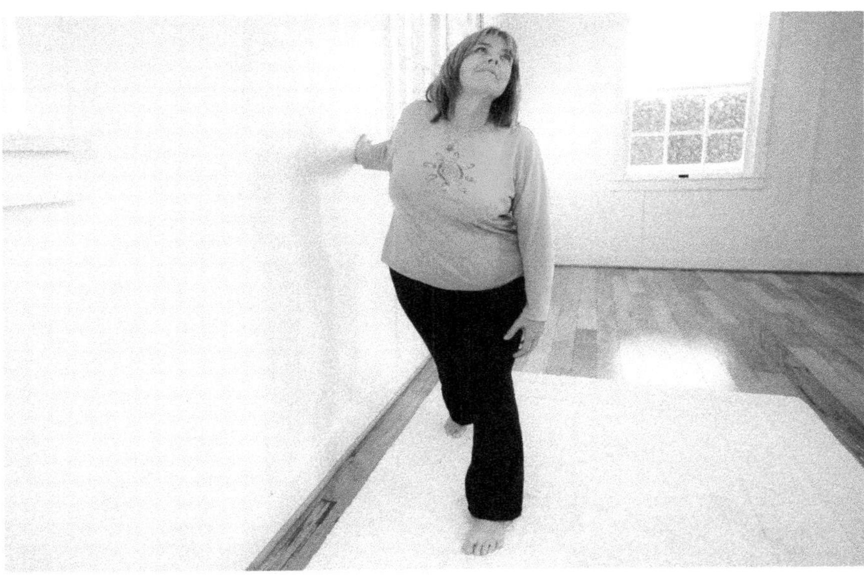

RESISTANCE FLEXIBILITY: Your right arm pushes forwards into the wall to resist while you turn your body to the left and move slightly left. Return to the starting position and repeat 10 times on each arm.

HELPFUL REMINDERS

1. Reverse movement for strengthening.
2. The Balancing Stretch muscles help you get into the stretch position.
3. The Opposing Stretch muscles help you get the necessary rotation.
4. Your stretch occurs only while you contract and resist.
5. Your breathing is different in every *type* of stretch.
6. Get perspective from others on how each stretch affects you.

#7 INTERMEDIATE (HEART)

BENEFITS

Health: Heart
Body Part: Upper Arm
Joint: Shoulder Joint
Movement: Push
Good Looks: Lovely, Joyful
Life: Political, Mediation

MUSCLES

Biceps, Pornator Teres, Brachialis, Forearm Flexors, Pronator Quadratus, Abductor Digit Minimi, Flexor Digiti Minimi Brevis, Lumbricals

Action: Flexion / Adduction / Inward
Stretch: Extension / Abduction / Outward

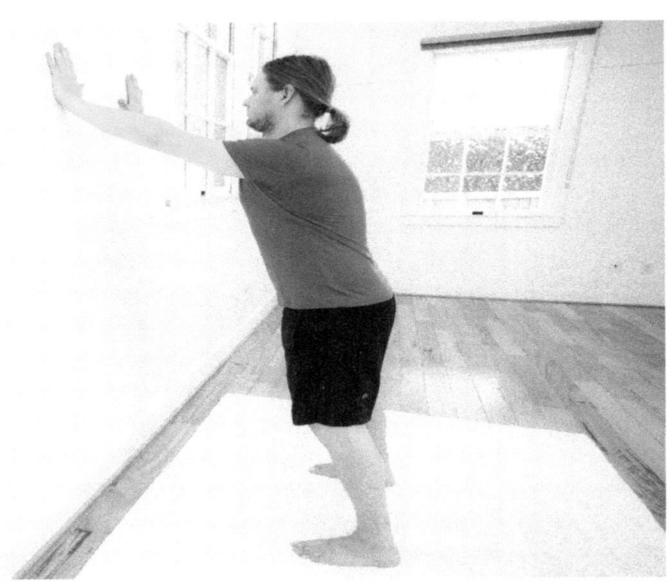

STARTING POSITION: Stand facing a wall. Place your palms against the wall above your head, arms shoulder width.

BALANCING STRETCH

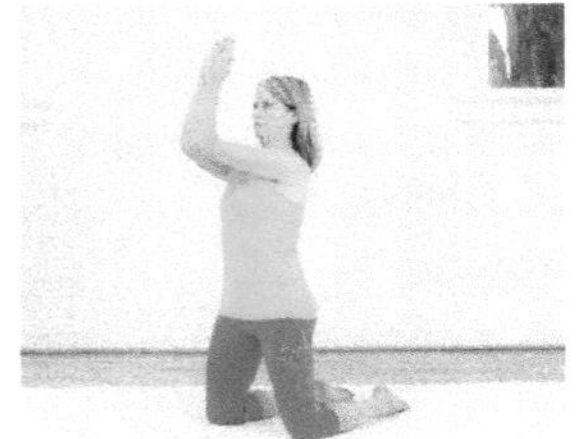

#8 Beginner (Small Intestine)

OPPOSING STRETCH

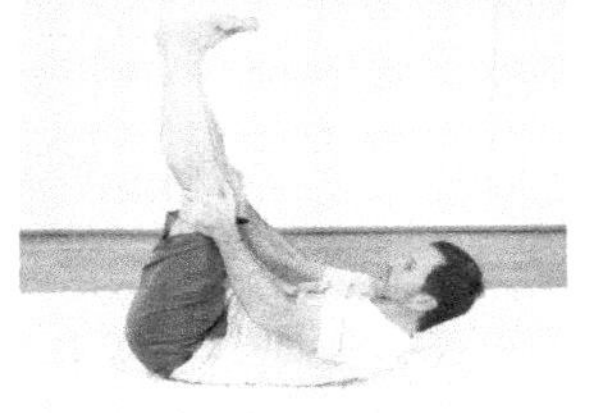

#1 Beginner (Gall Bladder)

HEART BOTH ARMS AT WALL

(TCM)

Organ: Heart
Tissue: Arterial Blood Volume
Body Part: Arms
System: Circulation
Sensory: Exteroceptive receptors
Yin/Yang Element: Yin Fire

PERSONALITY (GPT)

Time and Attention: Present and Inside
High Traits: Right Action, Love
Mediation, Political, Joy
Low Traits: Avoidant, Sloth
Instinct: Love/Anger

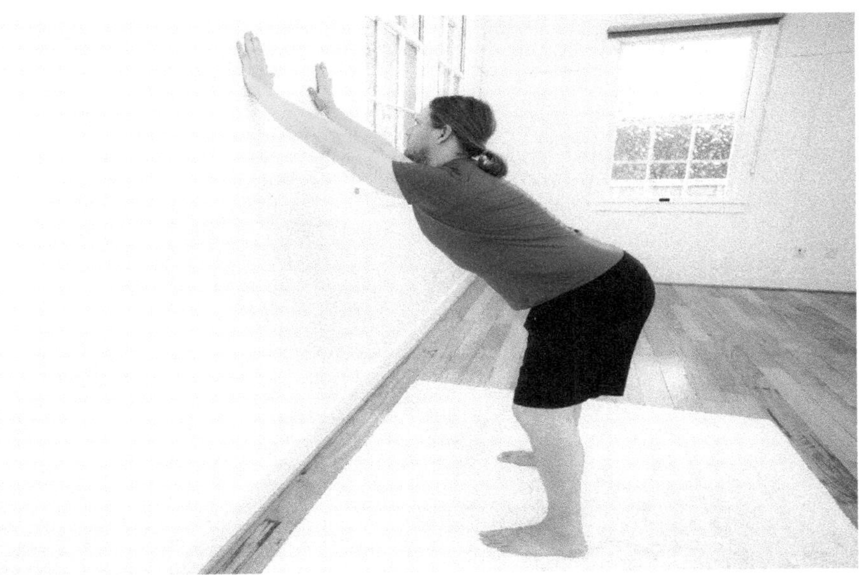

RESISTANCE FLEXIBILITY: Push your arms into the wall to resist as you bend forward at your hips and lower your chest towards the floor. Return to the starting position and repeat 10 times.

HELPFUL REMINDERS

1. Reverse movement for strengthening.
2. The Balancing Stretch muscles help you get into the stretch position.
3. The Opposing Stretch muscles help you get the necessary rotation.
4. Your stretch occurs only while you contract and resist.
5. Your breathing is different in every *type* of stretch.
6. Get perspective from others on how each stretch affects you.

#7 ADVANCED (HEART)

BENEFITS

Health: Heart
Body Part: Upper Arm
Joint: Shoulder Joint
Movement: Push
Good Looks: Lovely, Joyful
Life: Political, Mediation

MUSCLES

Biceps, Pornator Teres, Brachialis, Forearm Flexors, Pronator Quadratus, Abductor Digit Minimi, Flexor Digiti Minimi Brevis, Lumbricals

Action: Flexion/Adduction/Inward
Stretch: Extension/Abduction/Outward

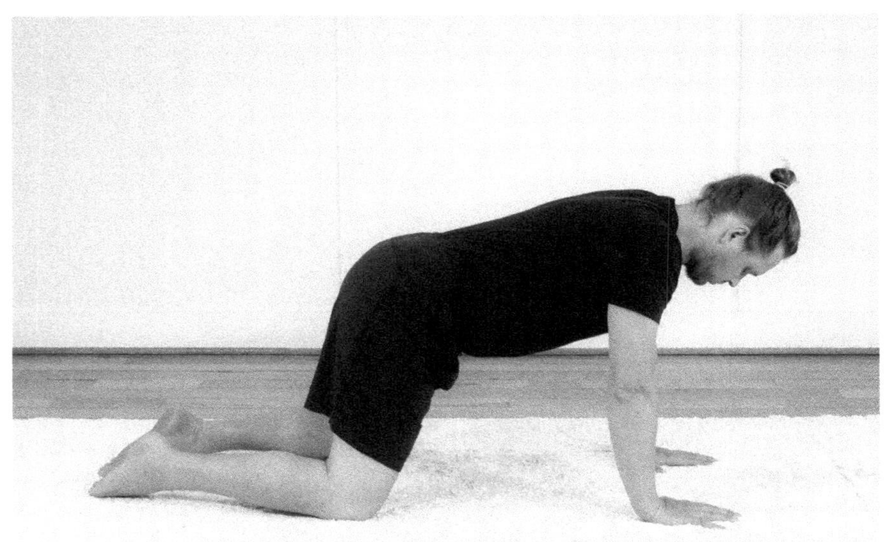

STARTING POSITION: Start on your hands and knees, arms shoulder width apart.

BALANCING STRETCH

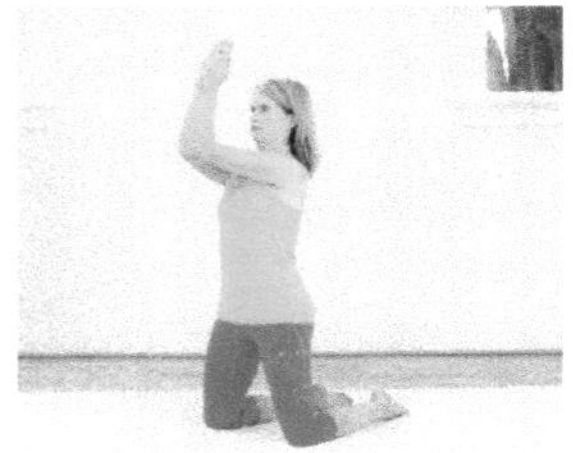

#8 Beginner (Small Intestine)

OPPOSING STRETCH

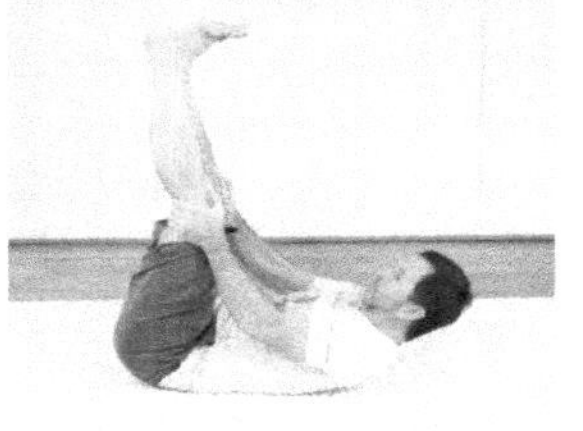

#1 Beginner (Gall Bladder)

HEART KNEELING

(TCM)

Organ: Heart
Tissue: Arterial Blood Volume
Body Part: Arms
System: Circulation
Sensory: Exteroceptive receptors
Yin/Yang Element: Yin Fire

PERSONALITY (GPT)

Time and Attention: Present and Inside
High Traits: Right Action, Love
Mediation, Political, Joy
Low Traits: Avoidant, Sloth
Instinct: Love/Anger

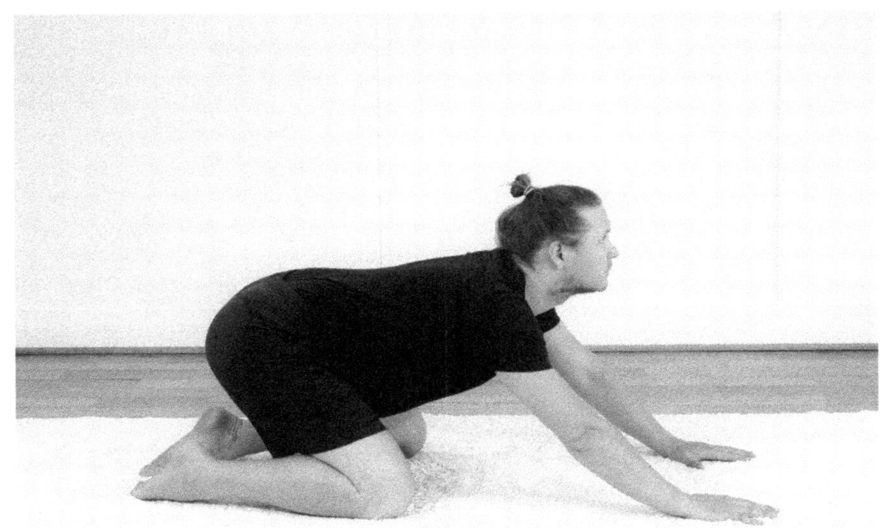

RESISTANCE FLEXIBILITY: Push your arms down into the floor to resist as you lower your hips backwards and lift your head. Return to the starting position and repeat 10 times.

HELPFUL REMINDERS

1. Reverse movement for strengthening.
2. The Balancing Stretch muscles help you get into the stretch position.
3. The Opposing Stretch muscles help you get the necessary rotation.
4. Your stretch occurs only while you contract and resist.
5. Your breathing is different in every *type* of stretch.
6. Get perspective from others on how each stretch affects you.

#7 ASSISTED (HEART)

BENEFITS

Health: Heart
Body Part: Upper Arm
Joint: Shoulder Joint
Movement: Push
Good Looks: Lovely, Joyful
Life: Political, Mediation

MUSCLES

Biceps, Pornator Teres, Brachialis, Forearm Flexors, Pronator Quadratus, Abductor Digit Minimi, Flexor Digiti Minimi Brevis, Lumbricals

Action: Flexion / Adduction / Inward
Stretch: Extension / Abduction / Outward

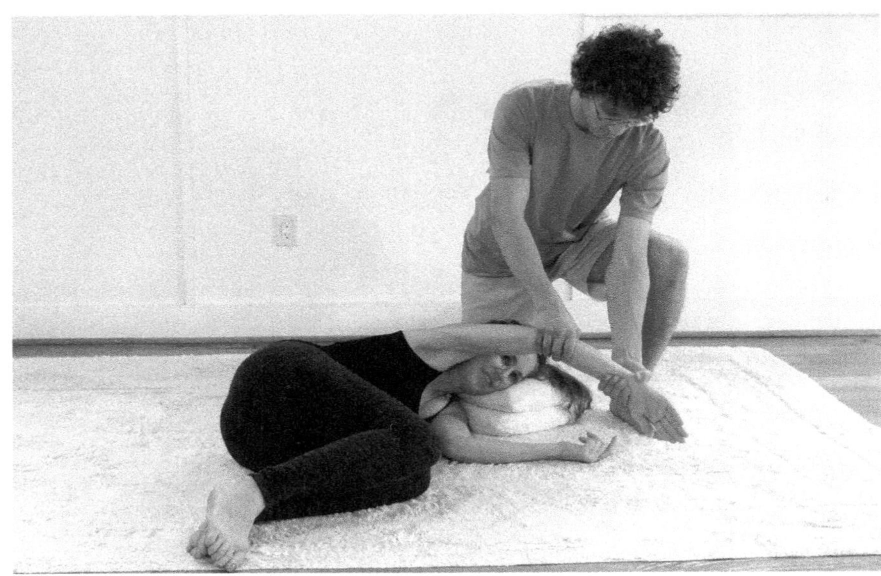

STARTING POSITION: Lie on your right side with a pillow under your head. The assister stands over you and grasps your left elbow and wrist with their hands, holding your arm forward.

BALANCING STRETCH

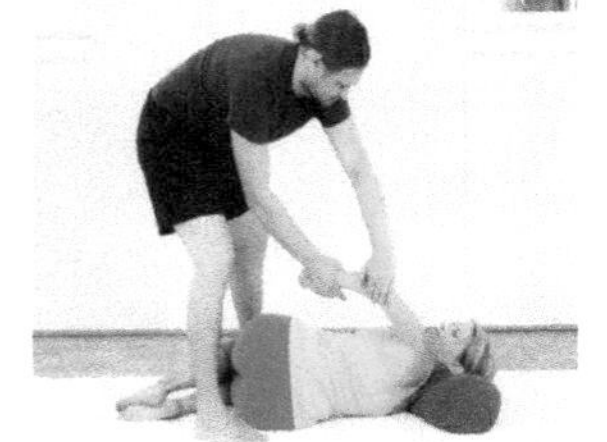

#8 Assisted (Small Intestine)

OPPOSING STRETCH

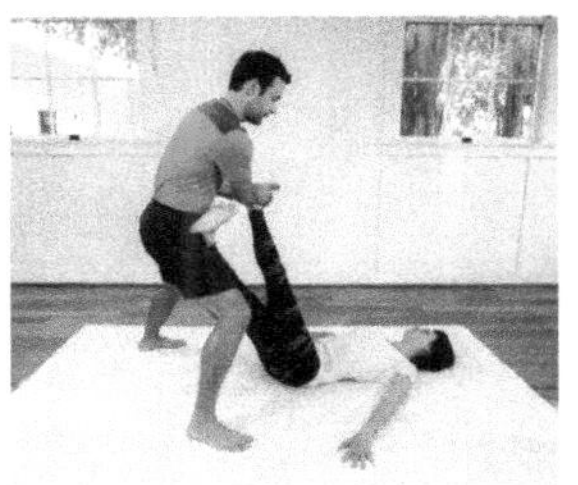

#1 Assisted (Gall Bladder)

ASSISTED SIDE LYING HEART

(TCM)

Organ: Heart
Tissue: Arterial Blood Volume
Body Part: Arms
System: Circulation
Sensory: Exteroceptive receptors
Yin/Yang Element: Yin Fire

PERSONALITY (GPT)

Time and Attention: Present and Inside
High Traits: Right Action, Love Mediation, Political, Joy
Low Traits: Avoidant, Sloth
Instinct: Love/Anger

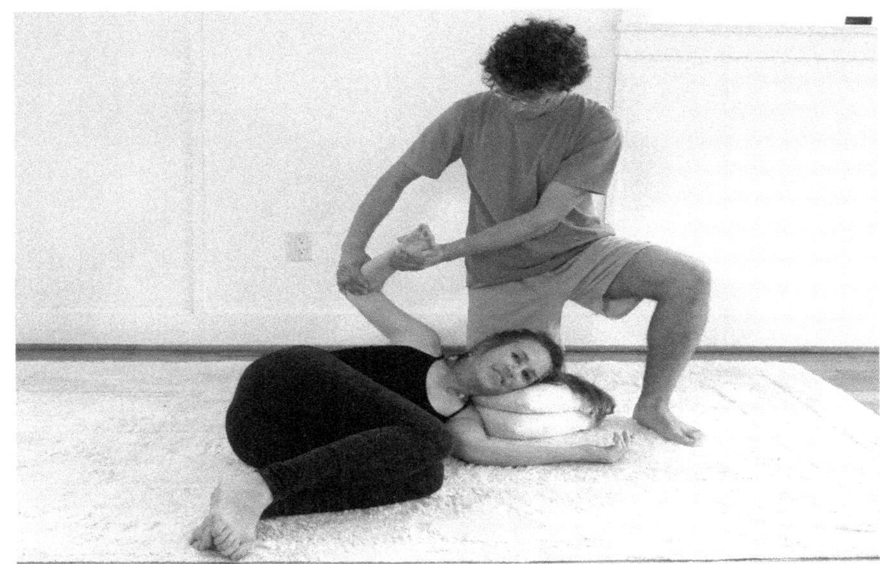

RESISTANCE FLEXIBILITY: Your left arm pushes forwards to resist while the assister pulls your elbow and wrist backwards. Return to the starting position and repeat 10 times on each arm.

HELPFUL REMINDERS

1. Reverse movement for strengthening.
2. The Balancing Stretch muscles help you get into the stretch position.
3. The Opposing Stretch muscles help you get the necessary rotation.
4. Your stretch occurs only while you contract and resist.
5. Your breathing is different in every *type* of stretch.
6. Get perspective from others on how each stretch affects you.

#8 BEGINNER (SMALL INTESTINE)

BENEFITS

Health: Protein Digestion
Body Part: Upper Arm
Joint: Shoulder Joint
Movement: Pull
Good Looks: Beautiful, Classy
Life: Artistic, Romantic

MUSCLES

Adductor Digiti Minimi, Extensor Carpi Ulnaris, Infraspinatus, Trapezius, Supraspinatus, Splenius, Scalene, SCM,
Action: Extension/Abduction/Outward
Stretch: Flexion/Adduction/Inward

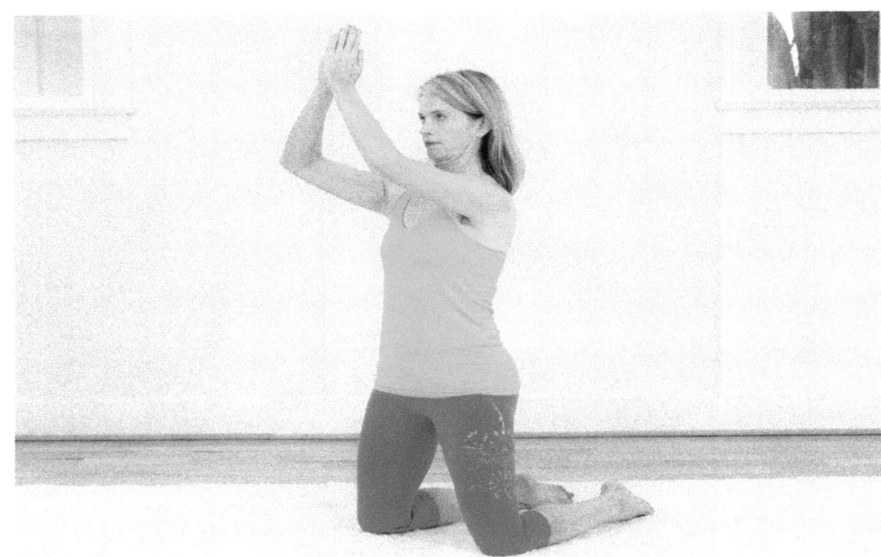

STARTING POSITION: While standing or kneeling, bring your arms up in front of you, palms together, bend your elbows to a 90 degree angle, and bring your elbows wide apart.

BALANCING STRETCH

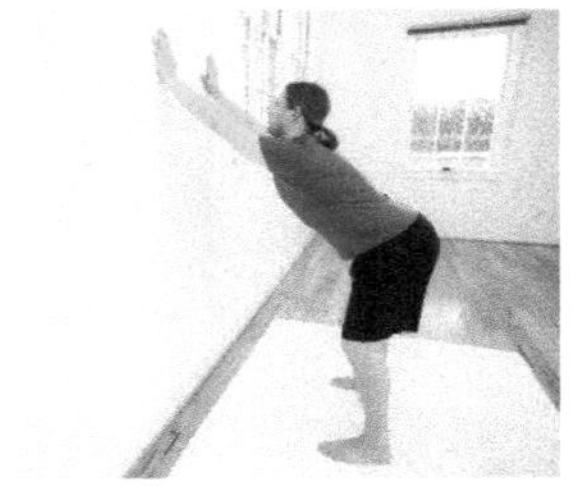

#7 Intermediate (Heart)

OPPOSING STRETCH

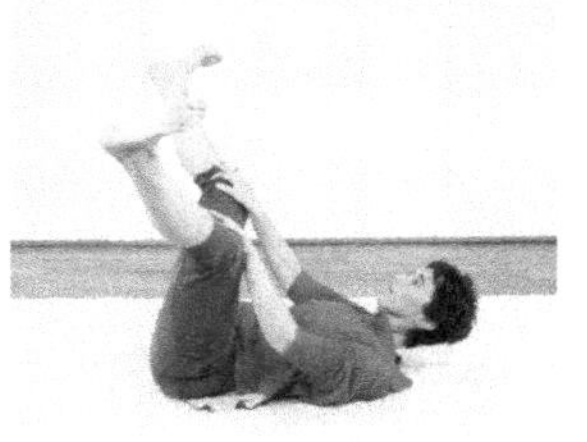

#2 Beginner (Liver)

PRAYER ARMS

(TCM)

Organ: Small Intestine
Tissue: CSF
Body Part: Face
System: Digestion
Sensory: Endocrine receptors
Yin/Yang Element: Yang Fire

PERSONALITY (GPT)

Group: Emotional
Time and Attention: Past and Outside
High Traits: Creative, Equanimity, Passion, Affirming, Classy
Low Traits: Hysterical, Depressed
Instinct: Excited/Anxiety

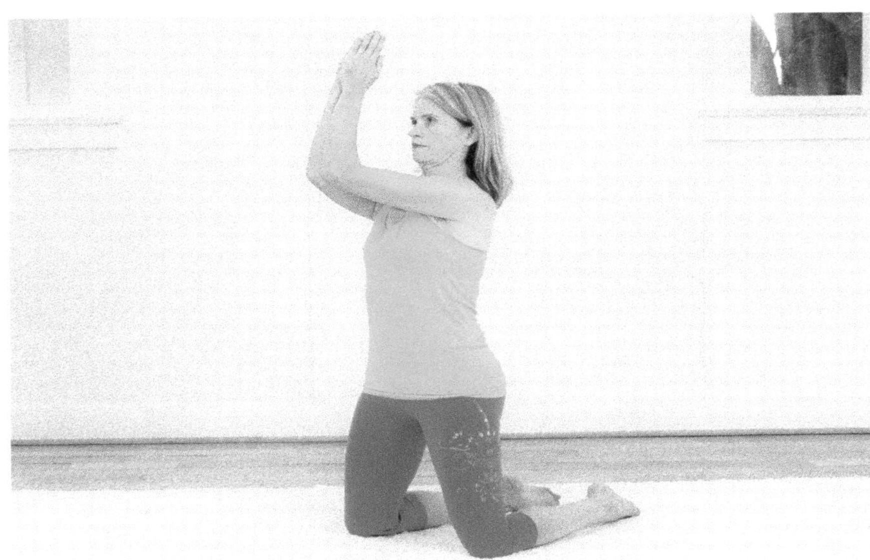

RESISTANCE FLEXIBILITY: Your elbows push outwards to resist while you bring your elbows together. Return to the starting position and repeat 10 times.

HELPFUL REMINDERS

1. Reverse movement for strengthening.
2. The Balancing Stretch muscles help you get into the stretch position.
3. The Opposing Stretch muscles help you get the necessary rotation.
4. Your stretch occurs only while you contract and resist.
5. Your breathing is different in every *type* of stretch.
6. Get perspective from others on how each stretch affects you.

#8 INTERMEDIATE (SMALL INTESTINE)

BENEFITS

Health: Protein Digestion
Body Part: Upper Arm
Joint: Shoulder Joint
Movement: Pull
Good Looks: Beautiful, Classy
Life: Artistic, Romantic

MUSCLES

Adductor Digiti Minimi, Extensor Carpi Ulnaris, Infraspinatus, Trapezius, Supraspinatus, Splenius, Scalene, SCM,
Action: Extension / Abduction / Outward
Stretch: Flexion / Adduction / Inward

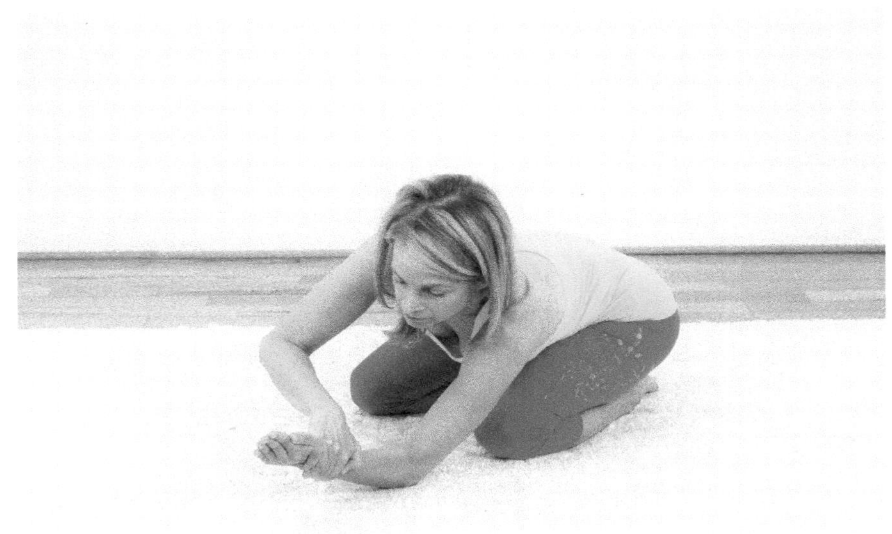

STARTING POSITION: Start on your hands and knees. Bend your knees and place your left elbow on the floor. Grasp your left wrist with your right hand and lean into the left elbow.

BALANCING STRETCH

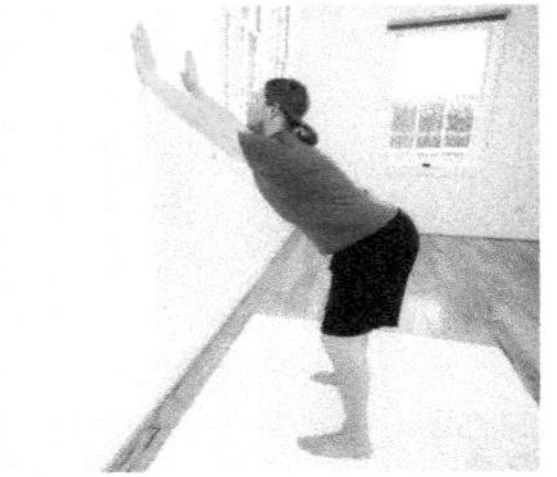

#7 Intermediate (Heart)

OPPOSING STRETCH

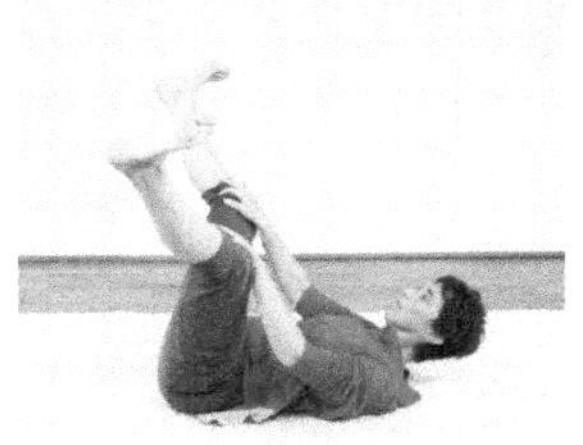

#2 Beginner (Liver)

BACK OF SHOULDER ON THE FLOOR

(TCM)

Organ: Small Intestine
Tissue: CSF
Body Part: Face
System: Digestion
Sensory: Endocrine receptors
Yin/Yang Element: Yang Fire

PERSONALITY (GPT)

Group: Emotional
Time and Attention: Past and Outside
High Traits: Creative, Equanimity, Passion, Affirming, Classy
Low Traits: Hysterical, Depressed
Instinct: Excited/Anxiety

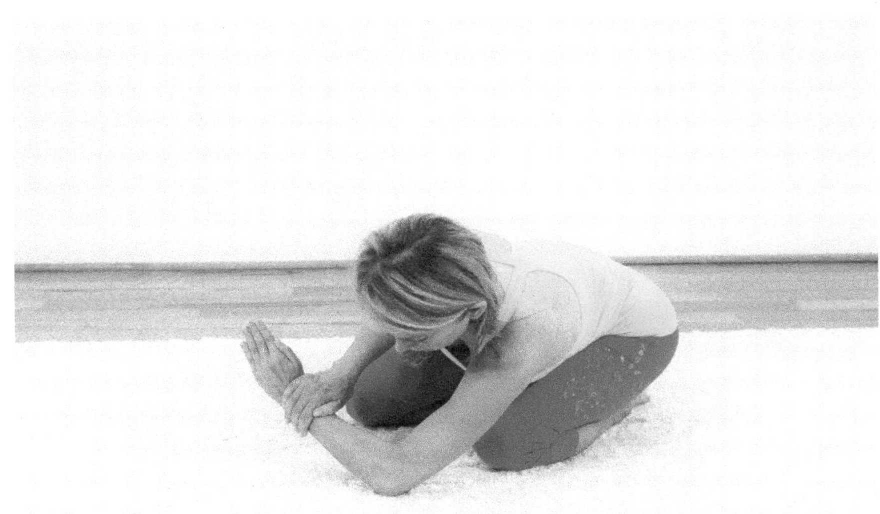

RESISTANCE FLEXIBILITY: Your left wrist pushes out to the left to resist while your right arms pulls the wrist across your body to the right. Return to the starting position and repeat 10 times on each arm.

HELPFUL REMINDERS

1. Reverse movement for strengthening.
2. The Balancing Stretch muscles help you get into the stretch position.
3. The Opposing Stretch muscles help you get the necessary rotation.
4. Your stretch occurs only while you contract and resist.
5. Your breathing is different in every *type* of stretch.
6. Get perspective from others on how each stretch affects you.

#8 ADVANCED (SMALL INTESTINE)

BENEFITS

Health: Protein Digestion
Body Part: Upper Arm
Joint: Shoulder Joint
Movement: Pull
Good Looks: Beautiful, Classy
Life: Artistic, Romantic

MUSCLES

Adductor Digiti Minimi, Extensor Carpi Ulnaris, Infraspinatus, Trapezius, Supraspinatus, Splenius, Scalene, SCM,
Action: Extension/Abduction/Outward
Stretch: Flexion/Adduction/Inward

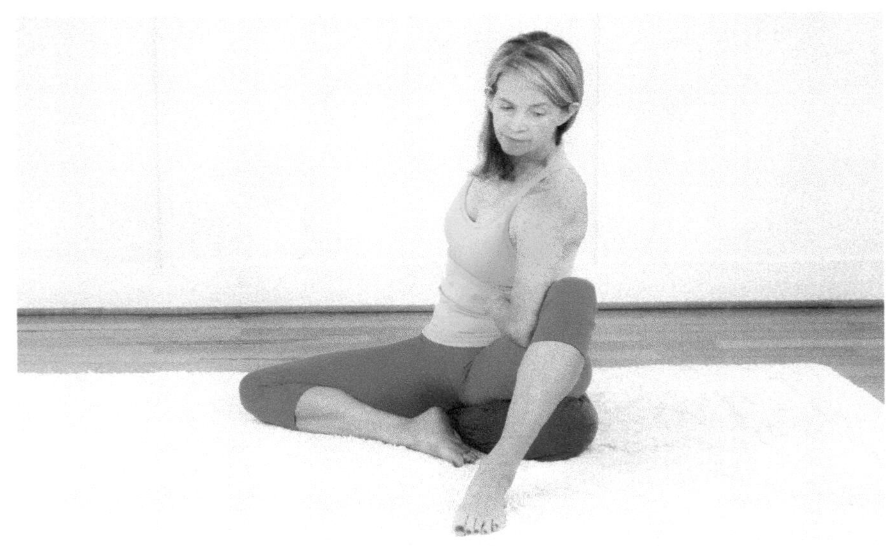

STARTING POSITION: Start on your hands and knees. Bend your knees and place your left elbow on the floor. Grasp your left wrist with your right hand and lean into the left elbow.

BALANCING STRETCH

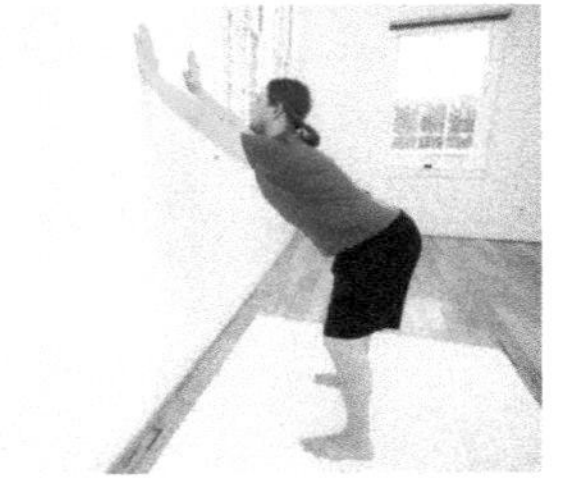

#7 Intermediate (Heart)

OPPOSING STRETCH

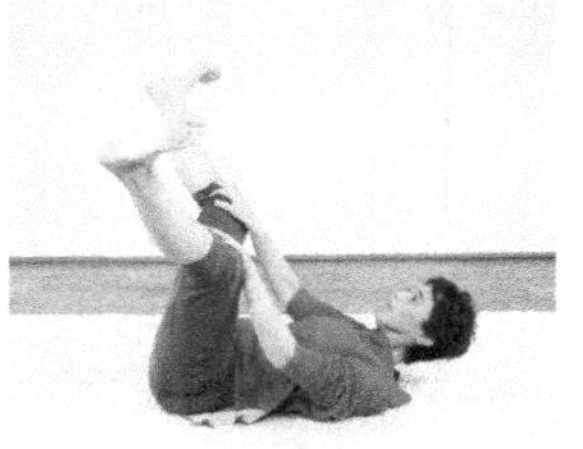

#2 Beginner (Liver)

BACK OF SHOULDER BLADE

(TCM)

Organ: Small Intestine
Tissue: CSF
Body Part: Face
System: Digestion
Sensory: Endocrine receptors
Yin/Yang Element: Yang Fire

PERSONALITY (GPT)

Group: Emotional
Time and Attention: Past and Outside
High Traits: Creative, Equanimity, Passion, Affirming, Classy
Low Traits: Hysterical, Depressed
Instinct: Excited/Anxiety

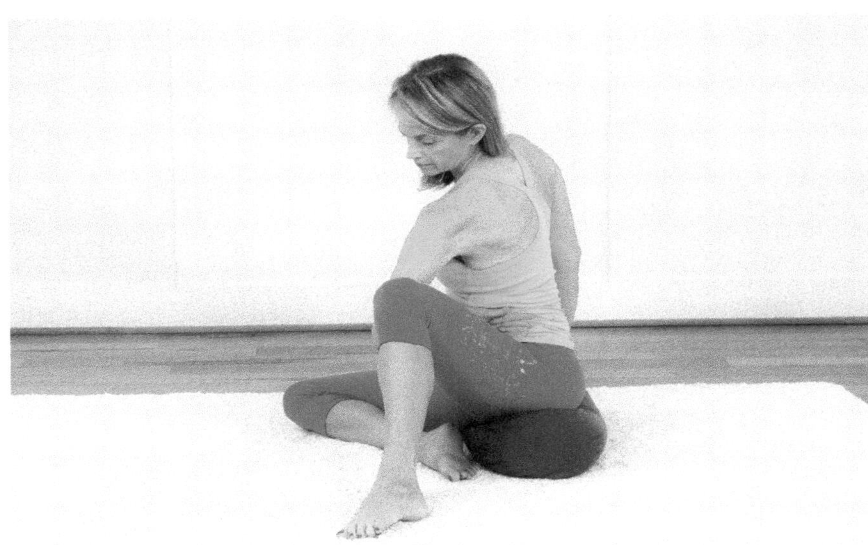

RESISTANCE FLEXIBILITY: Your left wrist pushes out to the left to resist while your right arms pulls the wrist across your body to the right. Return to the starting position and repeat 10 times on each arm.

HELPFUL REMINDERS

1. Reverse movement for strengthening.
2. The Balancing Stretch muscles help you get into the stretch position.
3. The Opposing Stretch muscles help you get the necessary rotation.
4. Your stretch occurs only while you contract and resist.
5. Your breathing is different in every *type* of stretch.
6. Get perspective from others on how each stretch affects you.

#8 ASSISTED (SMALL INTESTINE)

BENEFITS

Health: Protein Digestion
Body Part: Upper Arm
Joint: Shoulder Joint
Movement: Pull
Good Looks: Beautiful, Classy
Life: Artistic, Romantic

MUSCLES

Adductor Digiti Minimi, Extensor Carpi Ulnaris, Infraspinatus, Trapezius, Supraspinatus, Splenius, Scalene, SCM,
Action: Extension/Abduction/Outward
Stretch: Flexion/Adduction/Inward

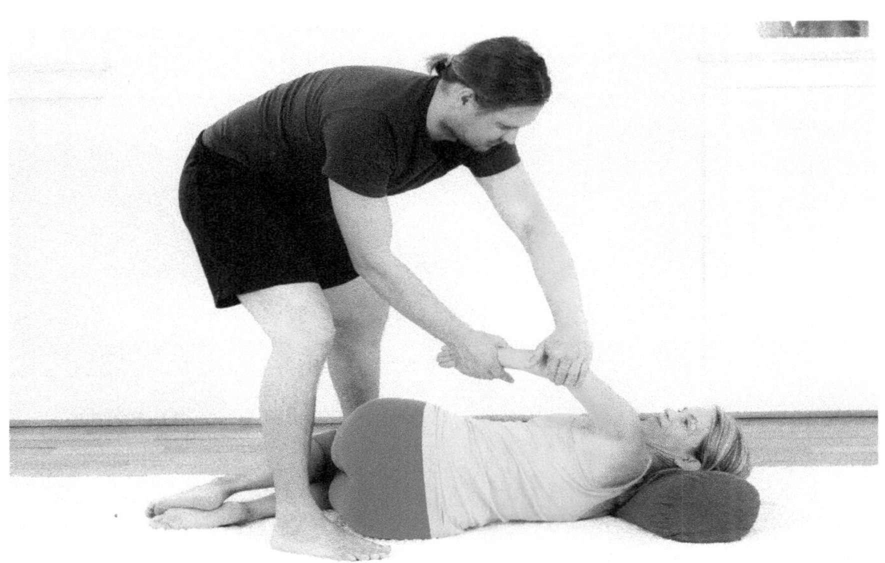

STARTING POSITION: Lie on your right side with a pillow under your head. The assister stands over you and grasps your left elbow and wrist with their hands, holding your arm behind you.

BALANCING STRETCH

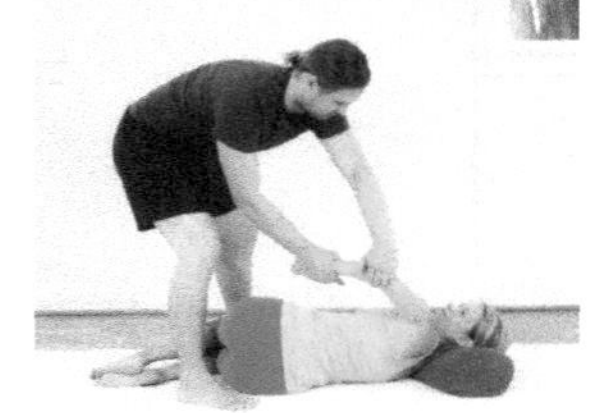

#7 Assisted (Heart)

OPPOSING STRETCH

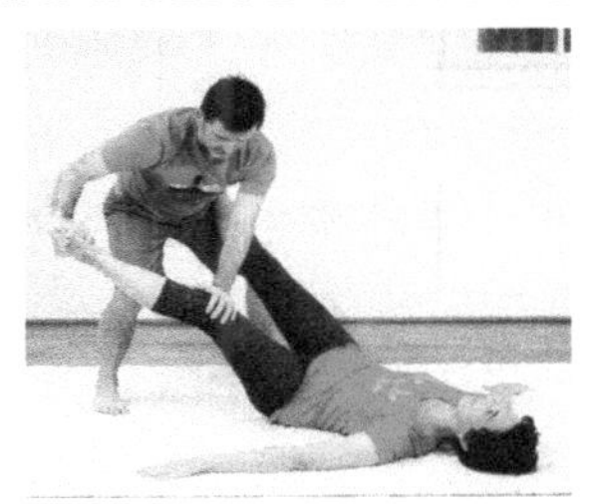

#2 Assited Leg Opener (Liver)

ASSISTED BACK OF SHOULDER BLADE

(TCM)

Organ: Small Intestine
Tissue: CSF
Body Part: Face
System: Digestion
Sensory: Endocrine receptors
Yin/Yang Element: Yang Fire

PERSONALITY (GPT)

Group: Emotional
Time and Attention: Past and Outside
High Traits: Creative, Equanimity, Passion, Affirming, Classy
Low Traits: Hysterical, Depressed
Instinct: Excited/Anxiety

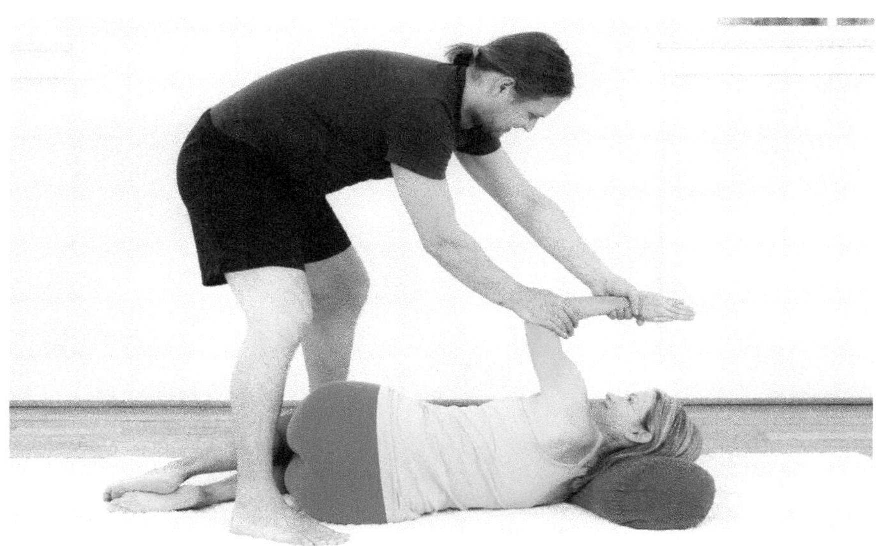

RESISTANCE FLEXIBILITY: Your left arm pulls backwards to resist while the assister pulls your elbow and wrist forwards. Return to the starting position and repeat 10 times on each arm.

HELPFUL REMINDERS

1. Reverse movement for strengthening.
2. The Balancing Stretch muscles help you get into the stretch position.
3. The Opposing Stretch muscles help you get the necessary rotation.
4. Your stretch occurs only while you contract and resist.
5. Your breathing is different in every *type* of stretch.
6. Get perspective from others on how each stretch affects you.

#9 BEGINNER (BRAIN)

BENEFITS

Health: Sleep
Body Part: Lower Leg
Joint: Knees
Movement: Twist
Good Looks: Aristocratic, Alluring
Life: Authoritative, Masterful

MUSCLES

Procerus, Frontalis, Erector Spinae, Spinal Rotators, Gluteus Maximus, Piriformus, Semitendosus, Gastrocnemius, Flexor Digitorium Brevis,
Action: Extension / Abduction / Inward
Stretch: Flexion / Adduction / Outward

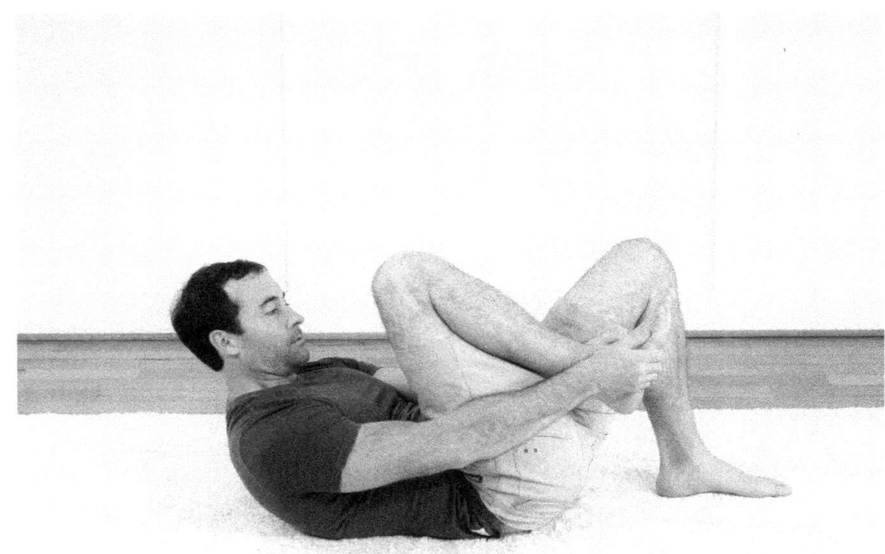

STARTING POSITION: Lie on your back with both knees bent. Bring your left knee up towards your chest and grasp your left ankle with both hands.

BALANCING STRETCH

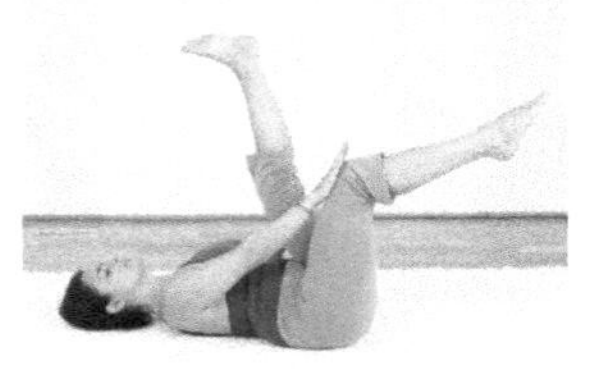

#10 Beginner (Sexual)

OPPOSING STRETCH

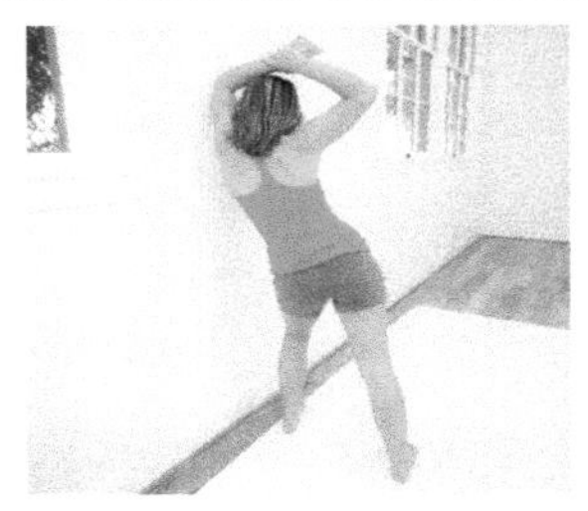

#15 Beginner (Appendix)

CENTRAL HAMSTRING

(TCM)

Organ: Brain
Tissue: CNS
Body Part: Legs
System: Central Nervous System
Sensory: Nervous system
Yin/Yang Element: Yang Air

PERSONALITY (GPT)

Group: Thinking
Time and Attention: Future and Inside
High Traits: Problem Solving, Trust, Mastery, Miracles, Superhero
Low Traits: Paranoid, Elitist
Instinct: Fearless/Fear

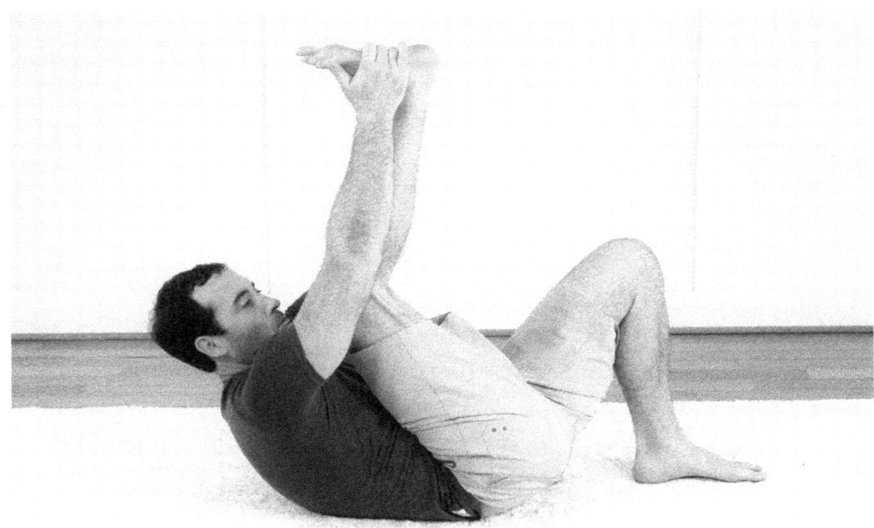

RESISTANCE FLEXIBILITY: Your left heel kicks down towards your butt to resist as your hands lift your leg up towards your head. Return to the starting position and repeat 10 times on each leg.

HELPFUL REMINDERS

1. Reverse movement for strengthening.
2. The Balancing Stretch muscles help you get into the stretch position.
3. The Opposing Stretch muscles help you get the necessary rotation.
4. Your stretch occurs only while you contract and resist.
5. Your breathing is different in every *type* of stretch.
6. Get perspective from others on how each stretch affects you.

#9 INTERMEDIATE (BRAIN)

BENEFITS

Health: Sleep
Body Part: Lower Leg
Joint: Knees
Movement: Twist
Good Looks: Aristocratic, Alluring
Life: Authoritative, Masterful

MUSCLES

Procerus, Frontalis, Erector Spinae, Spinal Rotators, Gluteus Maximus, Piriformus, Semitendosus, Gastrocnemius, Flexor Digitorium Brevis,
Action: Extension / Abduction / Inward
Stretch: Flexion / Adduction / Outward

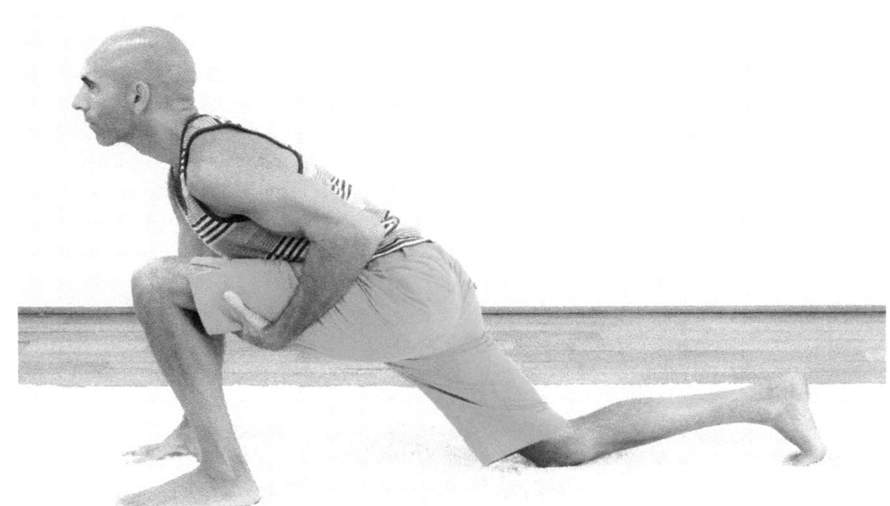

STARTING POSITION: Start on your hands and knees. Bring your left leg forward and lunge forward onto your left heel, bending the left knee. Place your left hand on the central back side of the left thigh in order to feel the upcoming stretch.

BALANCING STRETCH

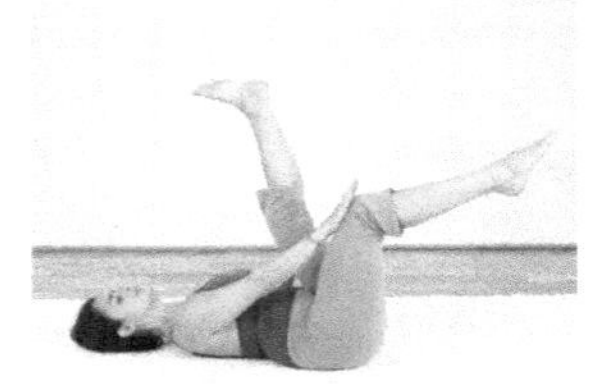

#10 Beginner (Sexual)

OPPOSING STRETCH

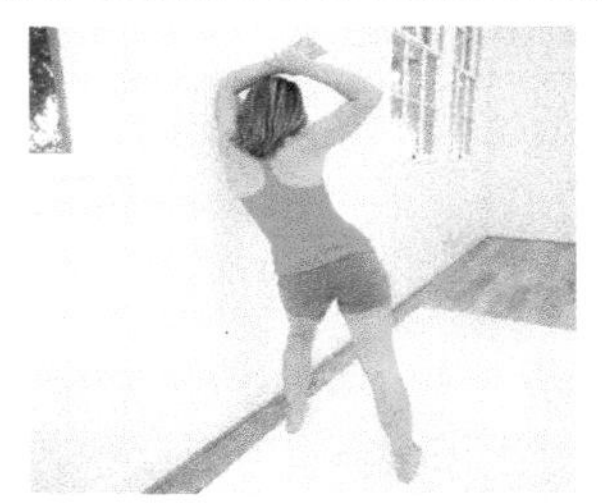

#15 Beginner (Appendix)

HALF SPLITS

(TCM)

Organ: Brain
Tissue: CNS
Body Part: Legs
System: Central Nervous System
Sensory: Nervous system
Yin/Yang Element: Yang Air

PERSONALITY (GPT)

Group: Thinking
Time and Attention: Future and Inside
High Traits: Problem Solving, Trust, Mastery, Miracles, Superhero
Low Traits: Paranoid, Elitist
Instinct: Fearless/Fear

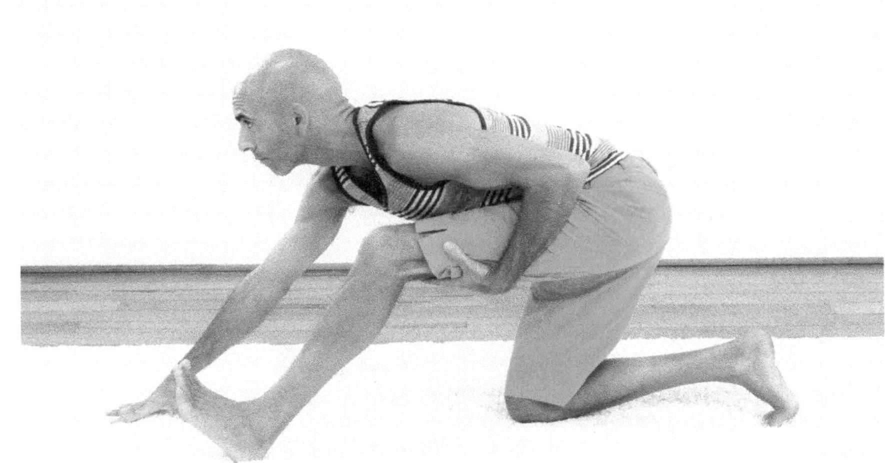

RESISTANCE FLEXIBILITY: Kick your left heel into the floor and scissor both thighs towards each other to resist while your right leg pulls and moves your hips backwards, straightening the left knee. Return to the starting position and repeat 10 times on each leg.

HELPFUL REMINDERS

1. Reverse movement for strengthening.
2. The Balancing Stretch muscles help you get into the stretch position.
3. The Opposing Stretch muscles help you get the necessary rotation.
4. Your stretch occurs only while you contract and resist.
5. Your breathing is different in every *type* of stretch.
6. Get perspective from others on how each stretch affects you.

#9 ADVANCED (BRAIN)

BENEFITS

Health: Sleep
Body Part: Lower Leg
Joint: Knees
Movement: Twist
Good Looks: Aristocratic, Alluring
Life: Authoritative, Masterful

MUSCLES

Procerus, Frontalis, Erector Spinae, Spinal Rotators, Gluteus Maximus, Piriformus, Semitendosus, Gastrocnemius, Flexor Digitorium Brevis,
Action: Extension/Abduction/Inward
Stretch: Flexion/Adduction/Outward

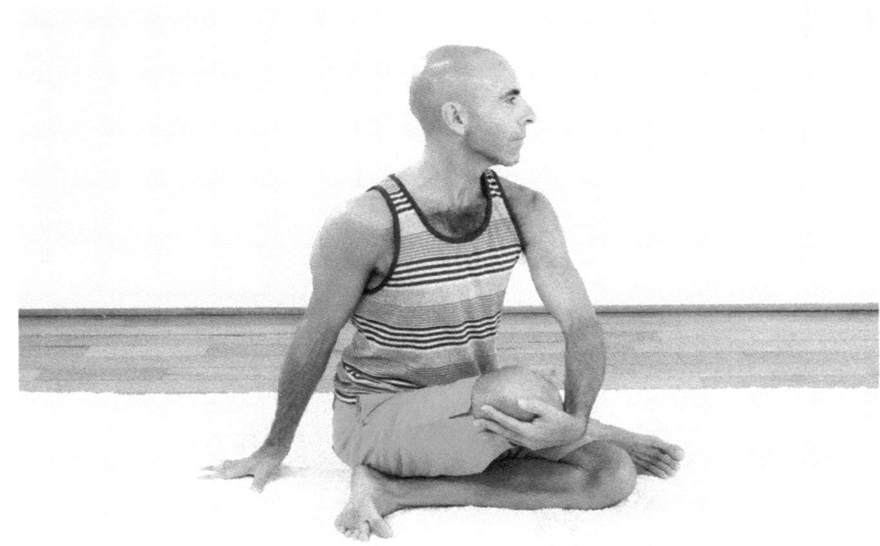

STARTING POSITION: Sit on the floor with one leg bent at the knee and brought down and out to the side. Your other leg steps up and across the first leg, its foot landing on the floor. Wrap your elbow and arm around your knee.

BALANCING STRETCH

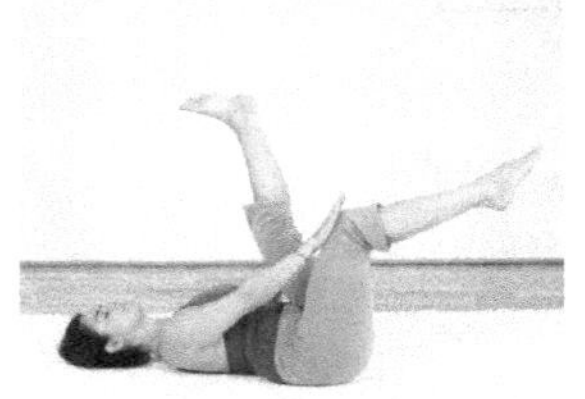

#10 Beginner (Sexual)

OPPOSING STRETCH

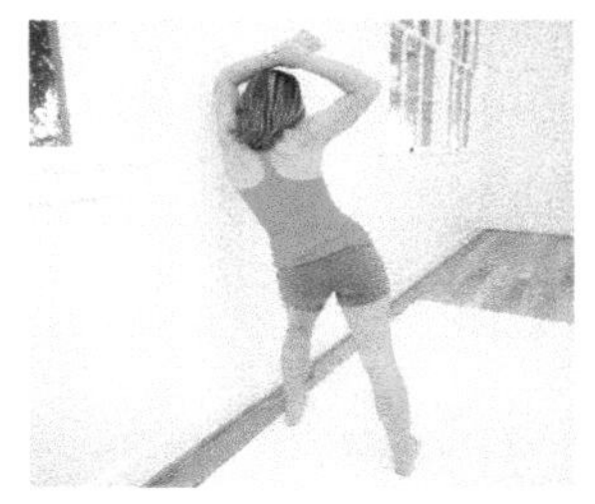

#15 Beginner (Appendix)

SEATED TWIST

(TCM)

Organ: Brain
Tissue: CNS
Body Part: Legs
System: Central Nervous System
Sensory: Nervous system
Yin/Yang Element: Yang Air

PERSONALITY (GPT)

Group: Thinking
Time and Attention: Future and Inside
High Traits: Problem Solving, Trust, Mastery, Miracles, Superhero
Low Traits: Paranoid, Elitist
Instinct: Fearless/Fear

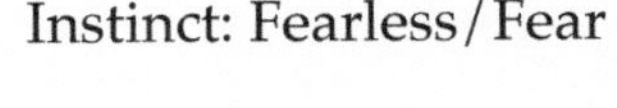

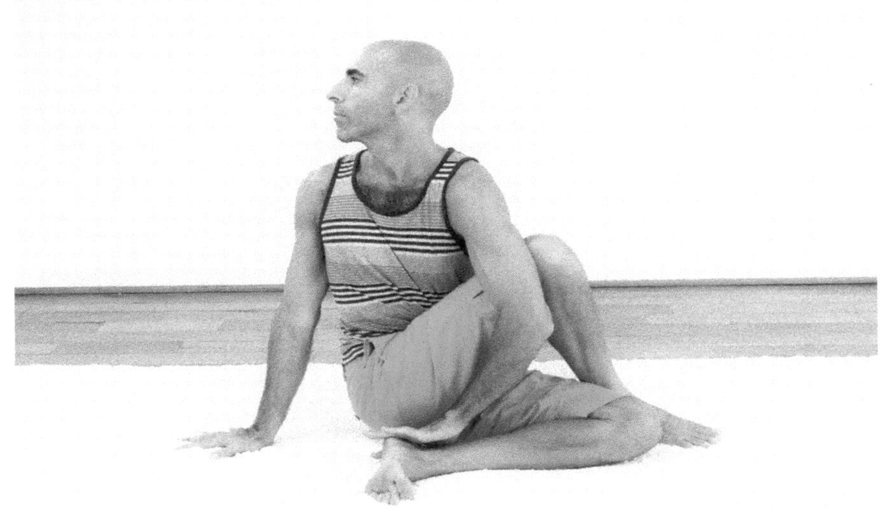

RESISTANCE FLEXIBILITY: Your vertical knee pushes out sideways to resist as your arm pulls it in and against your torso. Twist your torso backwards as you resist the twist in the opposite direction. Return to the starting position and repeat 10 times on each side.

HELPFUL REMINDERS

1. Reverse movement for strengthening.
2. The Balancing Stretch muscles help you get into the stretch position.
3. The Opposing Stretch muscles help you get the necessary rotation.
4. Your stretch occurs only while you contract and resist.
5. Your breathing is different in every *type* of stretch.
6. Get perspective from others on how each stretch affects you.

#9 ASSISTED (BRAIN)

BENEFITS

Health: Sleep
Body Part: Lower Leg
Joint: Knees
Movement: Twist
Good Looks: Aristocratic, Alluring
Life: Authoritative, Masterful

MUSCLES

Procerus, Frontalis, Erector Spinae, Spinal Rotators, Gluteus Maximus, Piriformus, Semitendosus, Gastrocnemius, Flexor Digitorium Brevis,
Action: Extension / Abduction / Inward
Stretch: Flexion / Adduction / Outward

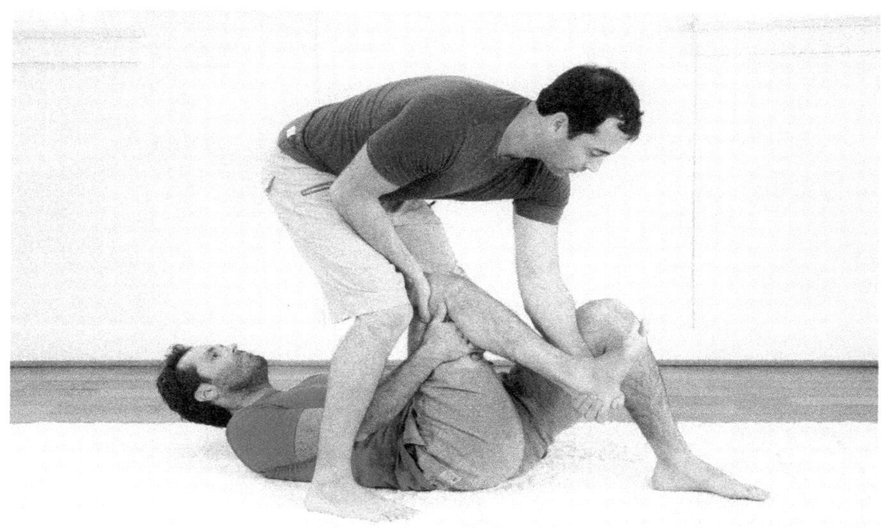

STARTING POSITION: Lie on your back with both knees bent. Bring your right knee up towards your chest with your hands behind that thigh. The assister stands over you, places one hand above your right knee and grasps your right heel with their other hand.

BALANCING STRETCH

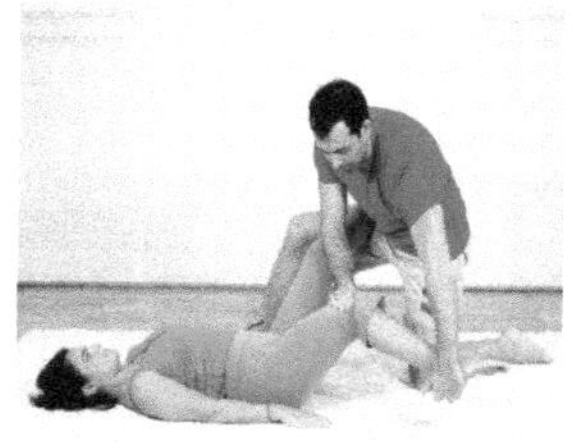

#10 Assisted (Sexual)

OPPOSING STRETCH

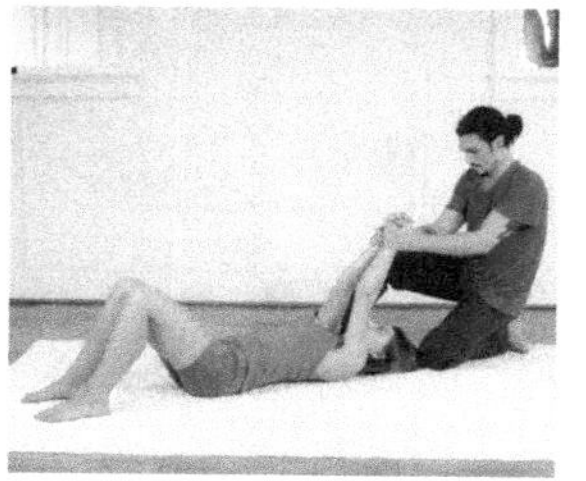

#15 Assisted (Appendix)

ASSISTED CENTRAL HAMSTRING

(TCM)

Organ: Brain
Tissue: CNS
Body Part: Legs
System: Central Nervous System
Sensory: Nervous system
Yin/Yang Element: Yang Air

PERSONALITY (GPT)

Group: Thinking
Time and Attention: Future and Inside
High Traits: Problem Solving, Trust, Mastery, Miracles, Superhero
Low Traits: Paranoid, Elitist
Instinct: Fearless/Fear

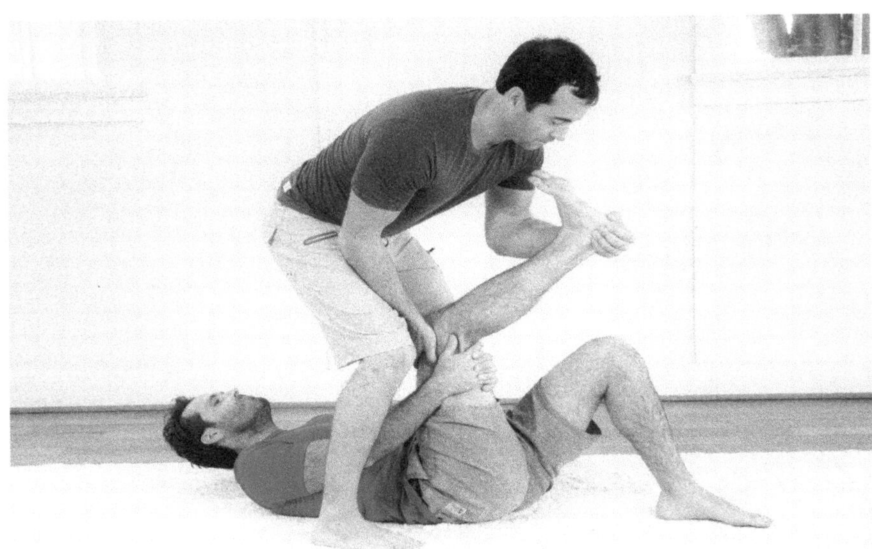

RESISTANCE FLEXIBILITY: Your right heel kicks down towards your butt to resist while the assister lifts your right heel to straighten your right leg. Return to the starting position and repeat 10 times on each leg.

HELPFUL REMINDERS

1. Reverse movement for strengthening.
2. The Balancing Stretch muscles help you get into the stretch position.
3. The Opposing Stretch muscles help you get the necessary rotation.
4. Your stretch occurs only while you contract and resist.
5. Your breathing is different in every *type* of stretch.
6. Get perspective from others on how each stretch affects you.

#10 BEGINNER (SEXUAL)

BENEFITS

Health: Endocrine
Body Part: Lower Leg
Joint: Knees
Movement: Untwist
Good Looks: Sexy, Gorgeous
Life: Stardom, Intimacy

MUSCLES

Extensor Digitorum Longus, Tibialis Anterior, Rectus Femoris, Psoas Major, Primidalis, Transverse Abdominals, Linea Alba

Action: Flexion / Adduction / Outward
Stretch: Extension / Abduction / Inward

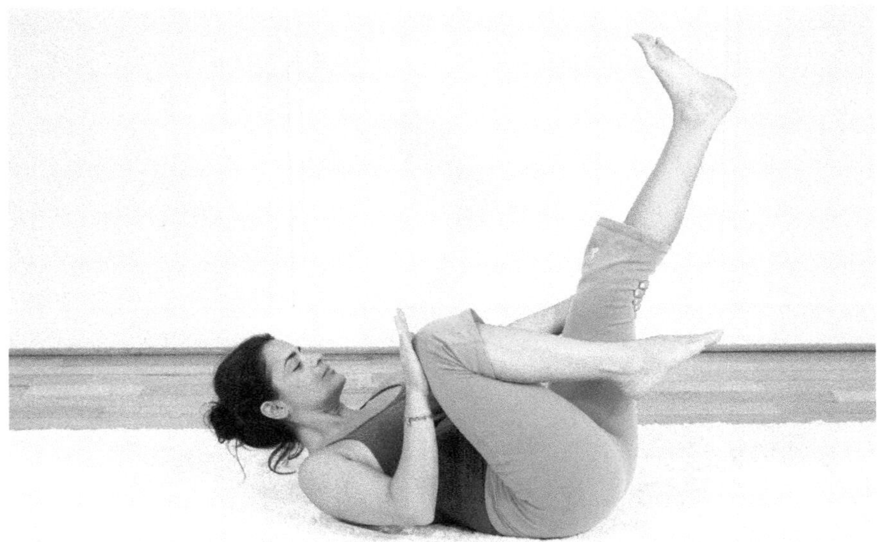

STARTING POSITION: Lie on your back with your right leg straight up perpendicular to the ground and your left knee pulled up to your chest and bent. Hold the back of your right knee with your right hand and put your left hand on your left knee.

BALANCING STRETCH

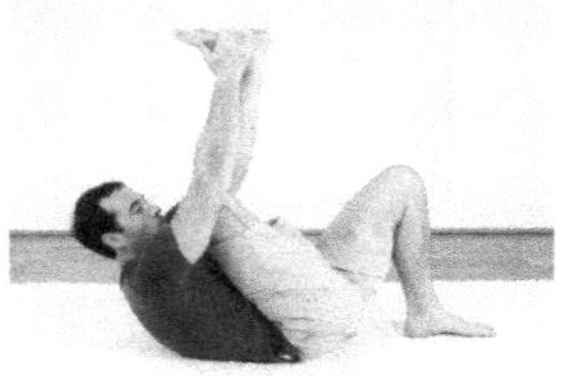

#9 Beginner (Brain)

OPPOSING STRETCH

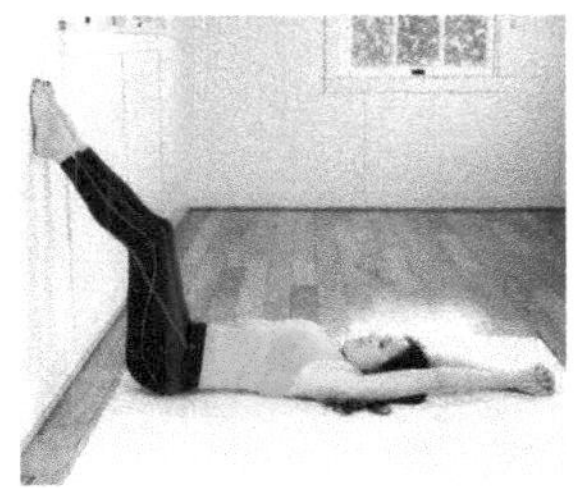

#16 Beginner (Thymus)

HIP FLEXOR

(TCM)

Organ: Sexual
Tissue: Hormones
Body Part: Face
System: Endocrine
Sensory: Hormonal receptors
Yin/Yang Element: Yin Air

PERSONALITY (GPT)

Group: Emotional
Time and Attention: Past and Outside
High Traits: Intimacy, Caring, Sexy, Respect, Willful
Low Traits: Mood Disorder/Self-Destructive
Instinct: Excited/Anxious

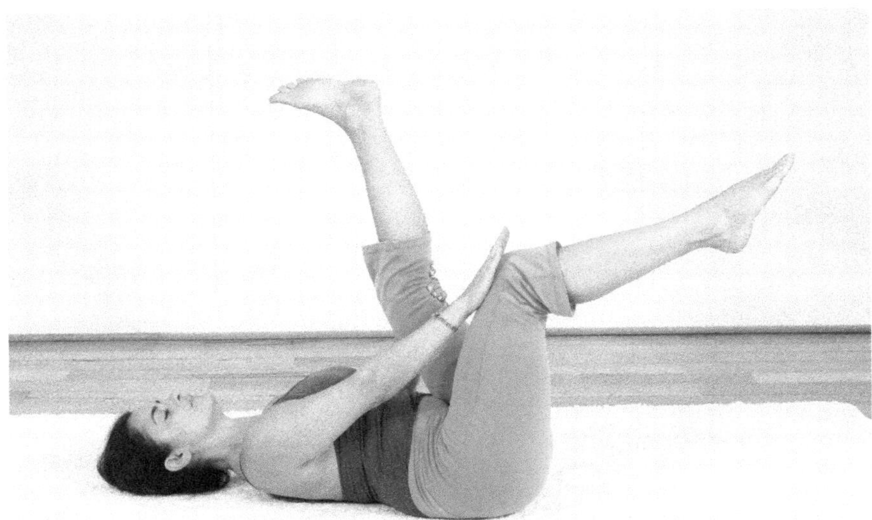

RESISTANCE FLEXIBILITY: While your right leg pushes into your right hand, your left knee kicks up towards your chest to resist as your left hand pushes that knee away from your chest. Return to the starting position and repeat 10 times on each leg.

HELPFUL REMINDERS

1. Reverse movement for strengthening.
2. The Balancing Stretch muscles help you get into the stretch position.
3. The Opposing Stretch muscles help you get the necessary rotation.
4. Your stretch occurs only while you contract and resist.
5. Your breathing is different in every *type* of stretch.
6. Get perspective from others on how each stretch affects you.

#10 INTERMEDIATE (SEXUAL)

BENEFITS

Health: Endocrine
Body Part: Lower Leg
Joint: Knees
Movement: Untwist
Good Looks: Sexy, Gorgeous
Life: Stardom, Intimacy

MUSCLES

Extensor Digitorum Longus, Tibialis Anterior, Rectus Femoris, Psoas Major, Primidalis, Transverse Abdominals, Linea Alba

Action: Flexion / Adduction / Outward

Stretch: Extension / Abduction / Inward

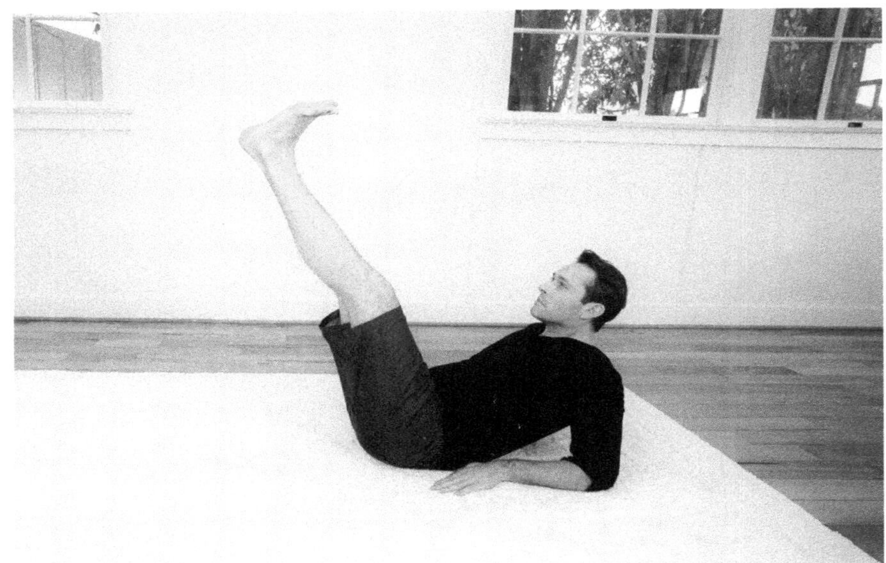

STARTING POSITION: Lie on your back, arms just underneath you and palms under your hips facing down. Bend your elbows to push yourself up onto your forearms. Raise your legs so they are perpendicular to the floor.

BALANCING STRETCH

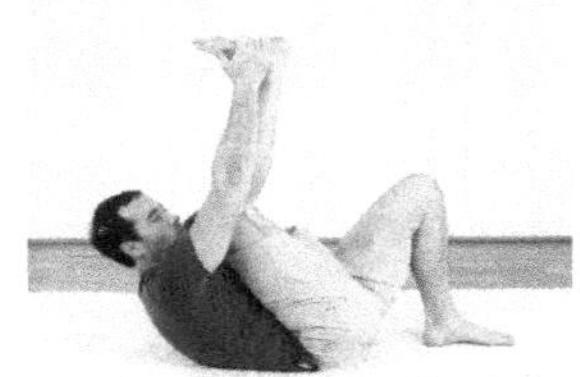

#9 Beginner (Brain)

OPPOSING STRETCH

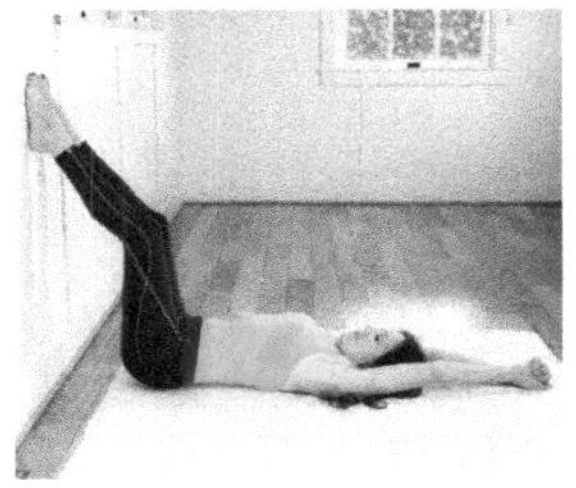

#16 Beginner (Thymus)

FISH ARCH

(TCM)

Organ: Sexual
Tissue: Hormones
Body Part: Face
System: Endocrine
Sensory: Hormonal receptors
Yin/Yang Element: Yin Air

PERSONALITY (GPT)

Group: Emotional
Time and Attention: Past and Outside
High Traits: Intimacy, Caring, Sexy, Respect, Willful
Low Traits: Mood Disorder/Self-Destructive
Instinct: Excited/Anxious

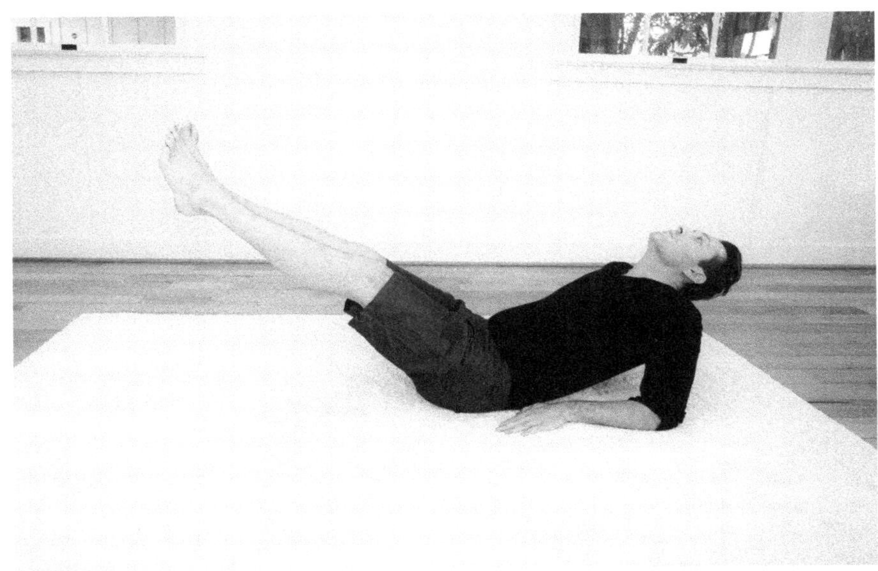

RESISTANCE FLEXIBILITY: Contract your abdominals to resist as you slowly lower your legs half way down to the floor. Return to the starting position and repeat 10 times.

HELPFUL REMINDERS

1. Reverse movement for strengthening.
2. The Balancing Stretch muscles help you get into the stretch position.
3. The Opposing Stretch muscles help you get the necessary rotation.
4. Your stretch occurs only while you contract and resist.
5. Your breathing is different in every *type* of stretch.
6. Get perspective from others on how each stretch affects you.

#10 ADVANCED (SEXUAL)

BENEFITS

Health: Endocrine
Body Part: Lower Leg
Joint: Knees
Movement: Untwist
Good Looks: Sexy, Gorgeous
Life: Stardom, Intimacy

MUSCLES

Extensor Digitorum Longus, Tibialis Anterior, Rectus Femoris, Psoas Major, Primidalis, Transverse Abdominals, Linea Alba

Action: Flexion / Adduction / Outward
Stretch: Extension / Abduction / Inward

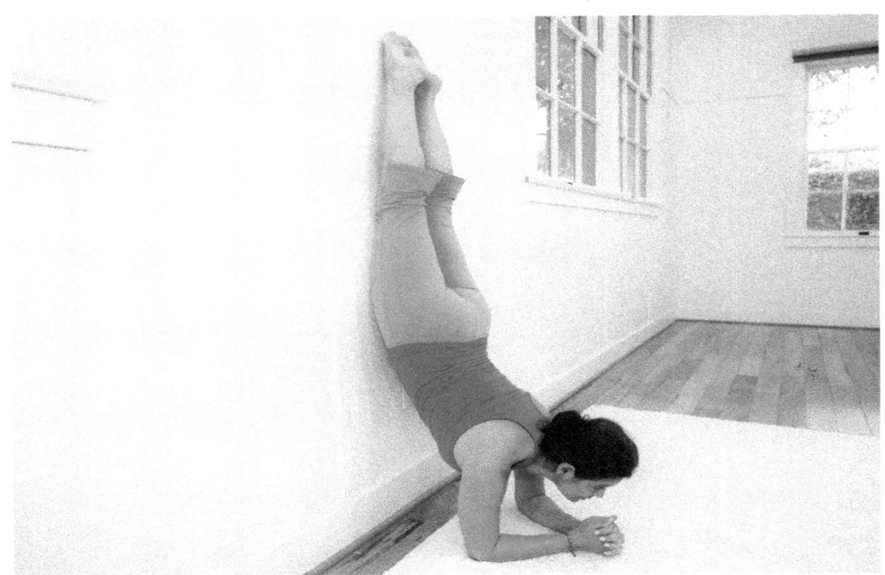

STARTING POSITION: Start on your hands and knees facing a wall. Clasp your hands together and place your elbows shoulder width apart. Kick your legs up onto the wall.

BALANCING STRETCH

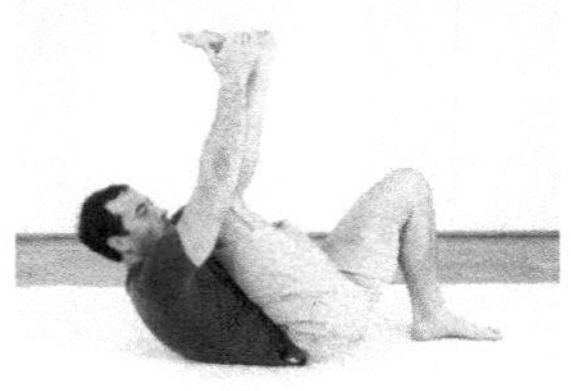

#9 Beginner (Brain)

OPPOSING STRETCH

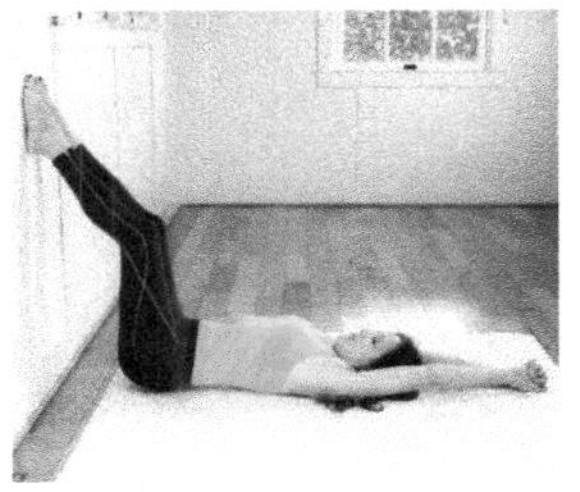

#16 Beginner (Thymus)

FOREARM ARCH

(TCM)

Organ: Sexual
Tissue: Hormones
Body Part: Face
System: Endocrine
Sensory: Hormonal receptors
Yin / Yang Element: Yin Air

PERSONALITY (GPT)

Group: Emotional
Time and Attention: Past and Outside
High Traits: Intimacy, Caring, Sexy, Respect, Willful
Low Traits: Mood Disorder / Self-Destructive
Instinct: Excited / Anxious

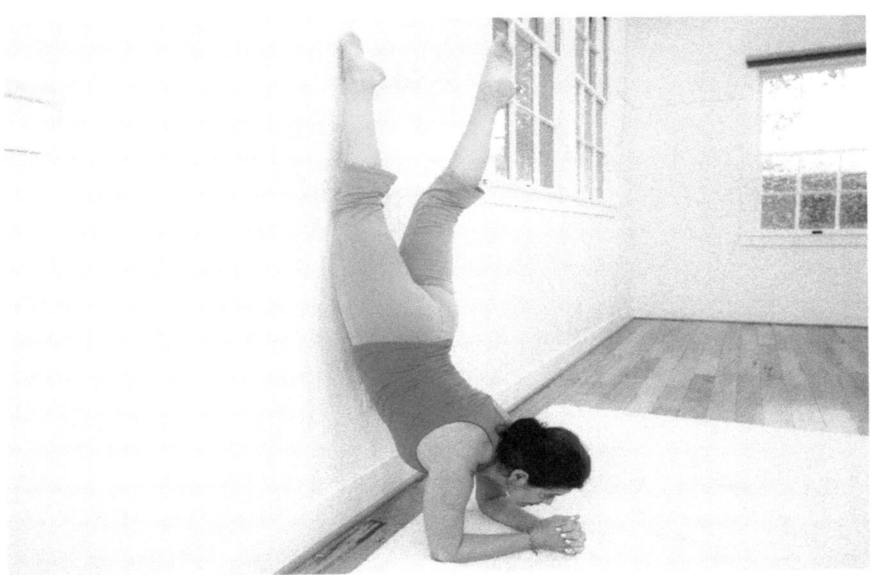

RESISTANCE FLEXIBILITY: Continuously contract the muscles on the front of your torso to resist while your arms press into the floor and outwards. Return to the starting position and repeat 10 times.

HELPFUL REMINDERS

1. Reverse movement for strengthening.
2. The Balancing Stretch muscles help you get into the stretch position.
3. The Opposing Stretch muscles help you get the necessary rotation.
4. Your stretch occurs only while you contract and resist.
5. Your breathing is different in every *type* of stretch.
6. Get perspective from others on how each stretch affects you.

#10 ASSISTED (SEXUAL)

BENEFITS

Health: Endocrine
Body Part: Lower Leg
Joint: Knees
Movement: Untwist
Good Looks: Sexy, Gorgeous
Life: Stardom, Intimacy

MUSCLES

Extensor Digitorum Longus, Tibialis Anterior, Rectus Femoris, Psoas Major, Primidalis, Transverse Abdominals, Linea Alba

Action: Flexion/Adduction/Outward
Stretch: Extension/Abduction/Inward

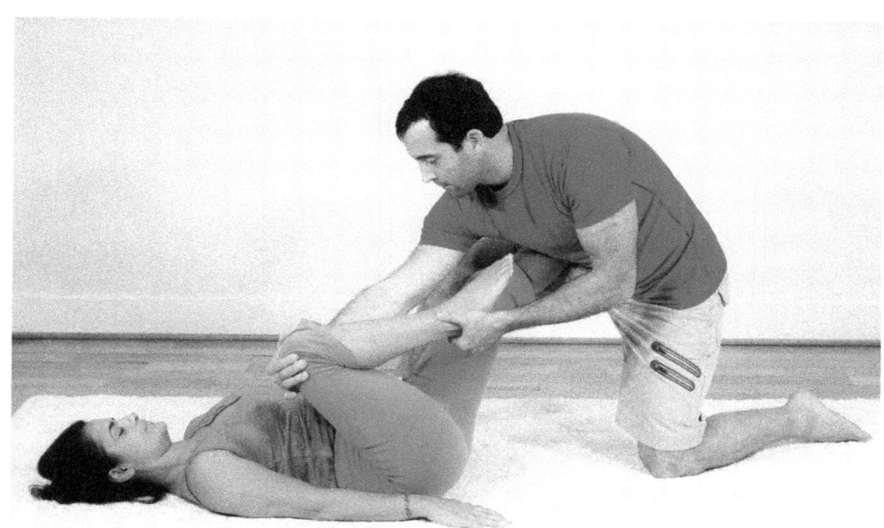

STARTING POSITION: Lie on your back with your right knee at your chest. Rest your left leg on your assister's right thigh. The assister places one hand above your right knee and grasps your right heel with their other hand.

BALANCING STRETCH

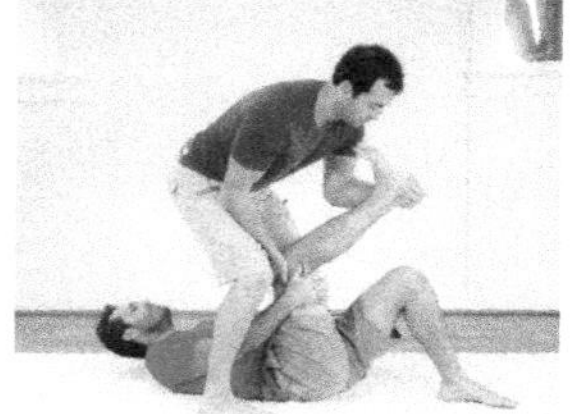

#9 Assisted (Brain)

OPPOSING STRETCH

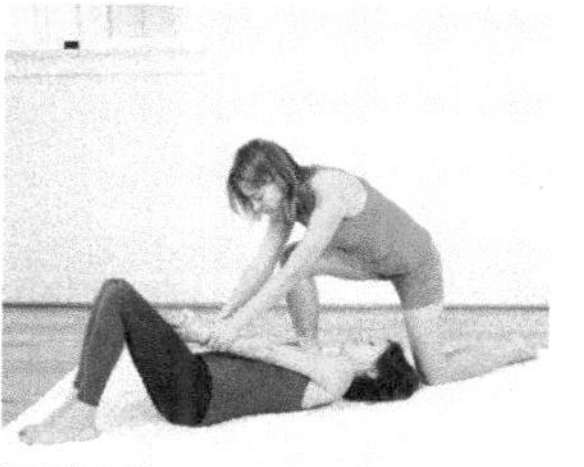

#16 Assisted (Thymus)

ASSISTED HIP FLEXOR

(TCM)

Organ: Sexual
Tissue: Hormones
Body Part: Face
System: Endocrine
Sensory: Hormonal receptors
Yin/Yang Element: Yin Air

PERSONALITY (GPT)

Group: Emotional
Time and Attention: Past and Outside
High Traits: Intimacy, Caring, Sexy, Respect, Willful
Low Traits: Mood Disorder/Self-Destructive
Instinct: Excited/Anxious

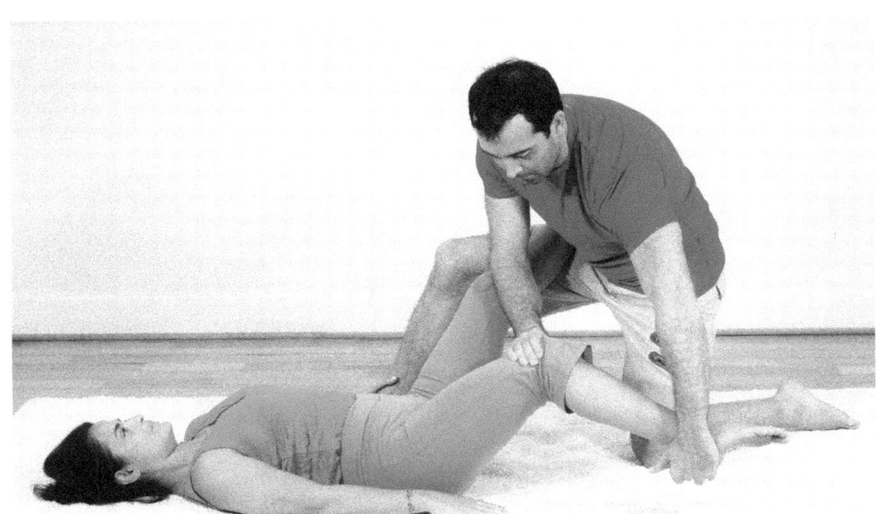

RESISTANCE FLEXIBILITY: Your right knee pulls up toward your chest to resist and your left leg pushes down on their thigh while the assister pulls your right leg away from your chest and midline. Return to the starting position and repeat 10 times on each leg.

HELPFUL REMINDERS

1. Reverse movement for strengthening.
2. The Balancing Stretch muscles help you get into the stretch position.
3. The Opposing Stretch muscles help you get the necessary rotation.
4. Your stretch occurs only while you contract and resist.
5. Your breathing is different in every *type* of stretch.
6. Get perspective from others on how each stretch affects you.

#11 BEGINNER (PERICARDIUM)

BENEFITS

Health: Circulation / Scar Tissue
Body Part: Forearm
Joint: Elbow
Movement: Close
Good Looks: Transparent, Magnificent
Life: Disciplined, Details

MUSCLES

Pectoralis Minor, Biceps Brachii, Brachialis, Coracobrachialis, Forearm Flexors, Palmaris Longus, Pronator Teres and Quadratus, Lumbricals

Action: Flexion / Abduction / Inward
Stretch: Extension / Adduction / Outward

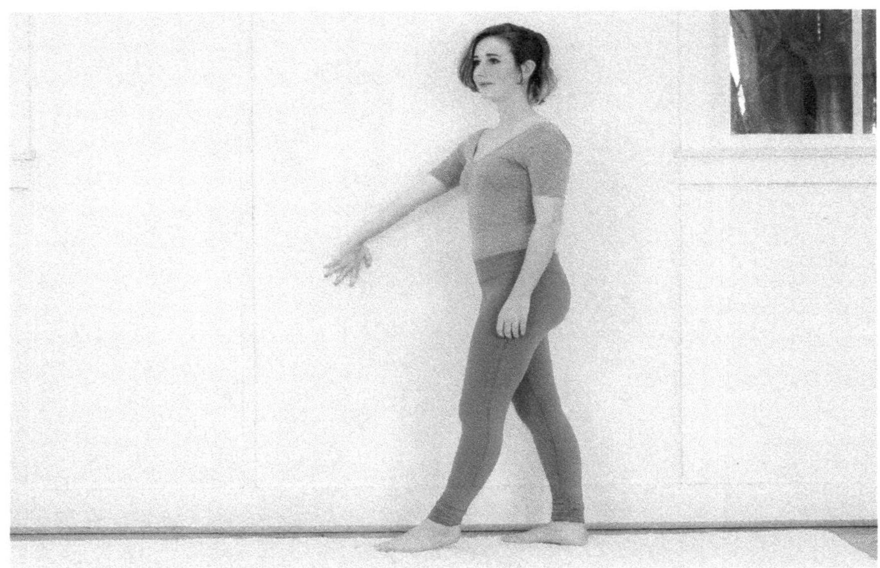

STARTING POSITION: Stand with a wall to your right. Bring your right arm slightly forward, turning it outwards, and place your palm against the wall.

BALANCING STRETCH

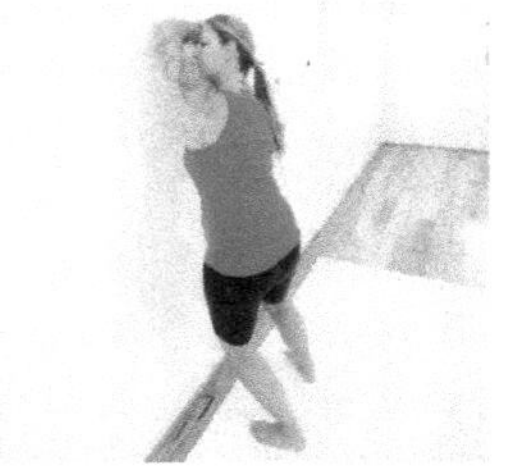

#12 Beginner (Skin)

OPPOSING STRETCH

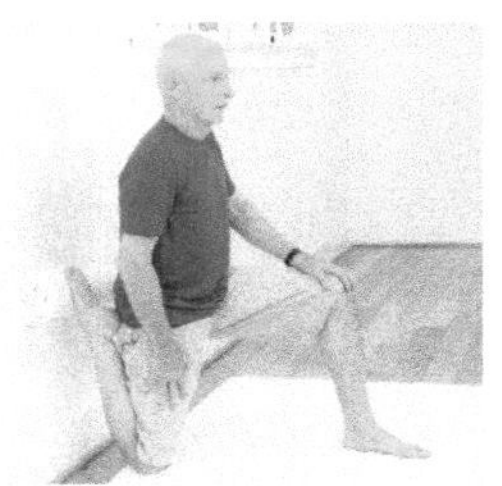

#5 Beginner (Stomach)

HEART OPENER AT WALL

(TCM)

Organ: Pericardium
Tissue: Epithelial
Body Part: Trunk
System: Blood Distribution
Sensory: Energetic receptors
Yin/Yang Element: Yin Electromagnetic

PERSONALITY (GPT)

Group: Spiritual
Time and Attention: Relative and Inside
High Traits: Judgment, Open, Disciplined, Philanthropy
Low Traits: Sabotaging, Arrogant
Instinct: Calm/Frightened

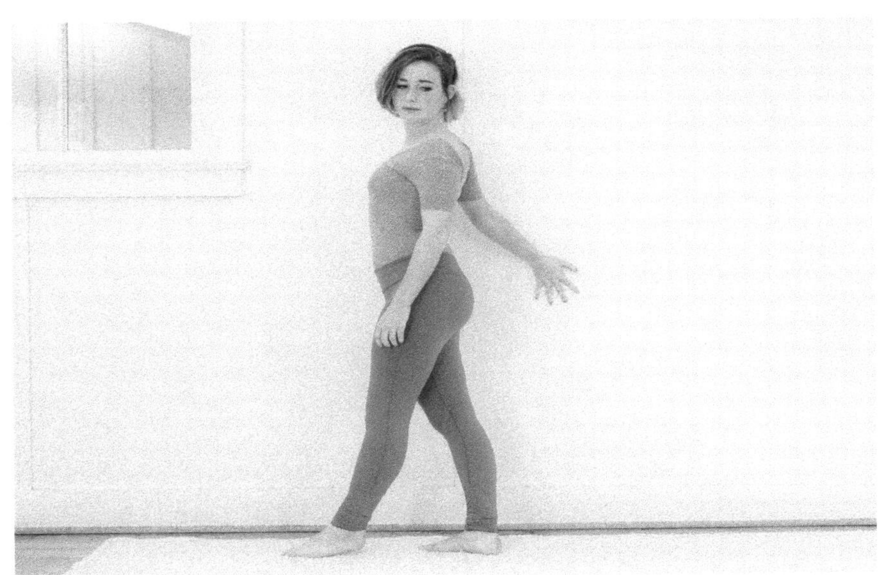

RESISTANCE FLEXIBILITY: Your right arm pushes forwards to resist as you walk your body forwards, holding on to the wall with your hand so that your right arm is pulled back behind you. Return to the starting position and repeat 10 times on each arm.

HELPFUL REMINDERS

1. Reverse movement for strengthening.
2. The Balancing Stretch muscles help you get into the stretch position.
3. The Opposing Stretch muscles help you get the necessary rotation.
4. Your stretch occurs only while you contract and resist.
5. Your breathing is different in every *type* of stretch.
6. Get perspective from others on how each stretch affects you.

#11 INTERMEDIATE (PERICARDIUM)

BENEFITS

Health: Circulation / Scar Tissue
Body Part: Forearm
Joint: Elbow
Movement: Close
Good Looks: Transparent, Magnificent
Life: Disciplined, Details

MUSCLES

Pectoralis Minor, Biceps Brachii, Brachialis, Coracobrachialis, Forearm Flexors, Palmaris Longus, Pronator Teres and Quadratus, Lumbricals

Action: Flexion / Abduction / Inward
Stretch: Extension / Adduction / Outward

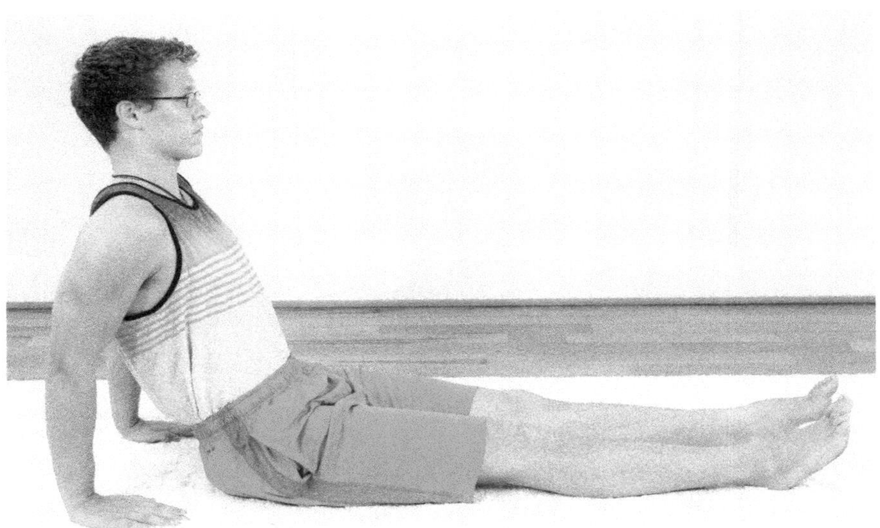

STARTING POSITION: Sit on the floor with your legs straight out in front of you. Place your arms behind you to support your torso, palms facing down and fingers pointing forward.

BALANCING STRETCH

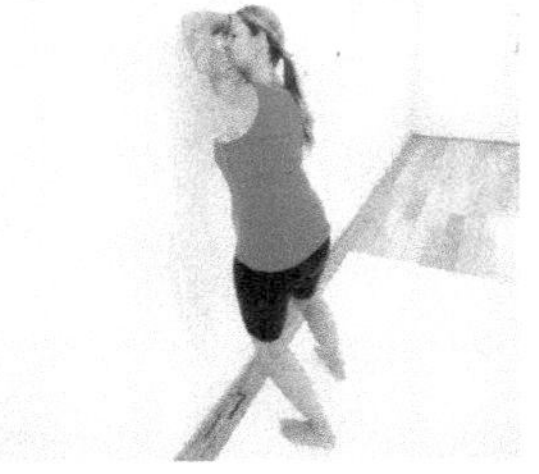

#12 Beginner (Skin)

OPPOSING STRETCH

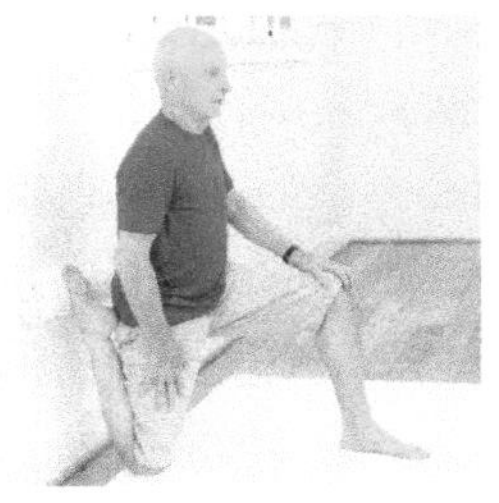

#5 Beginner (Stomach)

INCLINE PLANE

(TCM)

Organ: Pericardium
Tissue: Epithelial
Body Part: Trunk
System: Blood Distribution
Sensory: Energetic receptors
Yin/Yang Element: Yin Electromagnetic

PERSONALITY (GPT)

Group: Spiritual
Time and Attention: Relative and Inside
High Traits: Judgment, Open,
Disciplined, Philanthropy
Low Traits: Sabotaging, Arrogant
Instinct: Calm/Frightened

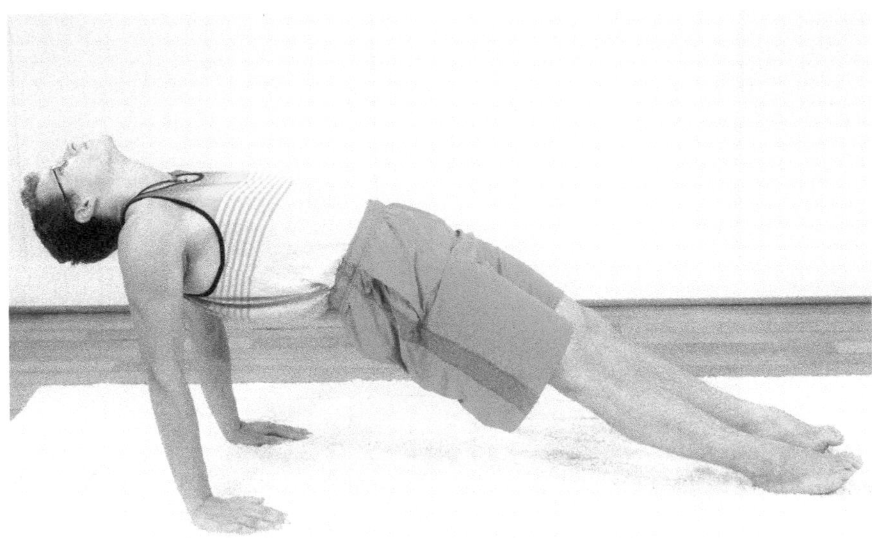

RESISTANCE FLEXIBILITY: Pull your arms forwards and up towards your chest to resist as you lift your hips off the floor and arch your spine backwards. Return to the starting position and repeat 10 times.

HELPFUL REMINDERS

1. Reverse movement for strengthening.
2. The Balancing Stretch muscles help you get into the stretch position.
3. The Opposing Stretch muscles help you get the necessary rotation.
4. Your stretch occurs only while you contract and resist.
5. Your breathing is different in every *type* of stretch.
6. Get perspective from others on how each stretch affects you.

#11 ADVANCED (PERICARDIUM)

BENEFITS

Health: Circulation / Scar Tissue
Body Part: Forearm
Joint: Elbow
Movement: Close
Good Looks: Transparent, Magnificent
Life: Disciplined, Details

MUSCLES

Pectoralis Minor, Biceps Brachii, Brachialis, Coracobrachialis, Forearm Flexors, Palmaris Longus, Pronator Teres and Quadratus, Lumbricals
Action: Flexion / Abduction / Inward
Stretch: Extension / Adduction / Outward

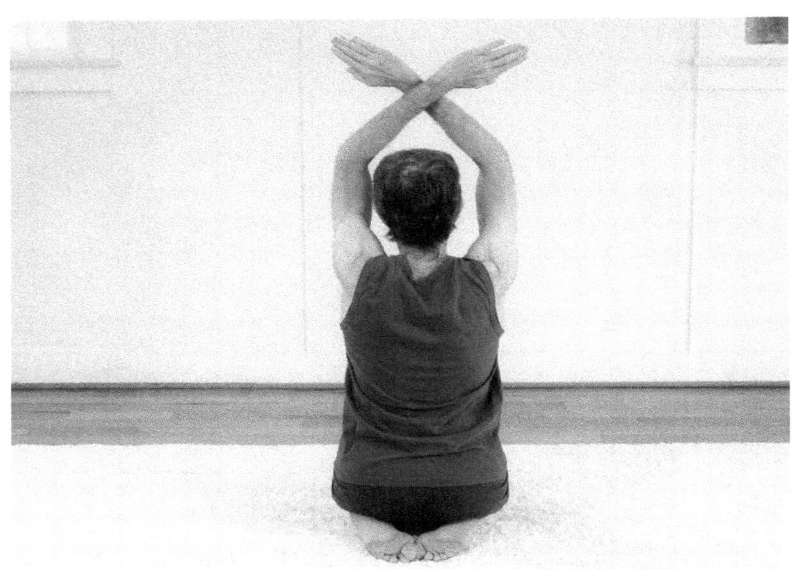

STARTING POSITION: Kneel on the floor with your arms above your head and forearms crossed.

BALANCING STRETCH

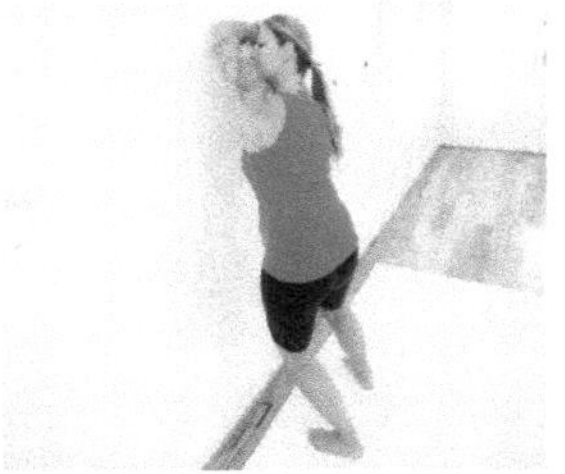

#12 Beginner (Skin)

OPPOSING STRETCH

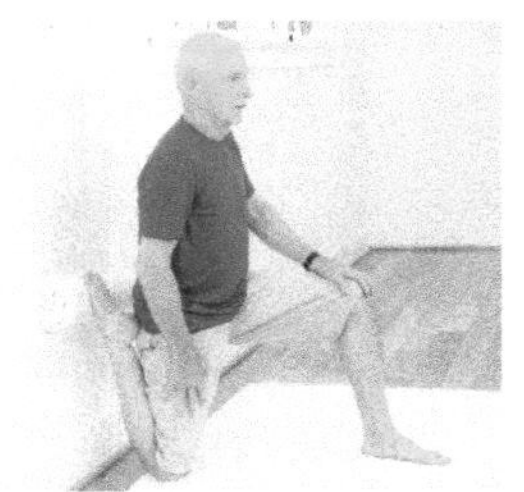

#5 Beginner (Stomach)

PRAYER ARMS BEHIND THE BACK

(TCM)

Organ: Pericardium
Tissue: Epithelial
Body Part: Trunk
System: Blood Distribution
Sensory: Energetic receptors
Yin/Yang Element: Yin Electromagnetic

PERSONALITY (GPT)

Group: Spiritual
Time and Attention: Relative and Inside
High Traits: Judgment, Open, Disciplined, Philanthropy
Low Traits: Sabotaging, Arrogant
Instinct: Calm/Frightened

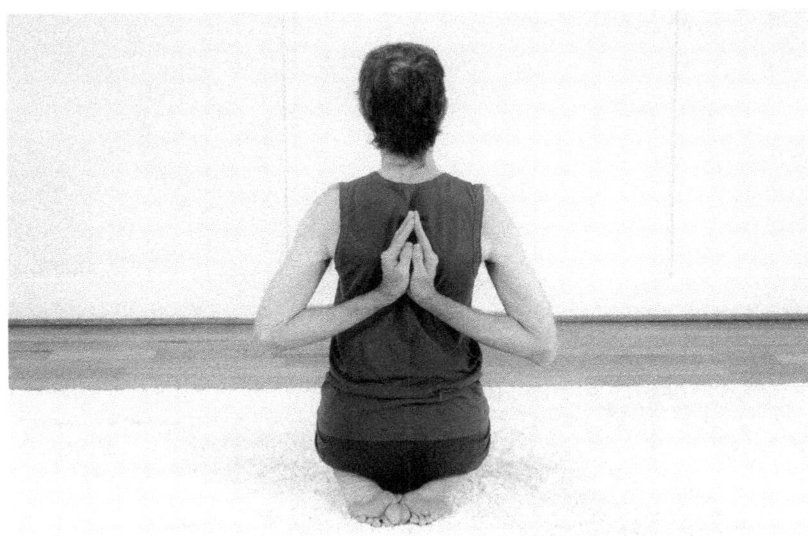

RESISTANCE FLEXIBILITY: Pull your elbows forwards to resist while you bring your hands behind your back with your palms touching. Return to the starting position and repeat 10 times.

HELPFUL REMINDERS

1. Reverse movement for strengthening.
2. The Balancing Stretch muscles help you get into the stretch position.
3. The Opposing Stretch muscles help you get the necessary rotation.
4. Your stretch occurs only while you contract and resist.
5. Your breathing is different in every *type* of stretch.
6. Get perspective from others on how each stretch affects you.

#11 ASSISTED (PERICARDIUM)

BENEFITS

Health: Circulation / Scar Tissue
Body Part: Forearm
Joint: Elbow
Movement: Close
Good Looks: Transparent, Magnificent
Life: Disciplined, Details

MUSCLES

Pectoralis Minor, Biceps Brachii, Brachialis, Coracobrachialis, Forearm Flexors, Palmaris Longus, Pronator Teres and Quadratus, Lumbricals

Action: Flexion / Abduction / Inward
Stretch: Extension / Adduction / Outward

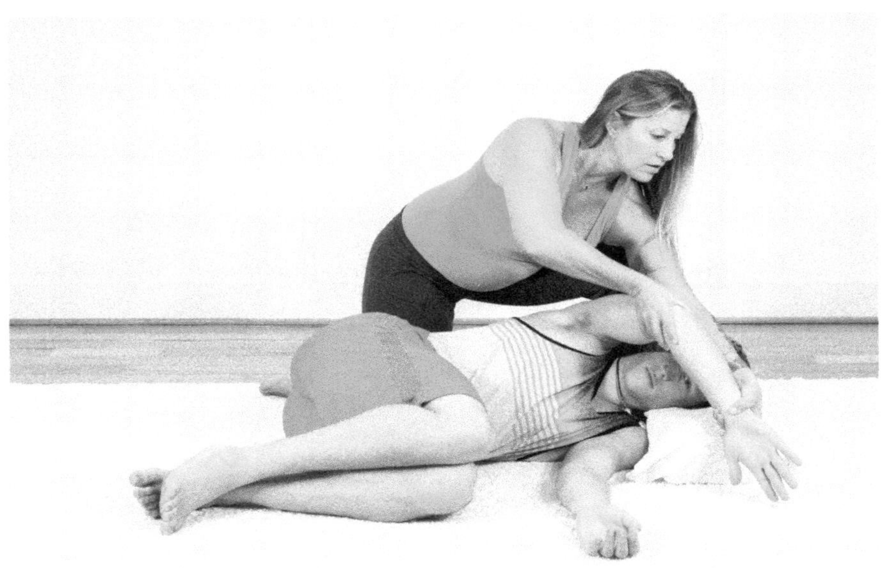

STARTING POSITION: Lie on your left side with a pillow under your head. The assister kneels behind you and grasps your right elbow and wrist with their hands, holding your arm straight and diagonally up across your body.

BALANCING STRETCH

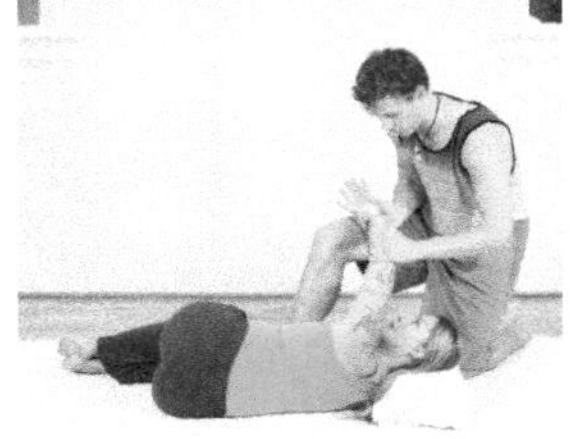

#12 Assisted (Skin)

OPPOSING STRETCH

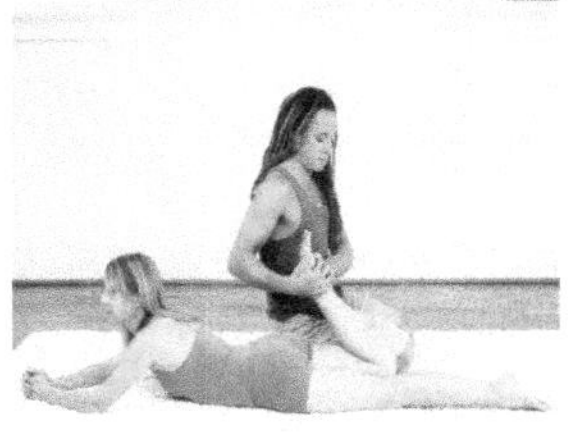

#5 Assisted (Stomach)

ASSISTED HEART OPENER

(TCM)

Organ: Pericardium
Tissue: Epithelial
Body Part: Trunk
System: Blood Distribution
Sensory: Energetic receptors
Yin/Yang Element: Yin Electromagnetic

PERSONALITY (GPT)

Group: Spiritual
Time and Attention: Relative and Inside
High Traits: Judgment, Open, Disciplined, Philanthropy
Low Traits: Sabotaging, Arrogant
Instinct: Calm/Frightened

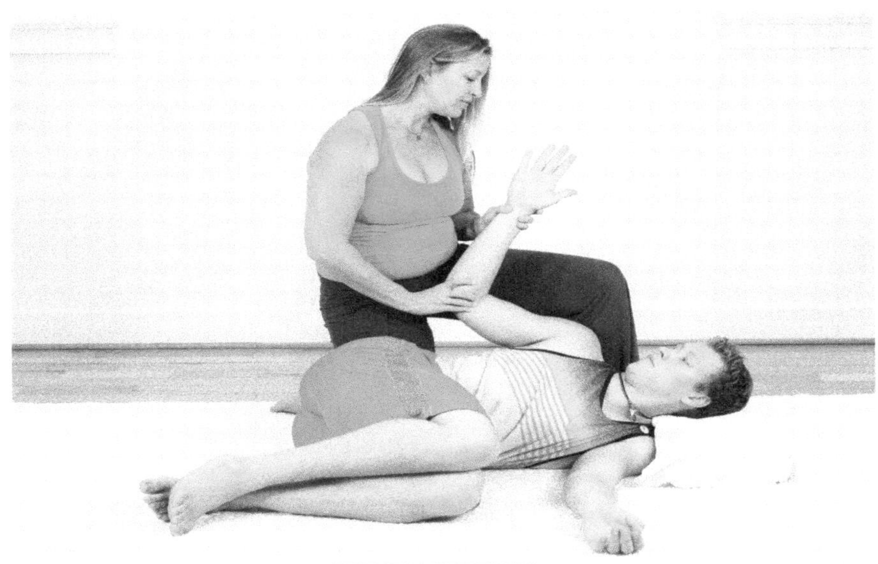

RESISTANCE FLEXIBILITY: Your right arm pushes forward to resist while the assister pulls your arm backwards and outwards. Return to the starting position and repeat 10 times on each arm.

HELPFUL REMINDERS

1. Reverse movement for strengthening.
2. The Balancing Stretch muscles help you get into the stretch position.
3. The Opposing Stretch muscles help you get the necessary rotation.
4. Your stretch occurs only while you contract and resist.
5. Your breathing is different in every *type* of stretch.
6. Get perspective from others on how each stretch affects you.

#12 BEGINNER (SKIN)

BENEFITS

Health: Recovery
Body Part: Forearm
Joint: Elbow
Movement: Open
Good Looks: Stylish, Delightful
Life: Athletic, Lucky

MUSCLES

Frontalis, Oribcularis Oculi, Solenius Capitis, SCM, Posterior Deltoid, Trapezius, Triceps Brachii, Forearm Extensors, Dorsal Interosseus

Action: Extension / Adduction / Outward
Stretch: Flexion / Abduction / Inward

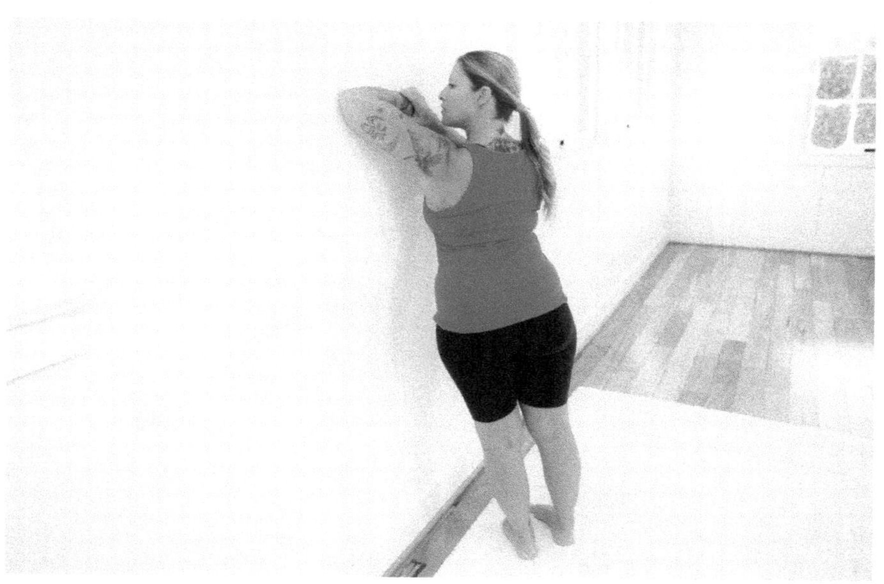

STARTING POSITION: Stand with a wall to your left. Bring your left elbow up onto the wall and grasp your left wrist with your right hand.

BALANCING STRETCH

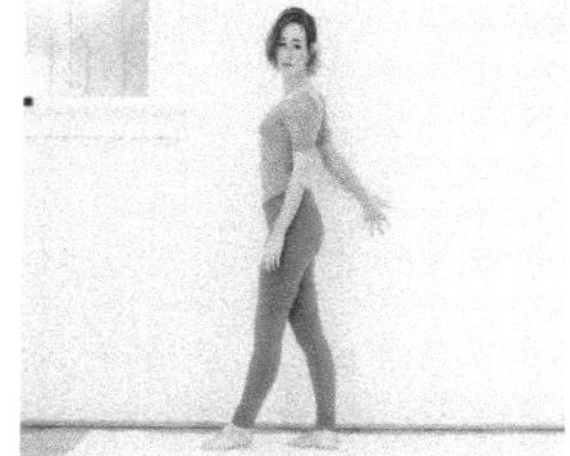

#11 Beginner (Skin)

OPPOSING STRETCH

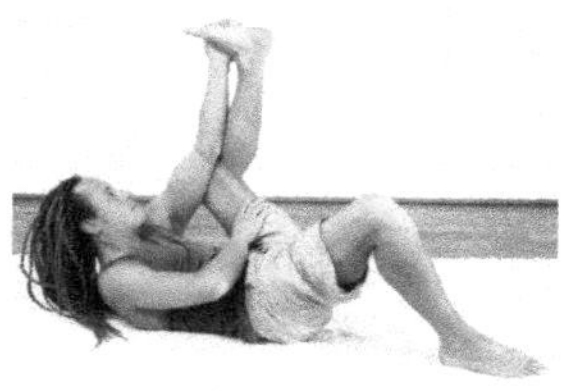

#6 Beginner (Pancreas)

CHALLENGER AT WALL

(TCM)

Organ: Skin
Tissue: External Immune
Body Part: Arms
System: Integumentary
Sensory: Energetic
Yin/Yang Element: Yang Electromagnetic

PERSONALITY (GPT)

Group: Physical
Time and Attention: Present and Outside
High Traits: Challenge, Conscience, Community, Luck, Defense
Low Traits: Antisocial,
Instinct: Love/Anger

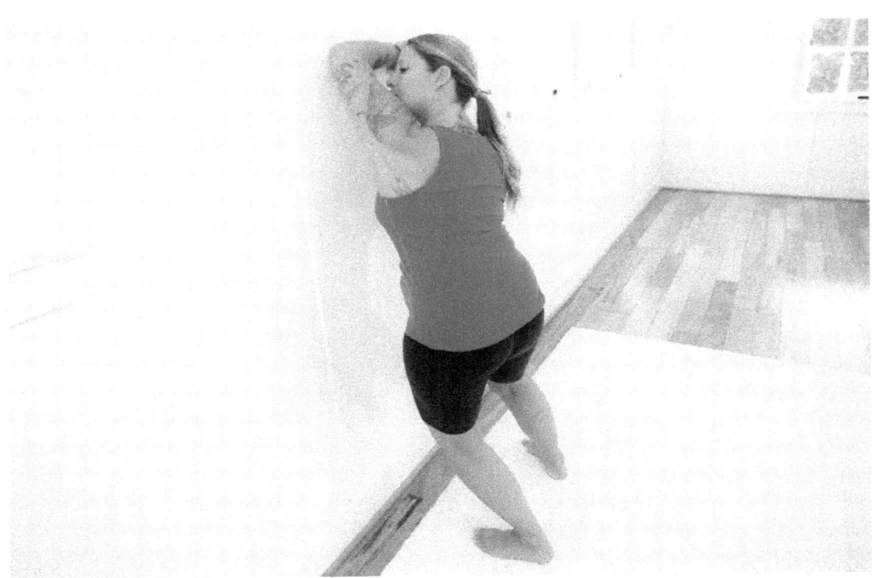

RESISTANCE FLEXIBILITY: Your left elbow pushes into the wall to resist as you fall backwards and turn your body to the left. Return to the starting position and repeat 10 times on each arm.

HELPFUL REMINDERS

1. Reverse movement for strengthening.
2. The Balancing Stretch muscles help you get into the stretch position.
3. The Opposing Stretch muscles help you get the necessary rotation.
4. Your stretch occurs only while you contract and resist.
5. Your breathing is different in every *type* of stretch.
6. Get perspective from others on how each stretch affects you.

#12 INTERMEDIATE (SKIN)

BENEFITS

Health: Recovery
Body Part: Forearm
Joint: Elbow
Movement: Open
Good Looks: Stylish, Delightful
Life: Athletic, Lucky

MUSCLES

Frontalis, Oribcularis Oculi, Solenius Capitis, SCM, Posterior Deltoid, Trapezius, Triceps Brachii, Forearm Extensors, Dorsal Interosseus

Action: Extension / Adduction / Outward
Stretch: Flexion / Abduction / Inward

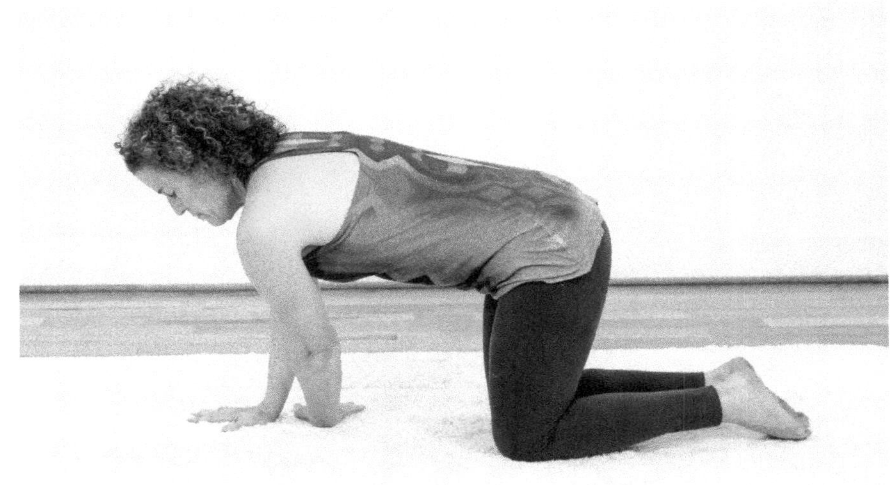

STARTING POSITION: Start on your hands and knees. Bring your left arm across your body behind the right hand and place your left hand on the floor, palm down.

BALANCING STRETCH

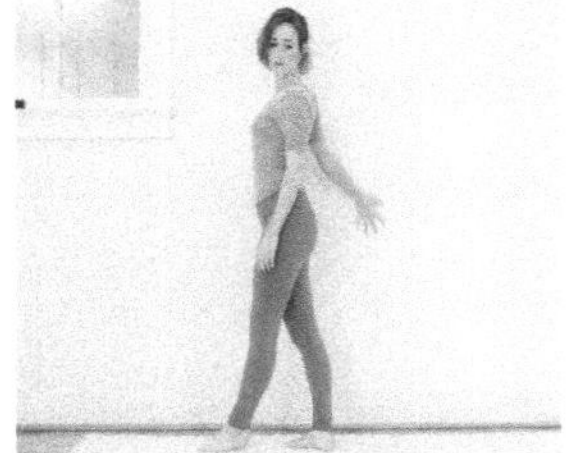

#11 Beginner (Skin)

OPPOSING STRETCH

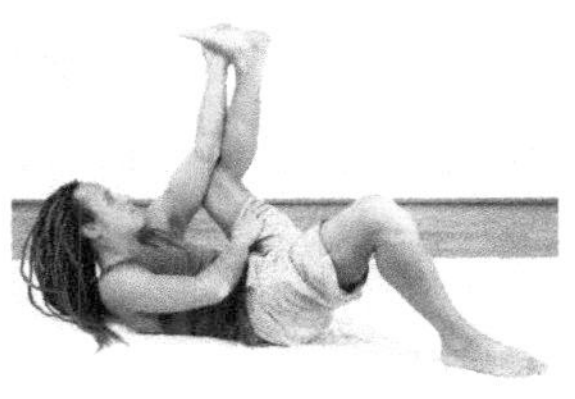

#6 Beginner (Pancreas)

CHALLENGING ON FLOOR

(TCM)

Organ: Skin
Tissue: External Immune
Body Part: Arms
System: Integumentary
Sensory: Energetic
Yin/Yang Element: Yang Electromagnetic

PERSONALITY (GPT)

Group: Physical
Time and Attention: Present and Outside
High Traits: Challenge, Conscience, Community, Luck, Defense
Low Traits: Antisocial,
Instinct: Love/Anger

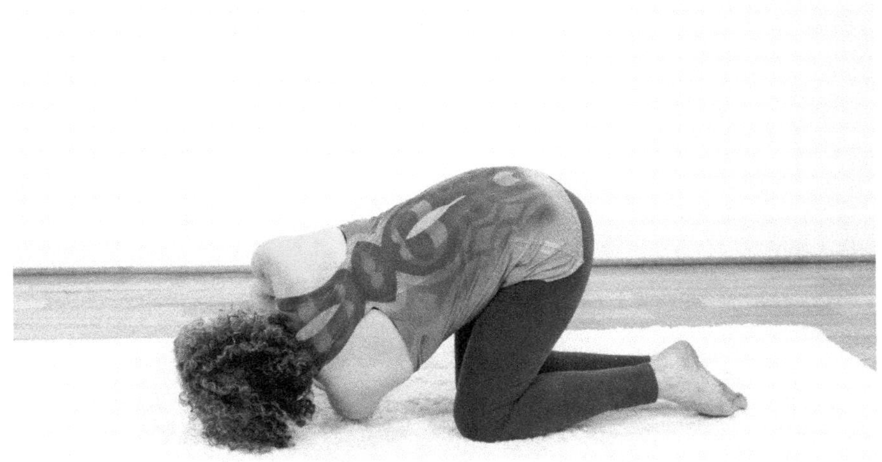

RESISTANCE FLEXIBILITY: Push your left arm down against the floor to resist as you lower your left shoulder down onto the floor. Return to the starting position and repeat 10 times on each arm. SIMPLE COBRA

HELPFUL REMINDERS

1. Reverse movement for strengthening.
2. The Balancing Stretch muscles help you get into the stretch position.
3. The Opposing Stretch muscles help you get the necessary rotation.
4. Your stretch occurs only while you contract and resist.
5. Your breathing is different in every *type* of stretch.
6. Get perspective from others on how each stretch affects you.

#12 ADVANCED (SKIN)

BENEFITS

Health: Recovery
Body Part: Forearm
Joint: Elbow
Movement: Open
Good Looks: Stylish, Delightful
Life: Athletic, Lucky

MUSCLES

Frontalis, Oribcularis Oculi, Solenius Capitis, SCM, Posterior Deltoid, Trapezius, Triceps Brachii, Forearm Extensors, Dorsal Interosseus

Action: Extension / Adduction / Outward
Stretch: Flexion / Abduction / Inward

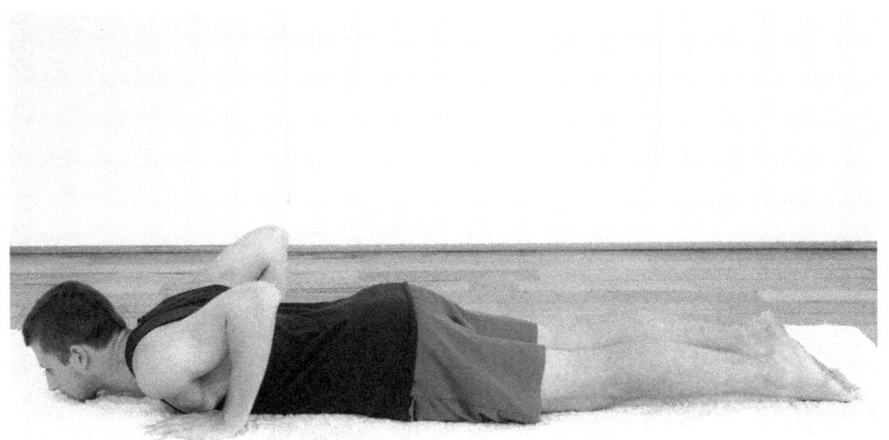

STARTING POSITION: Lie on your stomach and place your palms face down at your sides beside your pecs.

BALANCING STRETCH

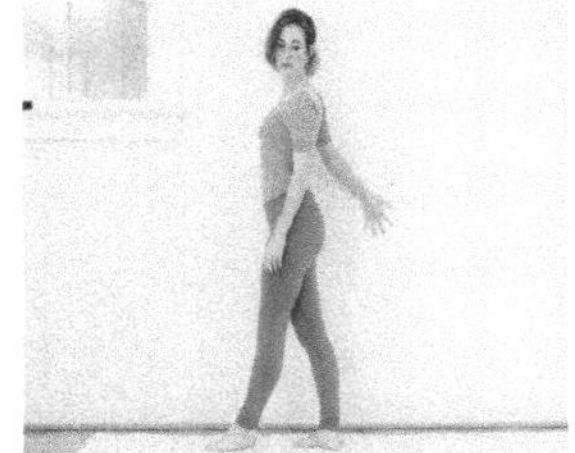

#11 Beginner (Skin)

OPPOSING STRETCH

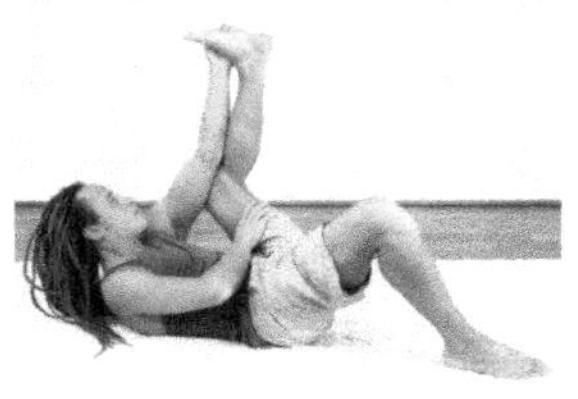

#6 Beginner (Pancreas)

SIMPLE COBRA

(TCM)

Organ: Skin
Tissue: External Immune
Body Part: Arms
System: Integumentary
Sensory: Energetic
Yin/Yang Element: Yang Electromagnetic

PERSONALITY (GPT)

Group: Physical
Time and Attention: Present and Outside
High Traits: Challenge, Conscience, Community, Luck, Defense
Low Traits: Antisocial,
Instinct: Love/Anger

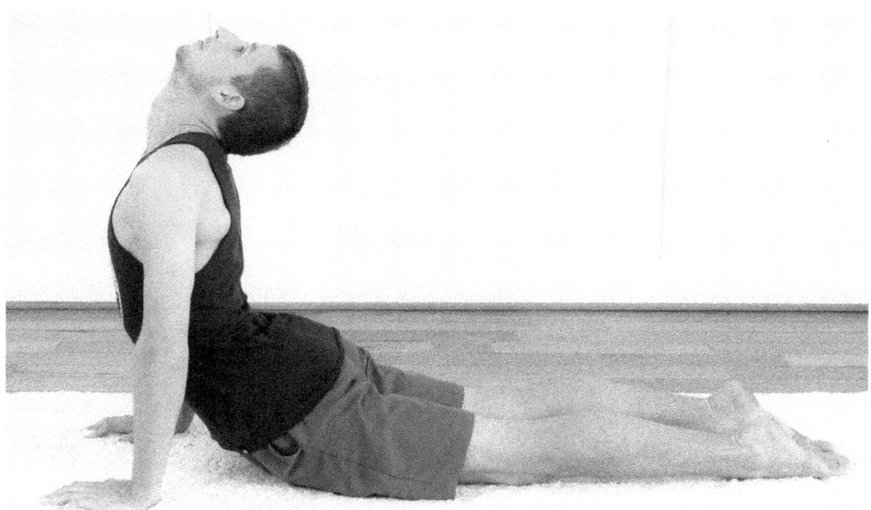

RESISTANCE FLEXIBILITY: Pull your arms backwards to resist as you arch your body, neck and head upward. Return to the starting position and repeat 10 times.

HELPFUL REMINDERS

1. Reverse movement for strengthening.
2. The Balancing Stretch muscles help you get into the stretch position.
3. The Opposing Stretch muscles help you get the necessary rotation.
4. Your stretch occurs only while you contract and resist.
5. Your breathing is different in every *type* of stretch.
6. Get perspective from others on how each stretch affects you.

#12 ASSISTED (SKIN)

BENEFITS

Health: Recovery
Body Part: Forearm
Joint: Elbow
Movement: Open
Good Looks: Stylish, Delightful
Life: Athletic, Lucky

MUSCLES

Frontalis, Oribcularis Oculi, Solenius Capitis, SCM, Posterior Deltoid, Trapezius, Triceps Brachii, Forearm Extensors, Dorsal Interosseus

Action: Extension / Adduction / Outward
Stretch: Flexion / Abduction / Inward

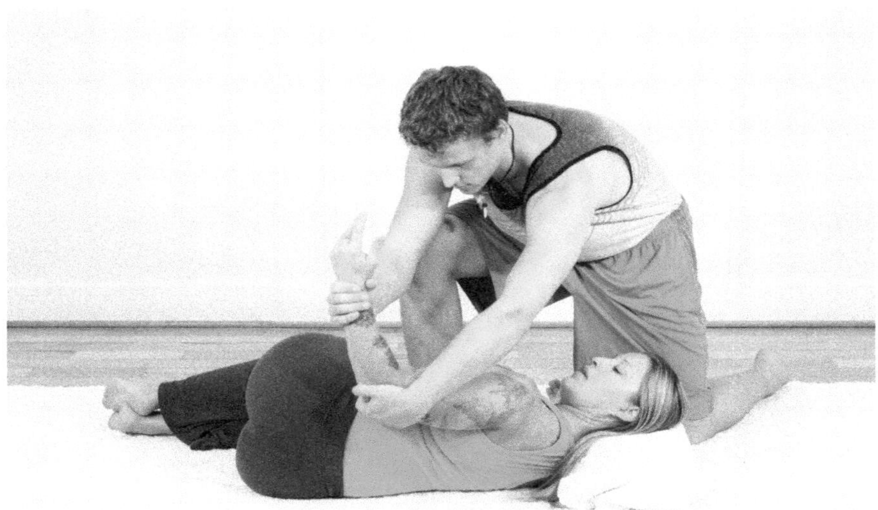

STARTING POSITION: Lie on your right side with a pillow under your head. The assister kneels before you and grasps your left elbow and wrist with their hands, holding your bent arm behind you and turned outward.

BALANCING STRETCH

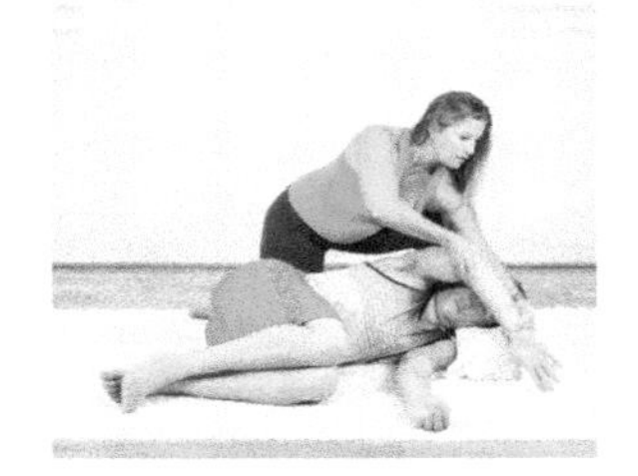

#11 Assisted (Pericardium)

OPPOSING STRETCH

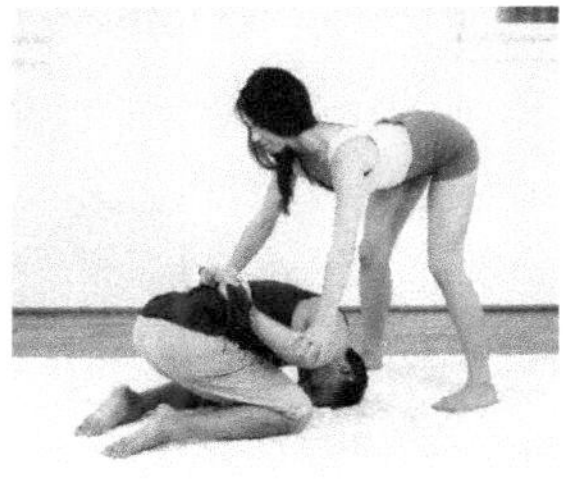

#6 Assisted (Pancreas)

ASSISTED CHALLENGING

(TCM)

Organ: Skin
Tissue: External Immune
Body Part: Arms
System: Integumentary
Sensory: Energetic
Yin/Yang Element: Yang Electromagnetic

PERSONALITY (GPT)

Group: Physical
Time and Attention: Present and Outside
High Traits: Challenge, Conscience, Community, Luck, Defense
Low Traits: Antisocial,
Instinct: Love/Anger

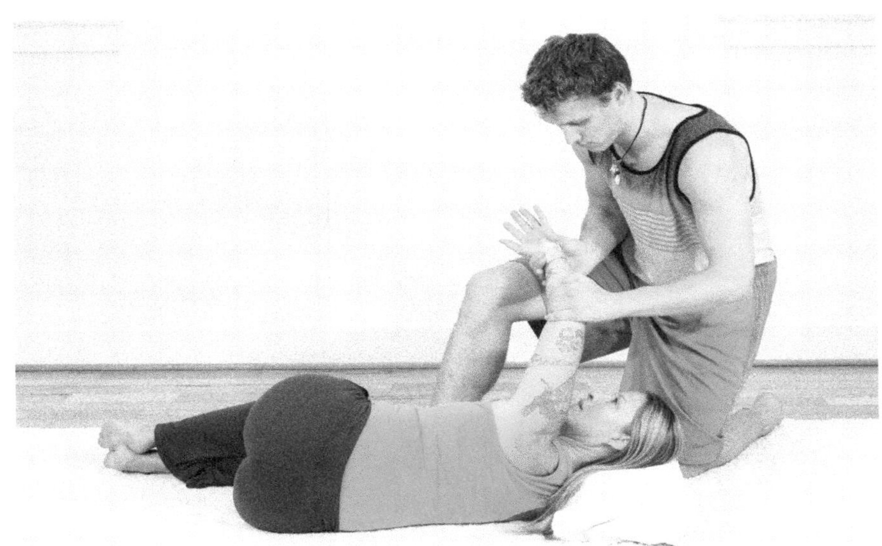

RESISTANCE FLEXIBILITY: Your left arm pulls backwards to resist while the assister pulls your arm towards your head and forward across you. Return to the starting position and repeat 10 times on each arm.

HELPFUL REMINDERS

1. Reverse movement for strengthening.
2. The Balancing Stretch muscles help you get into the stretch position.
3. The Opposing Stretch muscles help you get the necessary rotation.
4. Your stretch occurs only while you contract and resist.
5. Your breathing is different in every *type* of stretch.
6. Get perspective from others on how each stretch affects you.

13# BEGINNER (BLADDER)

BENEFITS

Health: Interferons
Body Part: Ankle, Feet
Joint: Ankle, Feet
Movement: Jump
Good Looks: Image, Statuesque
Life: Business, Team Work

MUSCLES

Frontalis, Upper Trapezius, Splenius Capiti,, Erector Spinae, Gluteus Maximus, Biceps Femoris, Gastrocnemius, Tibialis Posterior

Action: Extension/Abduction/Outward
Stretch: Flexion/Adduction/Inward

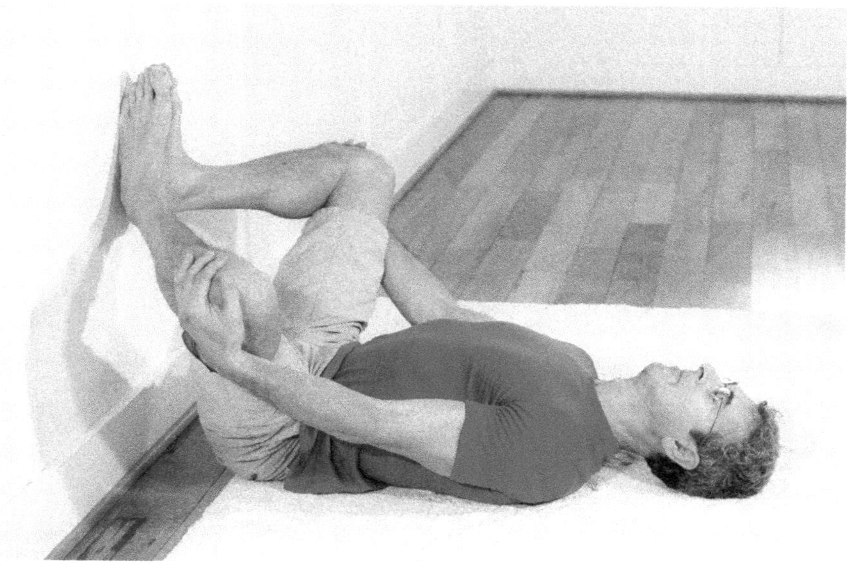

STARTING POSITION: Lie on your back with both legs up against a wall, knees bent and opened wide apart, feet together. Grasp the outside of your knees with your hands.

BALANCING STRETCH

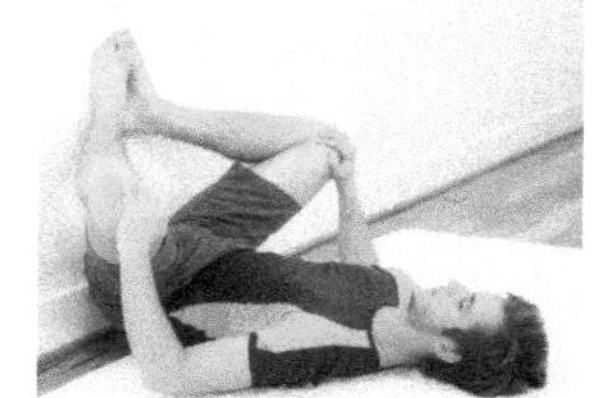

#14 Intermediate (Kidney)

OPPOSING STRETCH

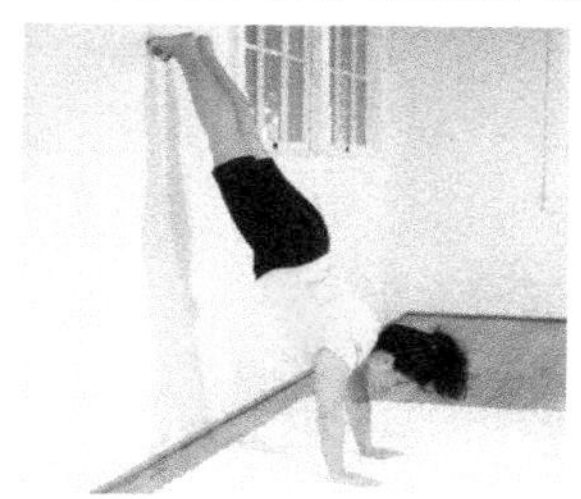

#3 Intermediate (Lung)

LATERAL HAMSTRING AT WALL

(TCM)

Organ: Bladder
Tissue: Bones
Body Part: Face
System: Urinary
Sensory: Hormonal receptors
Yin/Yang Element: Yang Water

PERSONALITY (GPT)

Group: Emotional
Time and Attention: Past and Outside
High Traits: Honesty, Diversity, Hopeful, Promotional, Esteem
Low Traits: Narcissism, Greed
Instinct: Excited/Anxiety

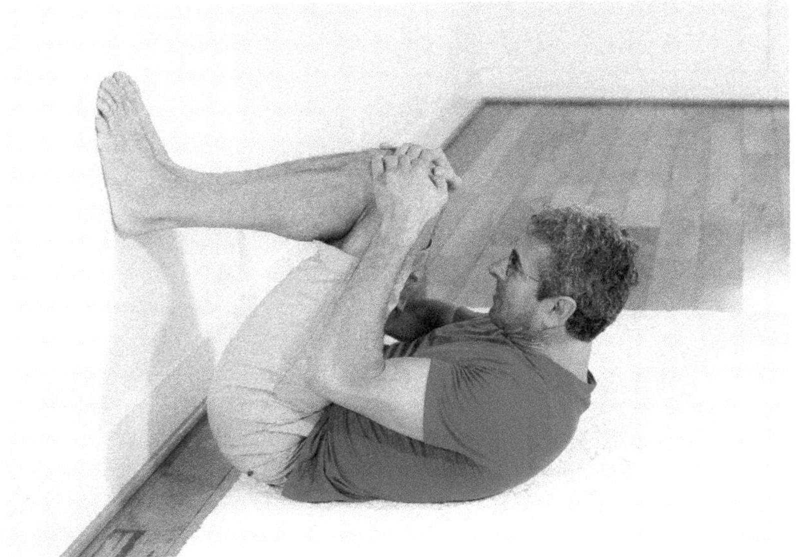

RESISTANCE FLEXIBILITY: Your knees push outwards to resist as your hands close your knees together. Return to the starting position and repeat 10 times.

HELPFUL REMINDERS

1. Reverse movement for strengthening.
2. The Balancing Stretch muscles help you get into the stretch position.
3. The Opposing Stretch muscles help you get the necessary rotation.
4. Your stretch occurs only while you contract and resist.
5. Your breathing is different in every *type* of stretch.
6. Get perspective from others on how each stretch affects you.

#13 INTERMEDIATE (BLADDER)

BENEFITS

Health: Interferons
Body Part: Ankle, Feet
Joint: Ankle, Feet
Movement: Jump
Good Looks: Image, Statuesque
Life: Business, Team Work

MUSCLES

Frontalis, Upper Trapezius, Splenius Capiti,, Erector Spinae, Gluteus Maximus, Biceps Femoris, Gastrocnemius, Tibialis Posterior
Action: Extension/Abduction/Outward
Stretch: Flexion/Adduction/Inward

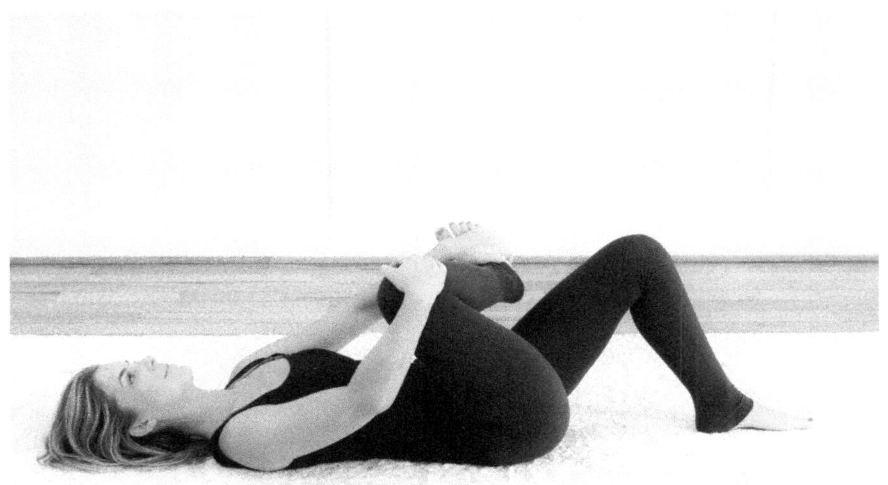

STARTING POSITION: Lie on your back with both knees bent. Lift your right knee up and out sideways to the right. With your left hand grasp the outside of the right ankle, then put your right hand on the outside of the right knee.

BALANCING STRETCH

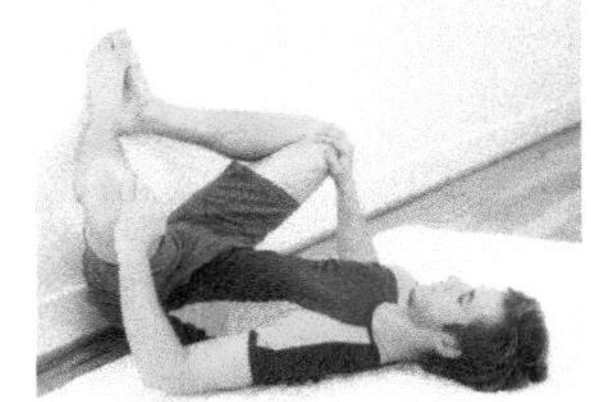

#14 Intermediate (Kidney)

OPPOSING STRETCH

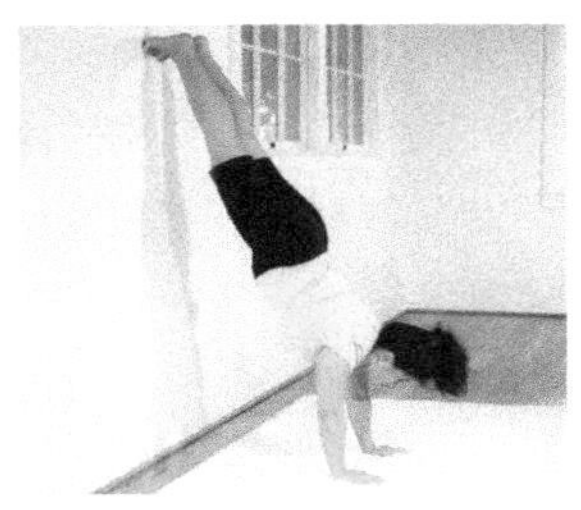

#3 Intermediate (Lung)

BACK LYING LATERAL HAMSTRING

(TCM)

Organ: Bladder
Tissue: Bones
Body Part: Face
System: Urinary
Sensory: Hormonal receptors
Yin/Yang Element: Yang Water

PERSONALITY (GPT)

Group: Emotional
Time and Attention: Past and Outside
High Traits: Honesty, Diversity, Hopeful, Promotional, Esteem
Low Traits: Narcissism, Greed
Instinct: Excited/Anxiety

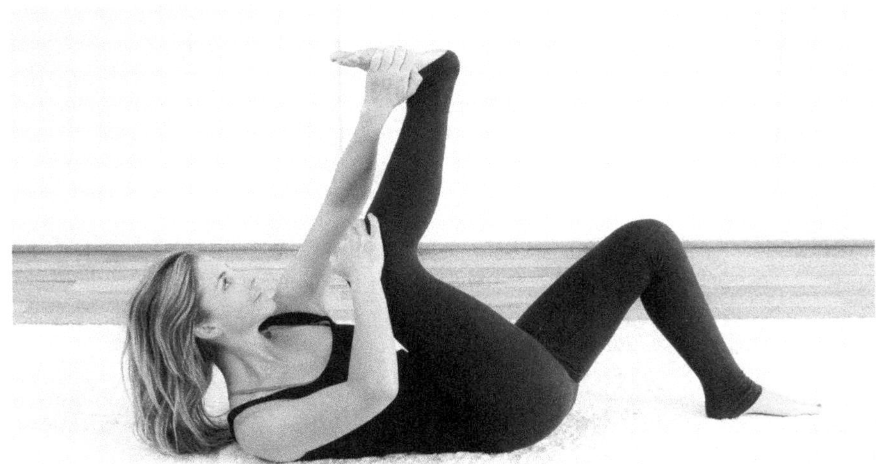

RESISTANCE FLEXIBILITY: Your right knee pushes out, away from your body, and your right heel kicks down towards your butt to resist while your right hand pulls the knee in and across your body and your left hand lifts the left foot upwards and to the left. Return to the starting position and repeat 10 times on each leg.

HELPFUL REMINDERS

1. Reverse movement for strengthening.
2. The Balancing Stretch muscles help you get into the stretch position.
3. The Opposing Stretch muscles help you get the necessary rotation.
4. Your stretch occurs only while you contract and resist.
5. Your breathing is different in every *type* of stretch.
6. Get perspective from others on how each stretch affects you.

#13 ADVANCED (BLADDER)

BENEFITS

Health: Interferons
Body Part: Ankle, Feet
Joint: Ankle, Feet
Movement: Jump
Good Looks: Image, Statuesque
Life: Business, Team Work

MUSCLES

Frontalis, Upper Trapezius, Splenius Capiti,, Erector Spinae, Gluteus Maximus, Biceps Femoris, Gastrocnemius, Tibialis Posterior

Action: Extension/Abduction/Outward
Stretch: Flexion/Adduction/Inward

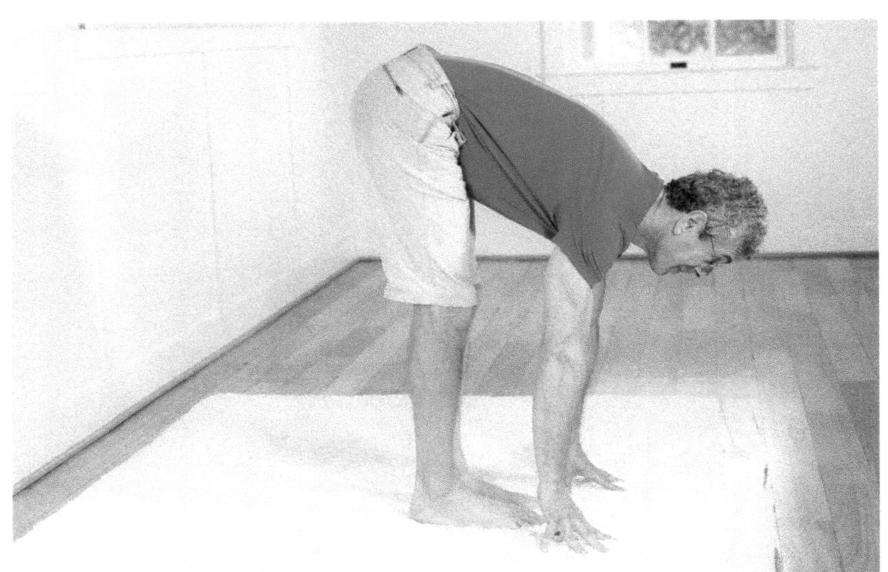

STARTING POSITION: Stand facing away from a wall. Bend forward and stand on one leg as you raise the other leg up onto the wall. Place a hand on the back outside of your standing leg's thigh.

BALANCING STRETCH

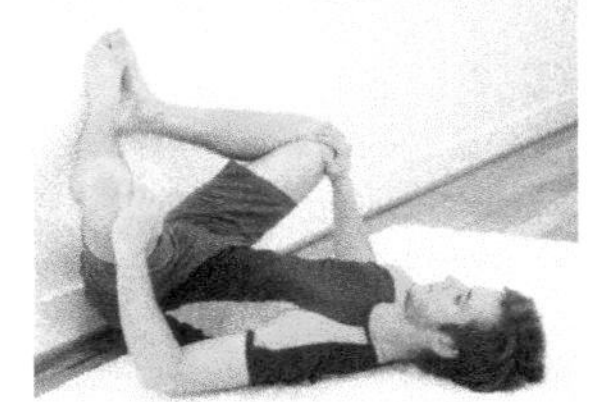

#14 Intermediate (Kidney)

OPPOSING STRETCH

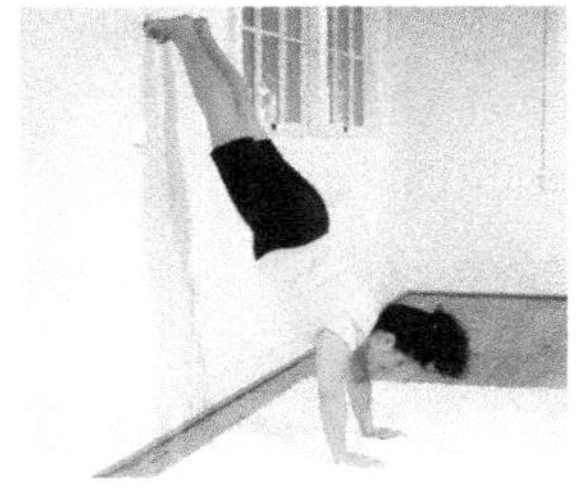

#3 Intermediate (Lung)

STANDING LATERAL HAMSTRING

(TCM)

Organ: Bladder
Tissue: Bones
Body Part: Face
System: Urinary
Sensory: Hormonal receptors
Yin/Yang Element: Yang Water

PERSONALITY (GPT)

Group: Emotional
Time and Attention: Past and Outside
High Traits: Honesty, Diversity, Hopeful, Promotional, Esteem
Low Traits: Narcissism, Greed
Instinct: Excited/Anxiety

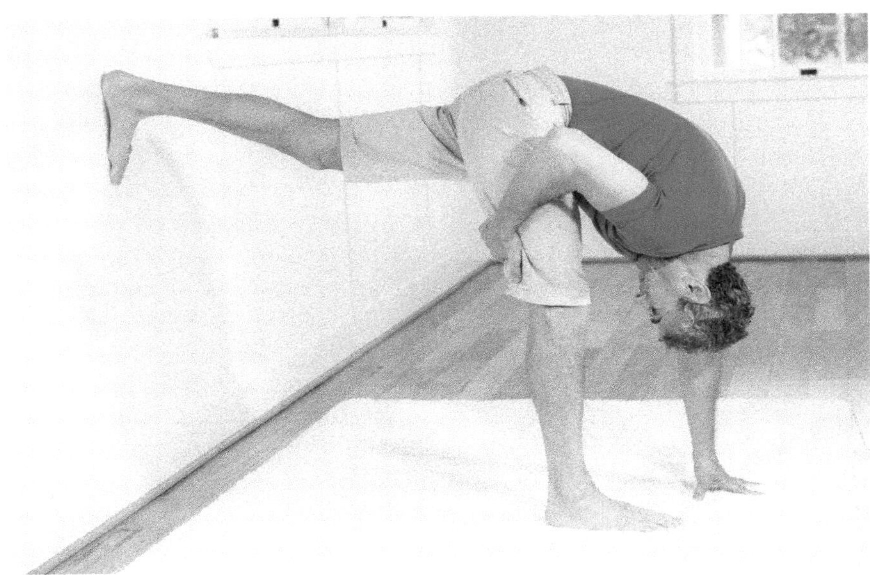

RESISTANCE FLEXIBILITY: Press your raised leg's foot into the wall and scissor your legs toward each other to resist. Return to the starting position and repeat 10 times on each leg.

HELPFUL REMINDERS

1. Reverse movement for strengthening.
2. The Balancing Stretch muscles help you get into the stretch position.
3. The Opposing Stretch muscles help you get the necessary rotation.
4. Your stretch occurs only while you contract and resist.
5. Your breathing is different in every *type* of stretch.
6. Get perspective from others on how each stretch affects you.

#13 ASSISTED (BLADDER)

BENEFITS

Health: Interferons
Body Part: Ankle, Feet
Joint: Ankle, Feet
Movement: Jump
Good Looks: Image, Statuesque
Life: Business, Team Work

MUSCLES

Frontalis, Upper Trapezius, Splenius Capiti,, Erector Spinae, Gluteus Maximus, Biceps Femoris, Gastrocnemius, Tibialis Posterior

Action: Extension / Abduction / Outward
Stretch: Flexion / Adduction / Inward

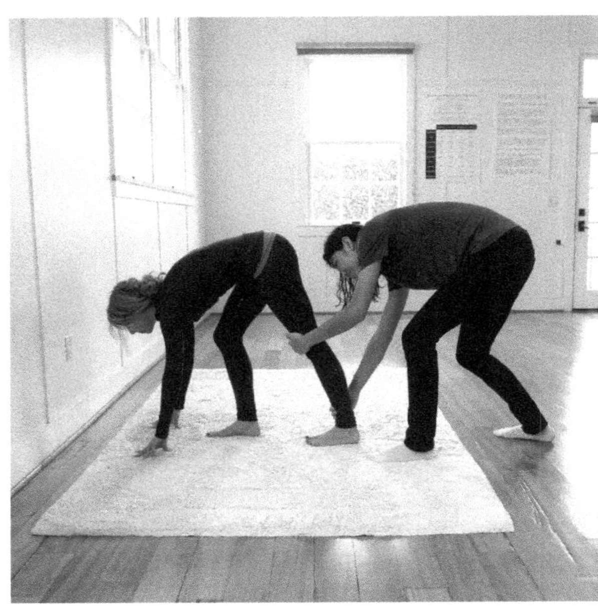

STARTING POSITION: Stand with your legs hip width, and then bring your palms to the floor. The assister squats behind you and grasps your right knee and ankle with their hands, holding your straight leg.

BALANCING STRETCH

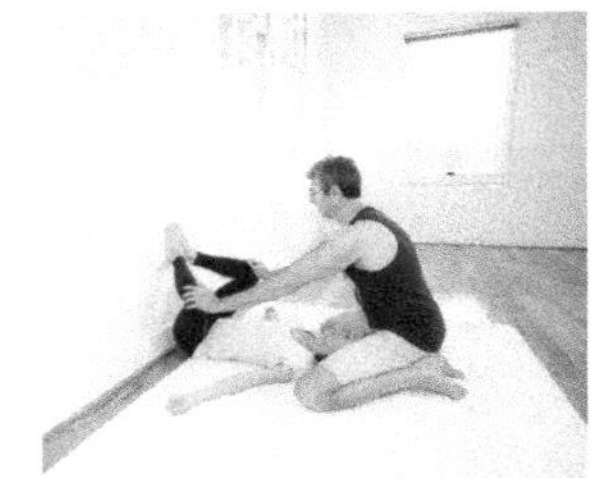

#14 Assisted (Kidney)

OPPOSING STRETCH

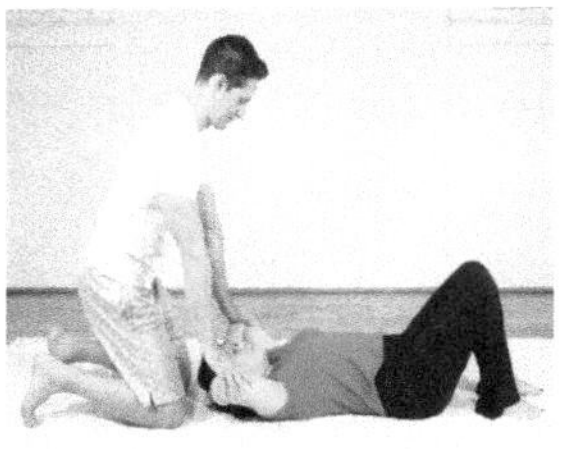

#3 Assisted (Lung)

ASSISTED STANDING LATERAL HAMSTRING

(TCM)

Organ: Bladder
Tissue: Bones
Body Part: Face
System: Urinary
Sensory: Hormonal receptors
Yin/Yang Element: Yang Water

PERSONALITY (GPT)

Group: Emotional
Time and Attention: Past and Outside
High Traits: Honesty, Diversity, Hopeful, Promotional, Esteem
Low Traits: Narcissism, Greed
Instinct: Excited/Anxiety

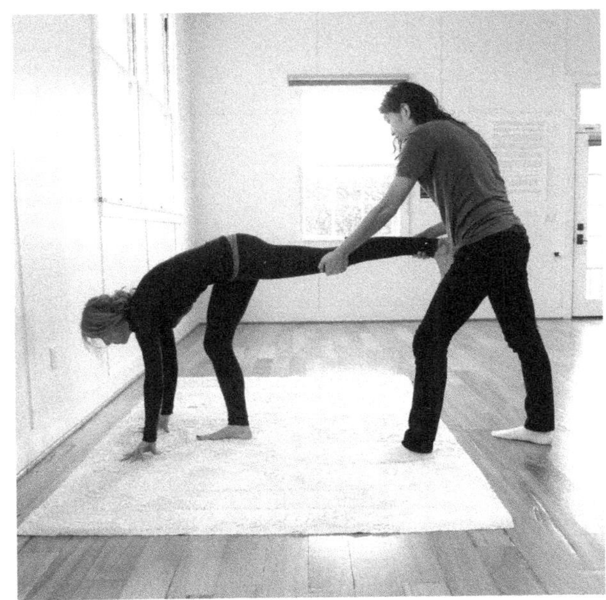

RESISTANCE FLEXIBILITY: Kick your right leg down and forwards and scissor your legs toward each other to resist while the assister lift your leg backwards. Return to the starting position and repeat 10 times on each leg.

HELPFUL REMINDERS

1. Reverse movement for strengthening.
2. The Balancing Stretch muscles help you get into the stretch position.
3. The Opposing Stretch muscles help you get the necessary rotation.
4. Your stretch occurs only while you contract and resist.
5. Your breathing is different in every *type* of stretch.
6. Get perspective from others on how each stretch affects you.

#14 BEGINNER (KIDNEY)

BENEFITS

Health: Adrenal
Body Part: Ankle, Feet
Joint: Ankle, Feet
Movement: Squat
Good Looks: Illuminated, Deep
Life: Humor, Confidant

MUSCLES

Flexor Digitorums, Lumbricalis, Interossious, Flexor Hallucis Longus, Gastrocnemius, Sartorius, Iliacus, Rectus Abdominals, Pectoralis Major
Action: Flexion / Adduction / Inward
Stretch: Extension / Abduction / Outward

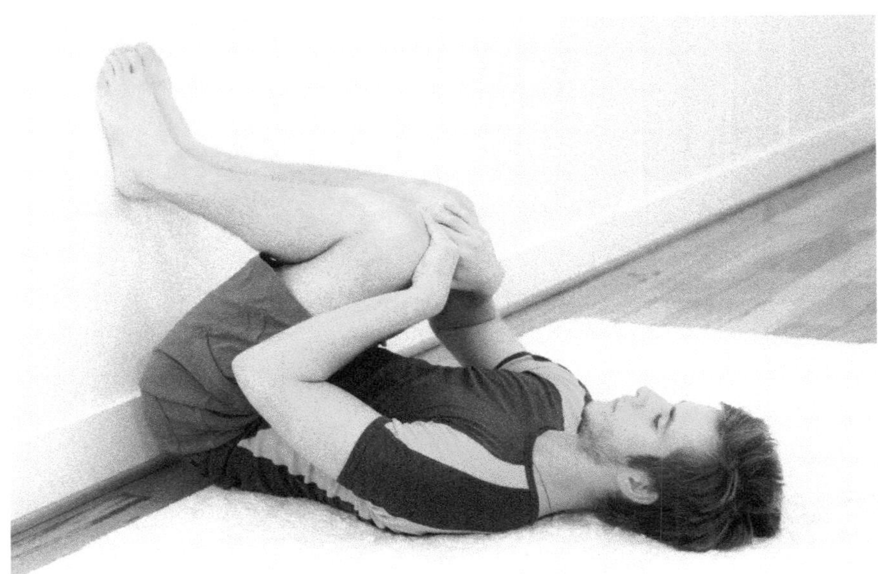

STARTING POSITION: Lie on your back with both legs up against a wall, knees bent and together, and feet together. Grasp the insides of your knees with your hands.

BALANCING STRETCH

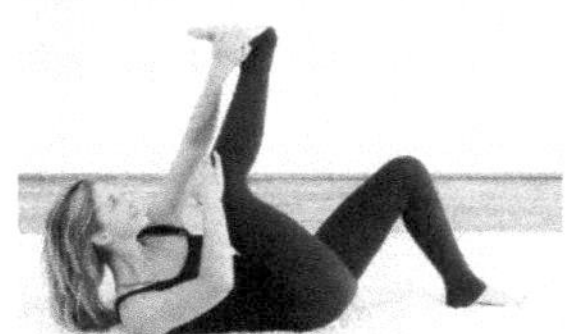

#13 Intermediate (Bladder)

OPPOSING STRETCH

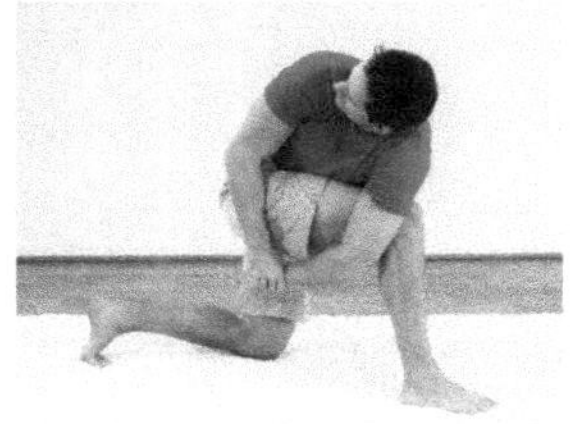

#4 Advanced (Large Intestine)

BACK LYING LOTUS

(TCM)

Organ: Kidney
Tissue: Joints
Body Part: Legs
System: Urinary
Sensory: Nervous System
Yin/Yang Element: Yin Water

PERSONALITY (GPT)

Group: Thinking
Time and Attention: Future and Inside
High Traits: Understanding, Humor, Compassion, Confidence, Intuition
Low Traits: Split, Withdrawn
Instinct: Fearless/ Fear

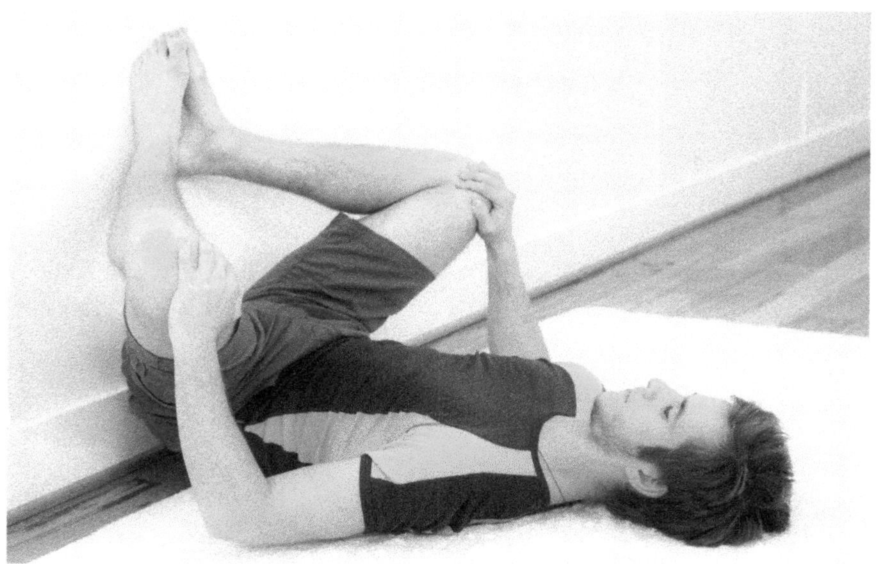

RESISTANCE FLEXIBILITY: Your knees squeeze together to resist as your hands pull your knees apart. Return to the starting position and repeat 10 times.

HELPFUL REMINDERS

1. Reverse movement for strengthening.
2. The Balancing Stretch muscles help you get into the stretch position.
3. The Opposing Stretch muscles help you get the necessary rotation.
4. Your stretch occurs only while you contract and resist.
5. Your breathing is different in every *type* of stretch.
6. Get perspective from others on how each stretch affects you.

#14 INTERMEDIATE (KIDNEY)

BENEFITS

Health: Adrenal
Body Part: Ankle, Feet
Joint: Ankle, Feet
Movement: Squat
Good Looks: Illuminated, Deep
Life: Humor, Confidant

MUSCLES

Flexor Digitorums, Lumbricalis, Interossious, Flexor Hallucis Longus, Gastrocnemius, Sartorius, Iliacus, Rectus Abdominals, Pectoralis Major
Action: Flexion / Adduction / Inward
Stretch: Extension / Abduction / Outward

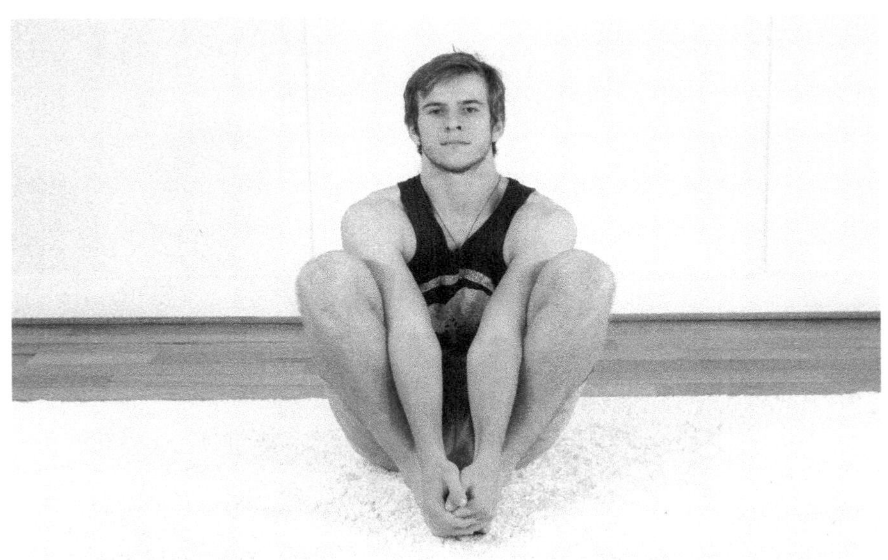

STARTING POSITION: Sit on the floor with your knees bent and together and the bottoms of your feet together. Grasp the insides of your ankles with your hands.

BALANCING STRETCH

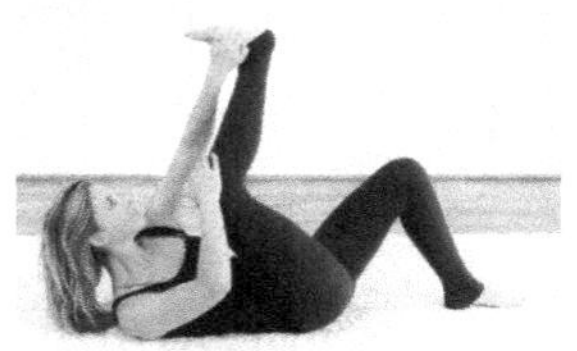

#13 Intermediate (Bladder)

OPPOSING STRETCH

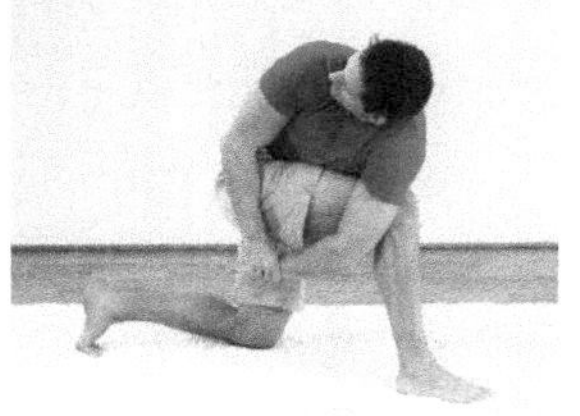

#4 Advanced (Large Intestine)

SEATED LOTUS

(TCM)

Organ: Kidney
Tissue: Joints
Body Part: Legs
System: Urinary
Sensory: Nervous System
Yin/Yang Element: Yin Water

PERSONALITY (GPT)

Group: Thinking
Time and Attention: Future and Inside
High Traits: Understanding, Humor, Compassion, Confidence, Intuition
Low Traits: Split, Withdrawn
Instinct: Fearless/ Fear

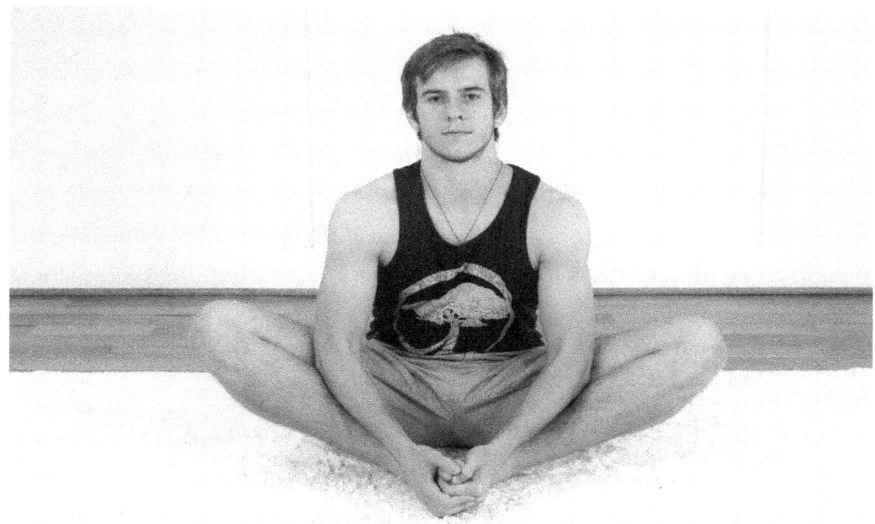

RESISTANCE FLEXIBILITY: Your knees squeeze together to resist while your arms both push your knees apart and pull your body forward. Return to the starting position and repeat 10 times.

HELPFUL REMINDERS

1. Reverse movement for strengthening.
2. The Balancing Stretch muscles help you get into the stretch position.
3. The Opposing Stretch muscles help you get the necessary rotation.
4. Your stretch occurs only while you contract and resist.
5. Your breathing is different in every *type* of stretch.
6. Get perspective from others on how each stretch affects you.

#14 ADVANCED (KIDNEY)

BENEFITS

Health: Adrenal
Body Part: Ankle, Feet
Joint: Ankle, Feet
Movement: Squat
Good Looks: Illuminated, Deep
Life: Humor, Confidant

MUSCLES

Flexor Digitorums, Lumbricalis, Interossious, Flexor Hallucis Longus, Gastrocnemius, Sartorius, Iliacus, Rectus Abdominals, Pectoralis Major
Action: Flexion/Adduction/Inward
Stretch: Extension/Abduction/Outward

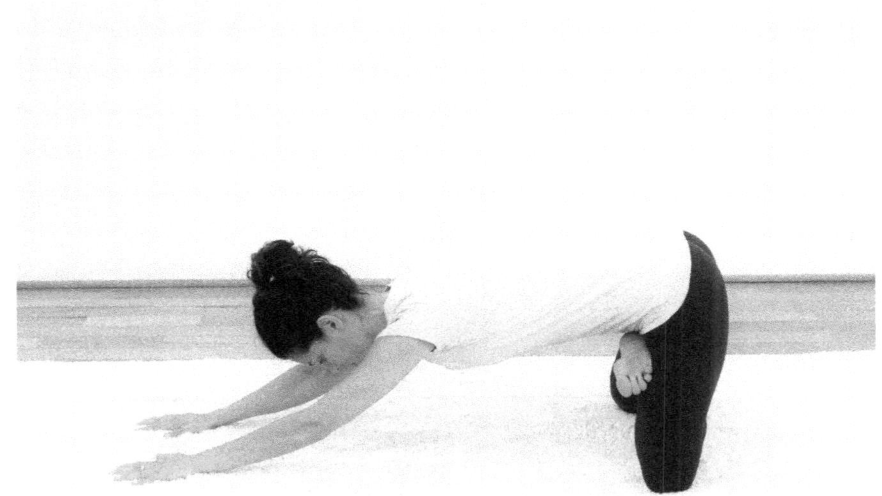

STARTING POSITION: Sit in lotus pose with either one or both legs locked across the other leg(s). Reach forward with your hands, going up onto your knees.

BALANCING STRETCH

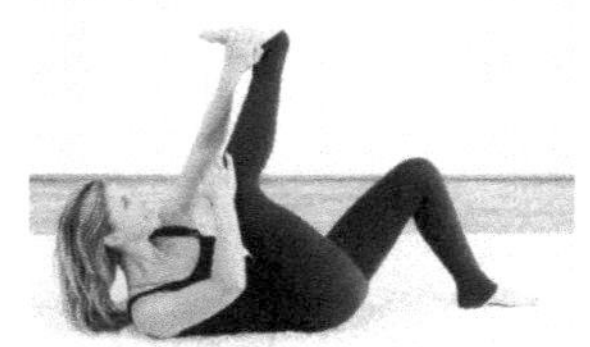

#13 Intermediate (Bladder)

OPPOSING STRETCH

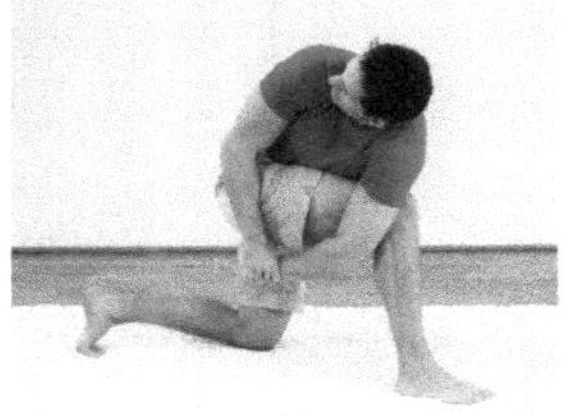

#4 Advanced (Large Intestine)

LOTUS ARCHING

(TCM)

Organ: Kidney
Tissue: Joints
Body Part: Legs
System: Urinary
Sensory: Nervous System
Yin/Yang Element: Yin Water

PERSONALITY (GPT)

Group: Thinking
Time and Attention: Future and Inside
High Traits: Understanding, Humor, Compassion, Confidence, Intuition
Low Traits: Split, Withdrawn
Instinct: Fearless/ Fear

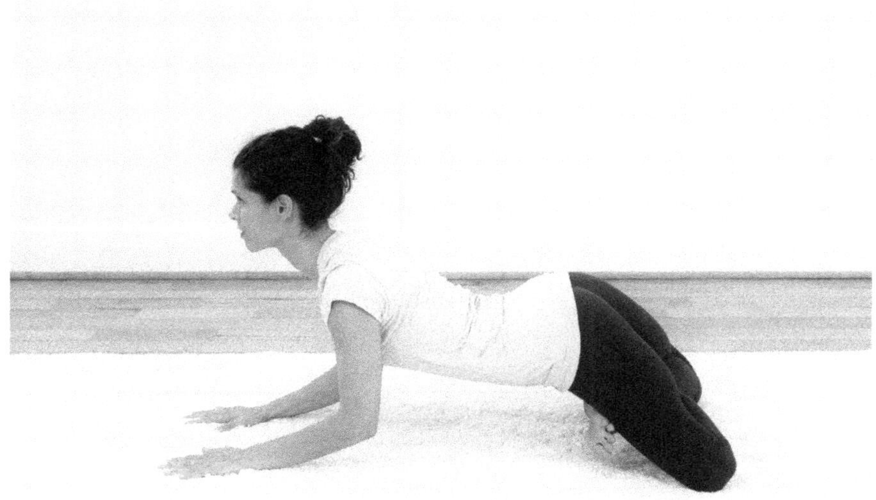

RESISTANCE FLEXIBILITY: Push your knees into the floor to resist as you arch your body up and pull it forwards. Return to the starting position and repeat 10 times.

HELPFUL REMINDERS

1. Reverse movement for strengthening.
2. The Balancing Stretch muscles help you get into the stretch position.
3. The Opposing Stretch muscles help you get the necessary rotation.
4. Your stretch occurs only while you contract and resist.
5. Your breathing is different in every *type* of stretch.
6. Get perspective from others on how each stretch affects you.

#14 ASSISTED (KIDNEY)

BENEFITS

Health: Adrenal
Body Part: Ankle, Feet
Joint: Ankle, Feet
Movement: Squat
Good Looks: Illuminated, Deep
Life: Humor, Confidant

MUSCLES

Flexor Digitorums, Lumbricalis, Interossious, Flexor Hallucis Longus, Gastrocnemius, Sartorius, Iliacus, Rectus Abdominals, Pectoralis Major
Action: Flexion / Adduction / Inward
Stretch: Extension / Abduction / Outward

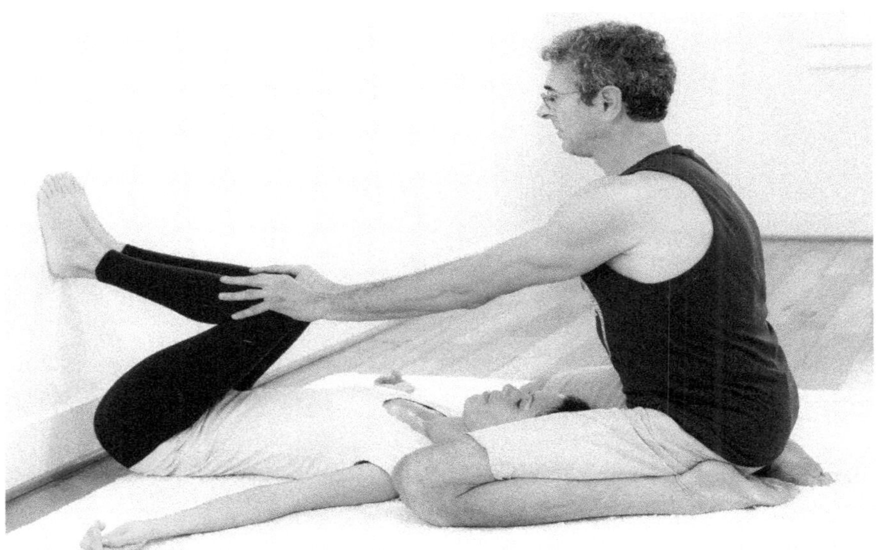

STARTING POSITION: Lie on your back with both legs up against a wall, knees bent and together, and feet together. The assister grasps the inside of your knees with their hands.

BALANCING STRETCH

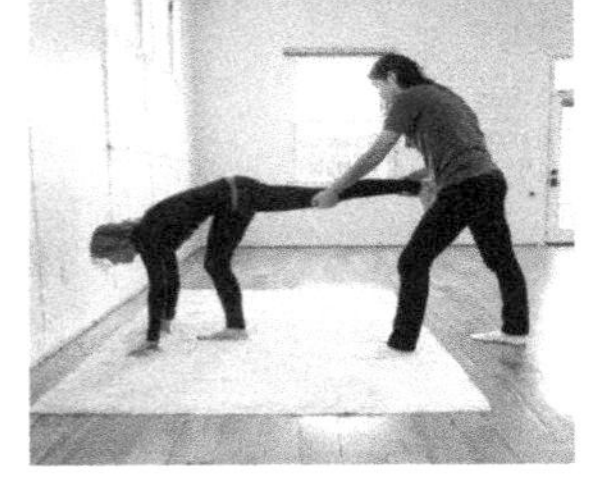

#13 Assisted (Bladder)

OPPOSING STRETCH

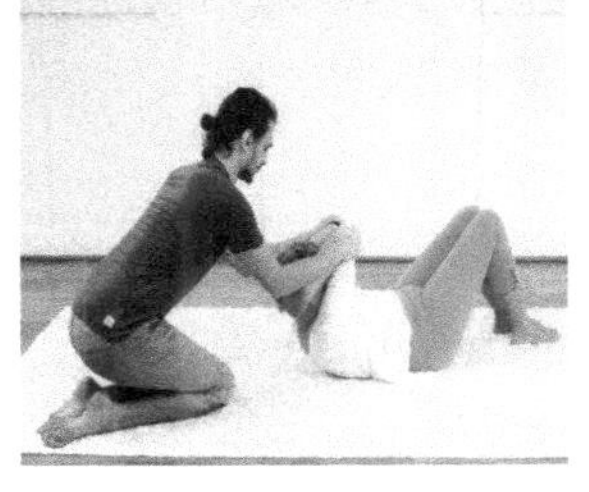

#14 Assisted (Large Intestine)

ASSISTED BACK LYING LOTUS

(TCM)

Organ: Kidney
Tissue: Joints
Body Part: Legs
System: Urinary
Sensory: Nervous System
Yin/Yang Element: Yin Water

PERSONALITY (GPT)

Group: Thinking
Time and Attention: Future and Inside
High Traits: Understanding, Humor, Compassion, Confidence, Intuition
Low Traits: Split, Withdrawn
Instinct: Fearless/ Fear

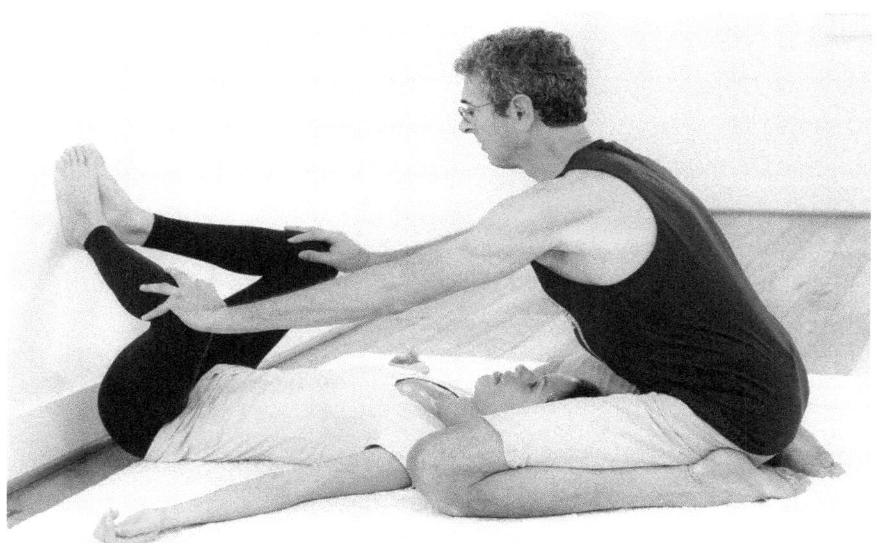

RESISTANCE FLEXIBILITY: Your knees squeeze together to resist while the assister pulls your knees apart. Return to the starting position and repeat 10 times.

HELPFUL REMINDERS

1. Reverse movement for strengthening.
2. The Balancing Stretch muscles help you get into the stretch position.
3. The Opposing Stretch muscles help you get the necessary rotation.
4. Your stretch occurs only while you contract and resist.
5. Your breathing is different in every *type* of stretch.
6. Get perspective from others on how each stretch affects you.

#15 BEGINNER (APPENDIX)

BENEFITS

Health: Prebiotics / Metal Detox
Body Part: Wrist, Hand
Joint: Wrist, Hand
Movement: Lowering
Good Looks: Iridescent, Extreme
Life: Change, Appreciation

MUSCLES

Wrist and Finger Flexors, Forearm Flexors, Biceps, Latissimus Dorsi, Platysma, Risorius, Buccinator,
Action: Extension / Adduction / Inward
Stretch: Flexion / Abduction / Outward

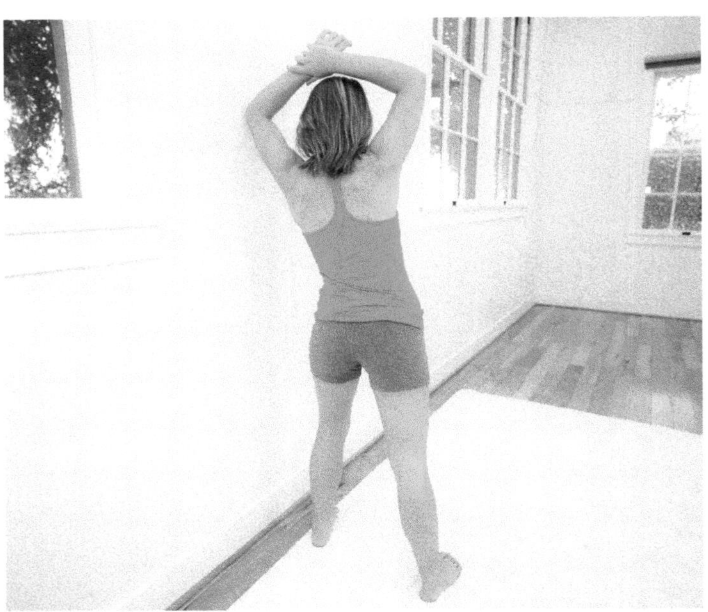

STARTING POSITION: Stand facing a wall, bend your left elbow and place it up high against the wall. With your right hand, grasp your left wrist.

BALANCING STRETCH

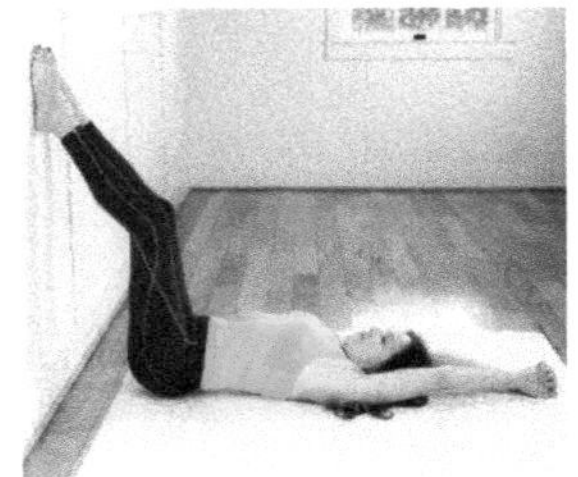

#16 Beginner (Thymus)

OPPOSING STRETCH

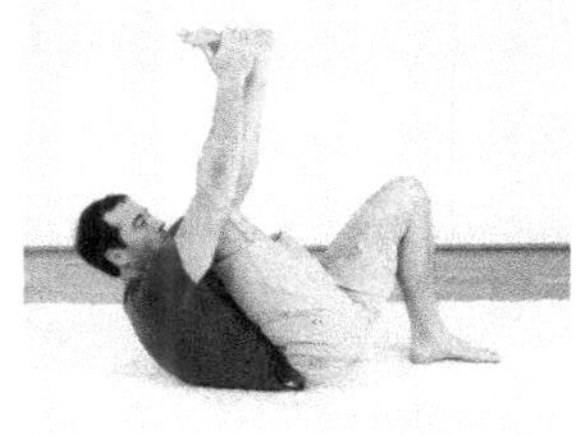

#9 Beginner (Brain)

TRICEPS AT WALL

(TCM)

Organ: Appendix
Tissue: Cartilage
Body Part: Trunk
System: Detoxification
Sensory: Energetic receptors
Yin/Yang Element: Yin Sentient Beings

PERSONALITY (GPT)

Group: Spiritual
Time and Attention: Relative and Outside
High Traits: Change, Integrity, Appreciation, Detox, Centered
Low Traits: Depersonalization, Frantic
Instinct: Calm/ Frightened

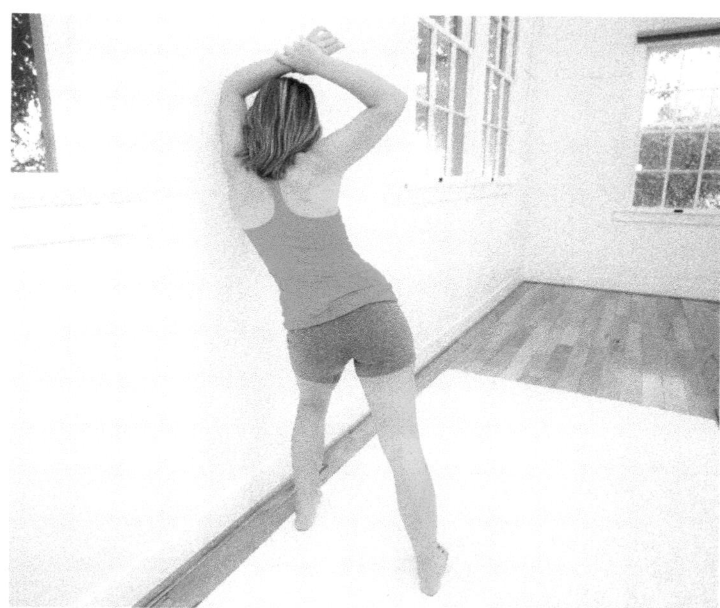

RESISTANCE FLEXIBILITY: Press your elbow into the wall to resist while you lean your body in closer to the wall. Return to the starting position and repeat 10 times on each arm.

HELPFUL REMINDERS

1. Reverse movement for strengthening.
2. The Balancing Stretch muscles help you get into the stretch position.
3. The Opposing Stretch muscles help you get the necessary rotation.
4. Your stretch occurs only while you contract and resist.
5. Your breathing is different in every *type* of stretch.
6. Get perspective from others on how each stretch affects you.

#15 INTERMEDIATE (APPENDIX)

BENEFITS

Health: Prebiotics / Metal Detox
Body Part: Wrist, Hand
Joint: Wrist, Hand
Movement: Lowering
Good Looks: Iridescent, Extreme
Life: Change, Appreciation

MUSCLES

Wrist and Finger Flexors, Forearm Flexors, Biceps, Latissimus Dorsi, Platysma, Risorius, Buccinator,
Action: Extension / Adduction / Inward
Stretch: Flexion / Abduction / Outward

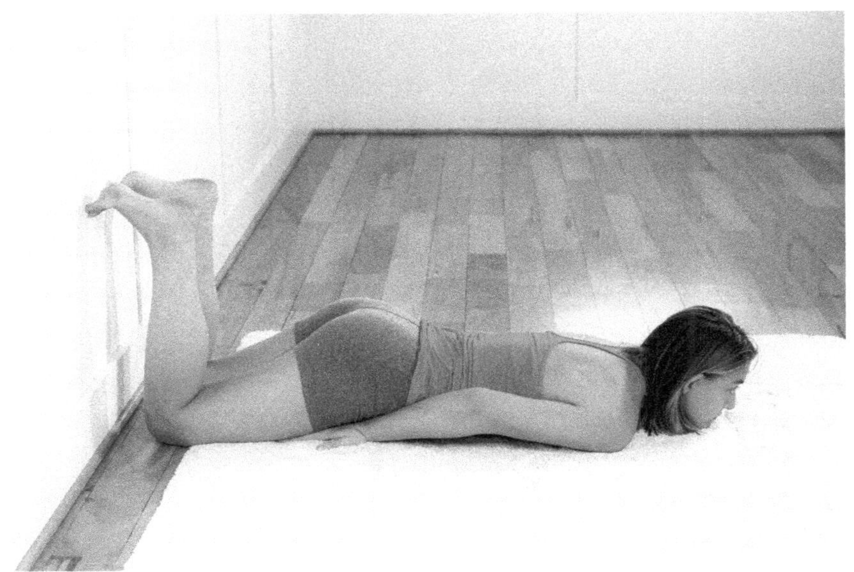

STARTING POSITION: Lie on your belly facing away from a wall. Your knees touch the wall and are bent so that your lowers legs and feet are vertical up against the wall. Your arms are straight and under your body, palms face down.

BALANCING STRETCH

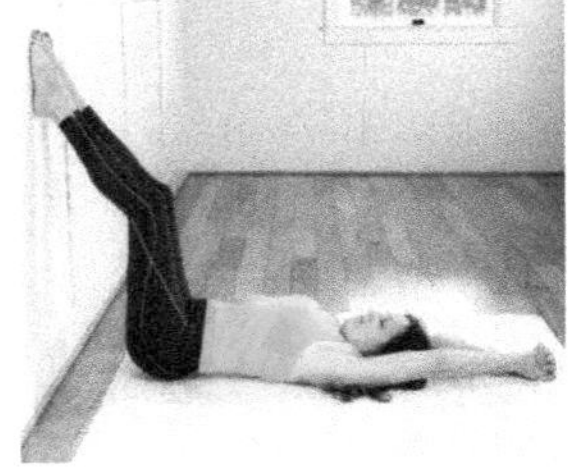

#16 Beginner (Thymus)

OPPOSING STRETCH

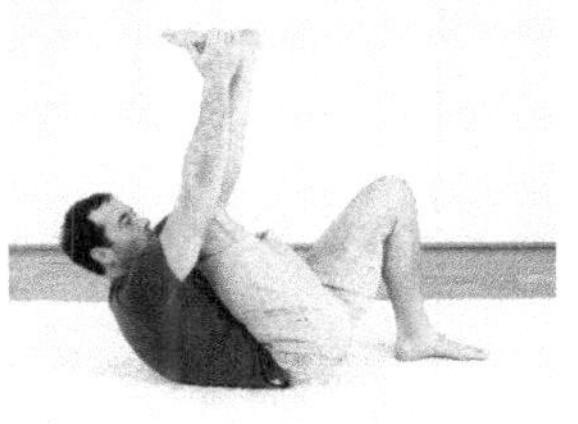

#9 Beginner (Brain)

LOCUST WALL

(TCM)

Organ: Appendix
Tissue: Cartilage
Body Part: Trunk
System: Detoxification
Sensory: Energetic receptors
Yin/Yang Element: Yin Sentient Beings

PERSONALITY (GPT)

Group: Spiritual
Time and Attention: Relative and Outside
High Traits: Change, Integrity, Appreciation, Detox, Centered
Low Traits: Depersonalization, Frantic
Instinct: Calm/ Frightened

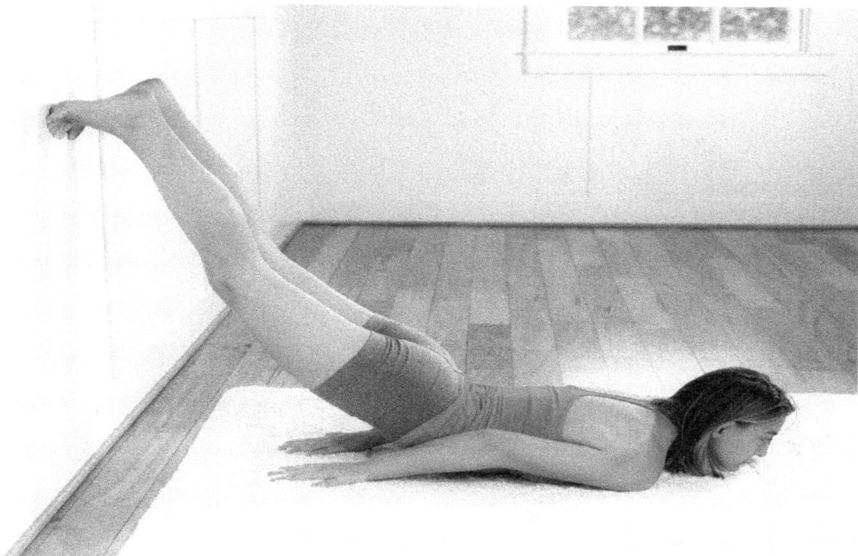

RESISTANCE FLEXIBILITY: Push your hands and arms into the floor to resist while walking your feet up the wall and pressing them against the wall. Return to the starting position and repeat 10 times.

HELPFUL REMINDERS

1. Reverse movement for strengthening.
2. The Balancing Stretch muscles help you get into the stretch position.
3. The Opposing Stretch muscles help you get the necessary rotation.
4. Your stretch occurs only while you contract and resist.
5. Your breathing is different in every *type* of stretch.
6. Get perspective from others on how each stretch affects you.

#15 ADVANCED (APPENDIX)

BENEFITS

Health: Prebiotics / Metal Detox
Body Part: Wrist, Hand
Joint: Wrist, Hand
Movement: Lowering
Good Looks: Iridescent, Extreme
Life: Change, Appreciation

MUSCLES

Wrist and Finger Flexors, Forearm Flexors, Biceps, Latissimus Dorsi, Platysma, Risorius, Buccinator,
Action: Extension / Adduction / Inward
Stretch: Flexion / Abduction / Outward

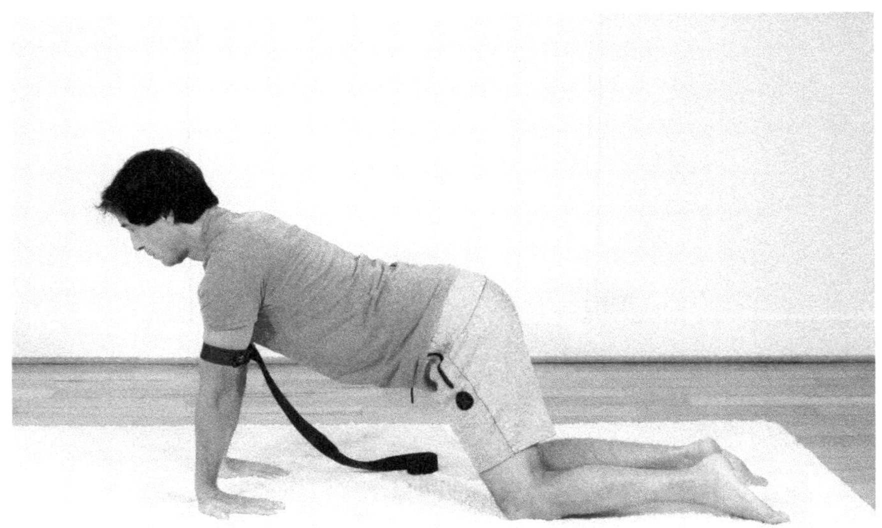

STARTING POSITION: Start on your hands and knees. Point your fingers backwards and lean your torso onto your arms.

BALANCING STRETCH

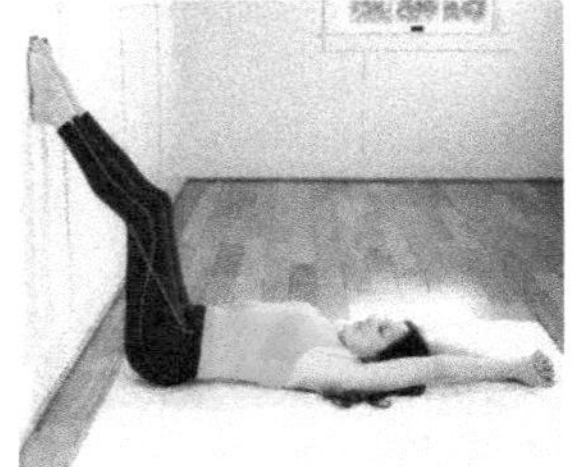

#16 Beginner (Thymus)

OPPOSING STRETCH

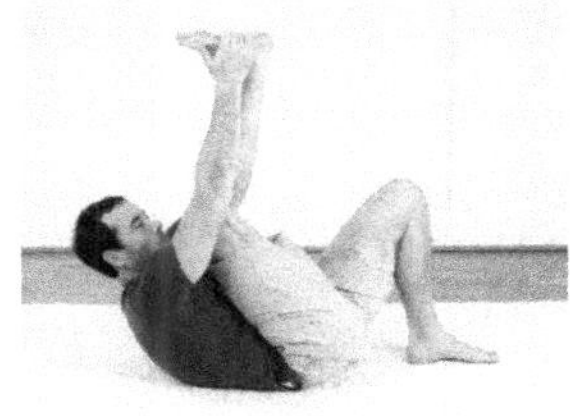

#9 Beginner (Brain)

FREE LOCUST

(TCM)

Organ: Appendix
Tissue: Cartilage
Body Part: Trunk
System: Detoxification
Sensory: Energetic receptors
Yin/Yang Element: Yin Sentient Beings

PERSONALITY (GPT)

Group: Spiritual
Time and Attention: Relative and Outside
High Traits: Change, Integrity, Appreciation, Detox, Centered
Low Traits: Depersonalization, Frantic
Instinct: Calm/ Frightened

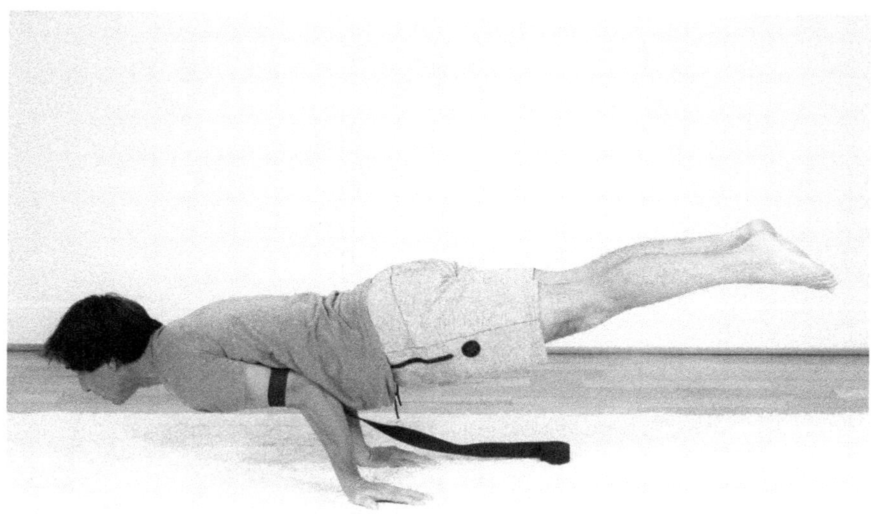

RESISTANCE FLEXIBILITY: Press your hands into the ground to resist while you resist your legs lifting up behind you. Return to the starting position and repeat 10 times.

HELPFUL REMINDERS

1. Reverse movement for strengthening.
2. The Balancing Stretch muscles help you get into the stretch position.
3. The Opposing Stretch muscles help you get the necessary rotation.
4. Your stretch occurs only while you contract and resist.
5. Your breathing is different in every *type* of stretch.
6. Get perspective from others on how each stretch affects you.

#15 ASSISTED (APPENDIX)

BENEFITS

Health: Prebiotics / Metal Detox
Body Part: Wrist, Hand
Joint: Wrist, Hand
Movement: Lowering
Good Looks: Iridescent, Extreme
Life: Change, Appreciation

MUSCLES

Wrist and Finger Flexors, Forearm Flexors, Biceps, Latissimus Dorsi, Platysma, Risorius, Buccinator,
Action: Extension / Adduction / Inward
Stretch: Flexion / Abduction / Outward

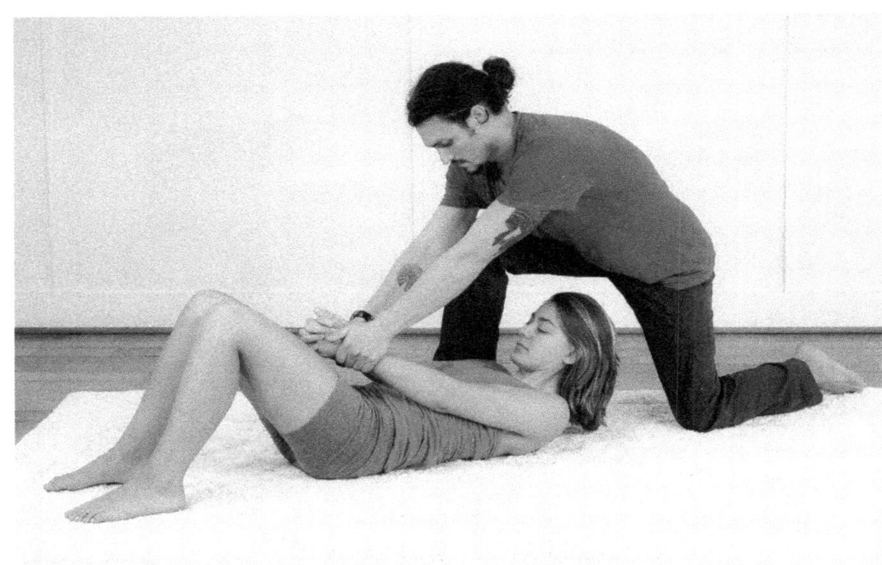

STARTING POSITION: Lie on your back with your arms straight and hands clasped at your waist. The assister is behind you and above your head and grasps your wrists with their hands.

BALANCING STRETCH

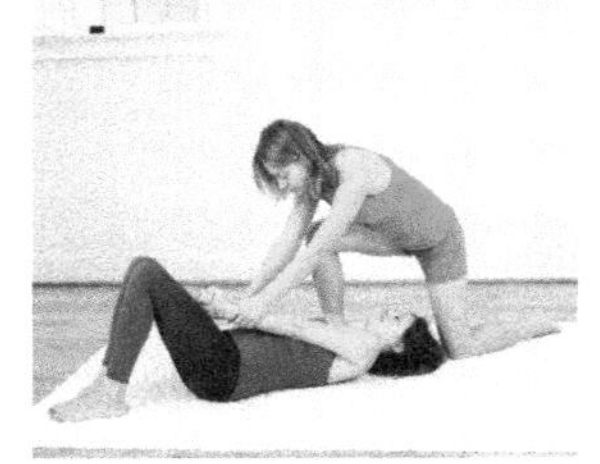

#16 Assisted (Thymus)

OPPOSING STRETCH

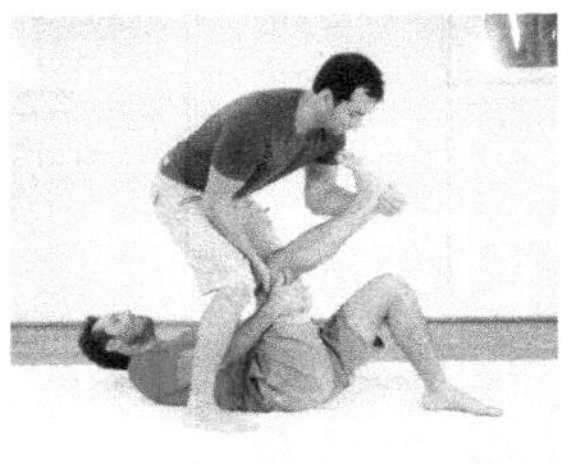

#9 Assisted (Brain)

ASSISTED LAT

(TCM)

Organ: Appendix
Tissue: Cartilage
Body Part: Trunk
System: Detoxification
Sensory: Energetic receptors
Yin/Yang Element: Yin Sentient Beings

PERSONALITY (GPT)

Group: Spiritual
Time and Attention: Relative and Outside
High Traits: Change, Integrity, Appreciation, Detox, Centered
Low Traits: Depersonalization, Frantic
Instinct: Calm/ Frightened

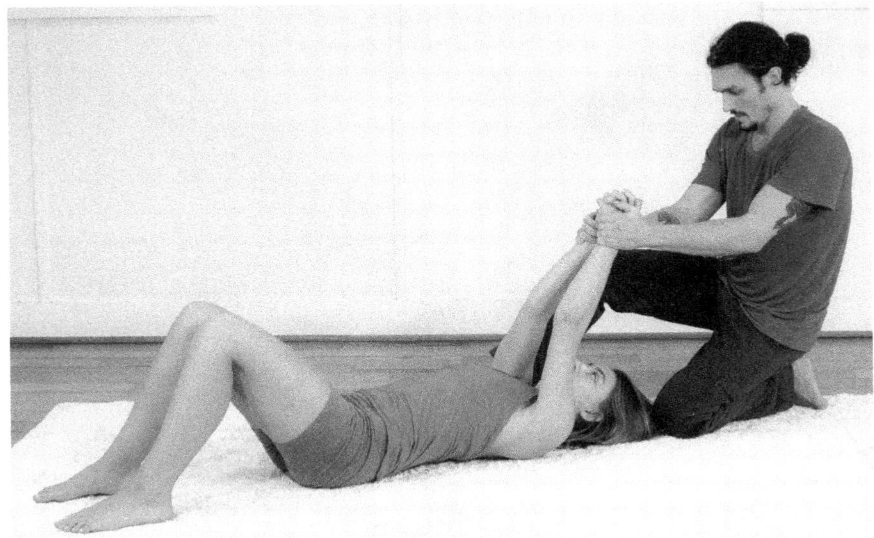

RESISTANCE FLEXIBILITY: Your arms push downwards to resist while the assister pulls your arms upward and over your head. Return to the starting position and repeat 10 times.

HELPFUL REMINDERS

1. Reverse movement for strengthening.
2. The Balancing Stretch muscles help you get into the stretch position.
3. The Opposing Stretch muscles help you get the necessary rotation.
4. Your stretch occurs only while you contract and resist.
5. Your breathing is different in every *type* of stretch.
6. Get perspective from others on how each stretch affects you.

#16 BEGINNER (THYMUS)

BENEFITS

Health: Immunity
Body Part: Wrist, Hand
Joint: Wrist, Hand
Movement: Lifting
Good Looks: Radiant, Healthy
Life: Healing, Diet

MUSCLES

Frontalis, Temporalis, Upper Trapezius, Supraspinas, Infraspinatus, Triceps, Wrist and Finger Extensors
Action: Flexion / Abduction / Outward
Stretch: Extension / Adduction / Inward

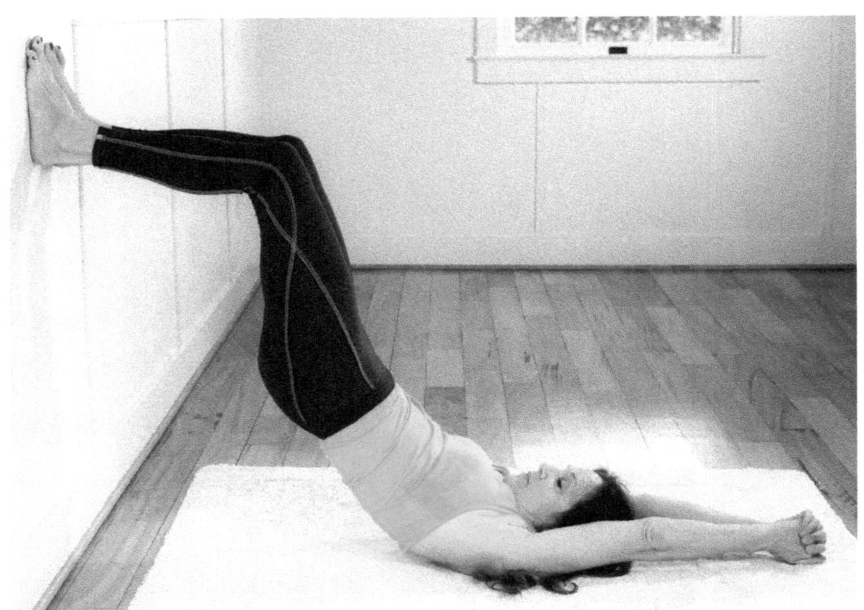

STARTING POSITION: Sit on the floor with a wall beside you. Roll onto your back, then rotate your hips toward the wall as you raise your feet up onto the wall. Lift your torso off the floor.

BALANCING STRETCH

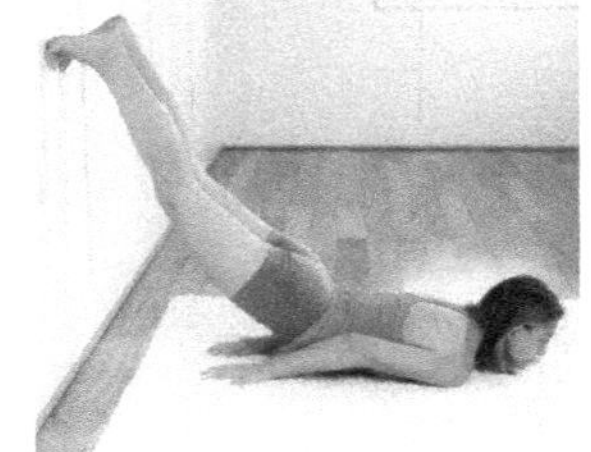

#15 Intermediate (Appendix)

OPPOSING STRETCH

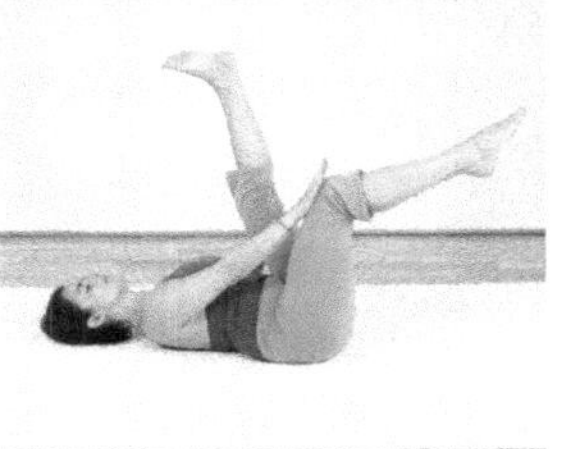

#10 Beginner (Sexual)

ROLLDOWNS

(TCM)

Organ: Thymus-Tonsils- Spleen
Tissue: Lymph Nodes
Body Part: Arms
System: Internal Immune
Sensory: Exteroceptive
Yin/Yang Element: Yang Sentient Beings

PERSONALITY (GPT)

Group: Physical
Time and Attention: Present and Inside
High Traits: Healing, Diet, Dreams, Flexibility, Forgiveness
Low Traits: Menticidal, Illness
Instinct: Love/ Anger

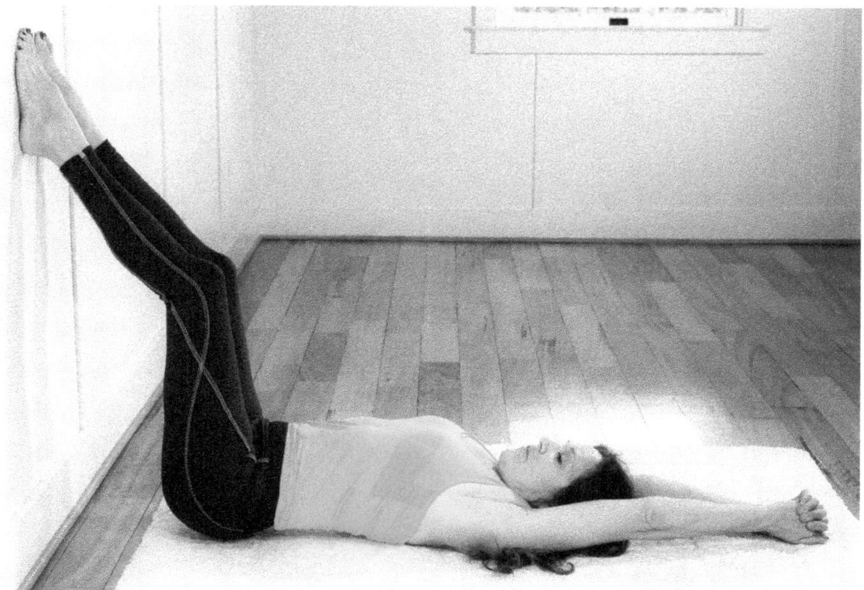

RESISTANCE FLEXIBILITY: Press your feet against the wall, push your arms above your head, and contract your abdominals to resist while you roll down onto the floor, keeping a slight arch in your lower back. Return to the starting position and repeat 10 times.

HELPFUL REMINDERS

1. Reverse movement for strengthening.
2. The Balancing Stretch muscles help you get into the stretch position.
3. The Opposing Stretch muscles help you get the necessary rotation.
4. Your stretch occurs only while you contract and resist.
5. Your breathing is different in every *type* of stretch.
6. Get perspective from others on how each stretch affects you.

#16 INTERMEDIATE (THYMUS)

BENEFITS

Health: Immunity
Body Part: Wrist, Hand
Joint: Wrist, Hand
Movement: Lifting
Good Looks: Radiant, Healthy
Life: Healing, Diet

MUSCLES

Frontalis, Temporalis, Upper Trapezius, Supraspinas, Infraspinatus, Triceps, Wrist and Finger Extensors
Action: Flexion / Abduction / Outward
Stretch: Extension / Adduction / Inward

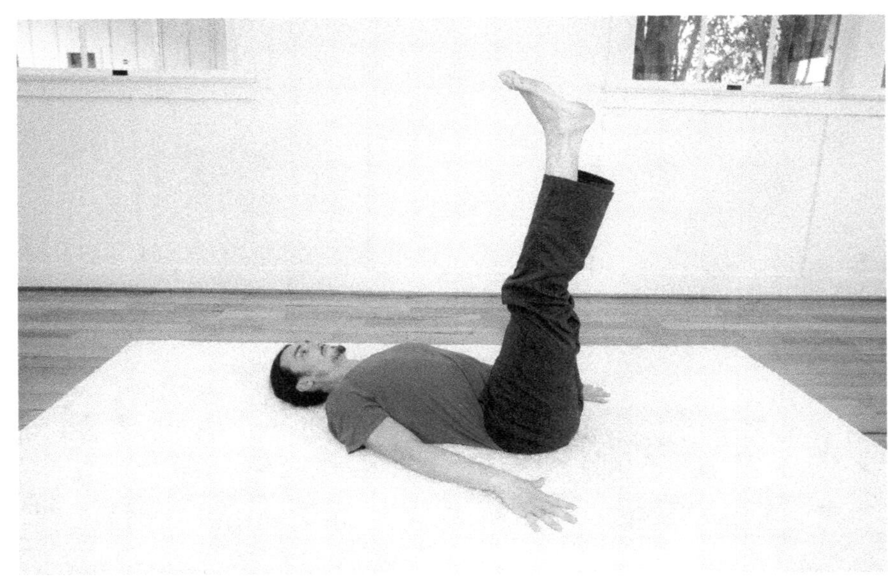

STARTING POSITION: Lie on your back with your legs together and perpendicular to the floor.

BALANCING STRETCH

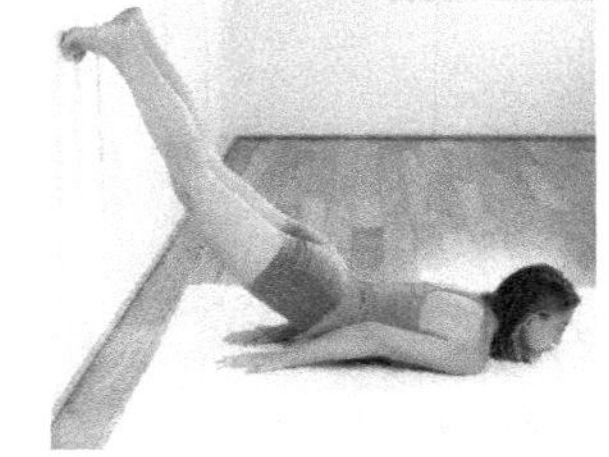

#15 Intermediate (Appendix)

OPPOSING STRETCH

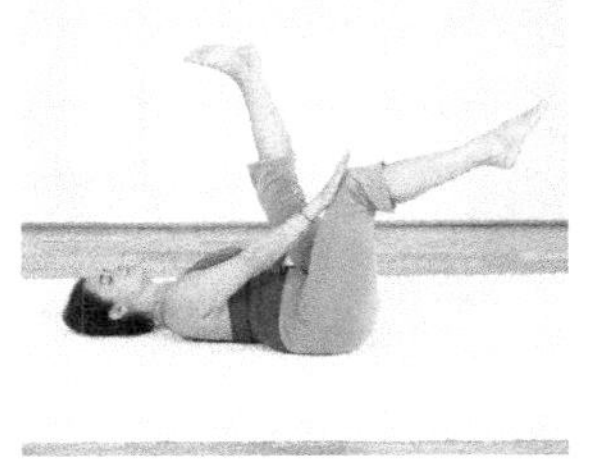

#10 Beginner (Sexual)

SHOULDER STAND

(TCM)

Organ: Thymus-Tonsils- Spleen
Tissue: Lymph Nodes
Body Part: Arms
System: Internal Immune
Sensory: Exteroceptive
Yin/Yang Element: Yang Sentient Beings

PERSONALITY (GPT)

Group: Physical
Time and Attention: Present and Inside
High Traits: Healing, Diet, Dreams, Flexibility, Forgiveness
Low Traits: Menticidal, Illness
Instinct: Love/ Anger

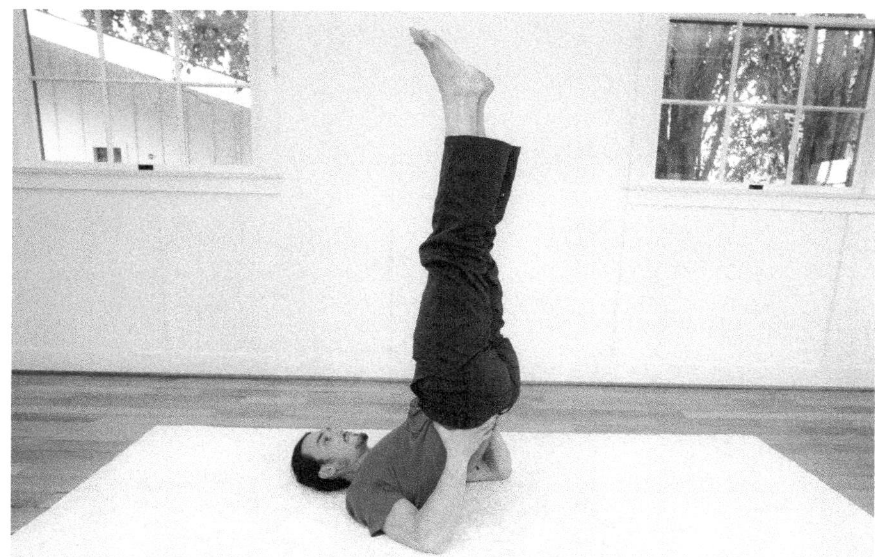

RESISTANCE FLEXIBILITY: Push your elbows into the floor to resist as you roll up onto your upper back, supporting your lower back with your hands. Reach your legs above your head. Return to the starting position and repeat 6 - 8 times.

HELPFUL REMINDERS

1. Reverse movement for strengthening.
2. The Balancing Stretch muscles help you get into the stretch position.
3. The Opposing Stretch muscles help you get the necessary rotation.
4. Your stretch occurs only while you contract and resist.
5. Your breathing is different in every *type* of stretch.
6. Get perspective from others on how each stretch affects you.

#16 ADVANCED (THYMUS)

BENEFITS

Health: Immunity
Body Part: Wrist, Hand
Joint: Wrist, Hand
Movement: Lifting
Good Looks: Radiant, Healthy
Life: Healing, Diet

MUSCLES

Frontalis, Temporalis, Upper Trapezius, Supraspinas, Infraspinatus, Triceps, Wrist and Finger Extensors
Action: Flexion/Abduction/Outward
Stretch: Extension/Adduction/Inward

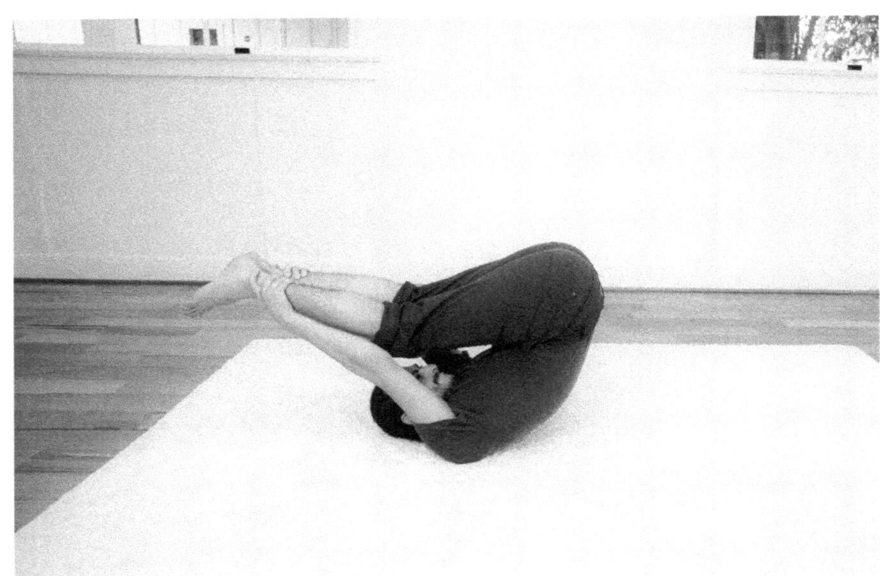

STARTING POSITION: Lie on your back with your legs straight and held above your head. Grasp your ankles with your hands.

BALANCING STRETCH

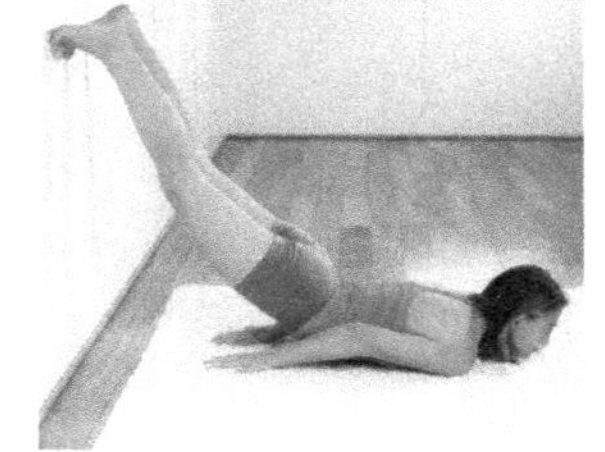

#15 Intermediate (Appendix)

OPPOSING STRETCH

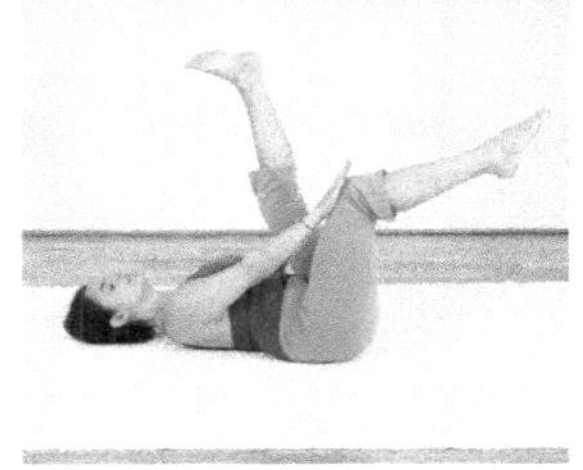

#10 Beginner (Sexual)

PLOUGH

(TCM)

Organ: Thymus-Tonsils- Spleen
Tissue: Lymph Nodes
Body Part: Arms
System: Internal Immune
Sensory: Exteroceptive
Yin/Yang Element: Yang Sentient Beings

PERSONALITY (GPT)

Group: Physical
Time and Attention: Present and Inside
High Traits: Healing, Diet, Dreams, Flexibility, Forgiveness
Low Traits: Menticidal, Illness
Instinct: Love/ Anger

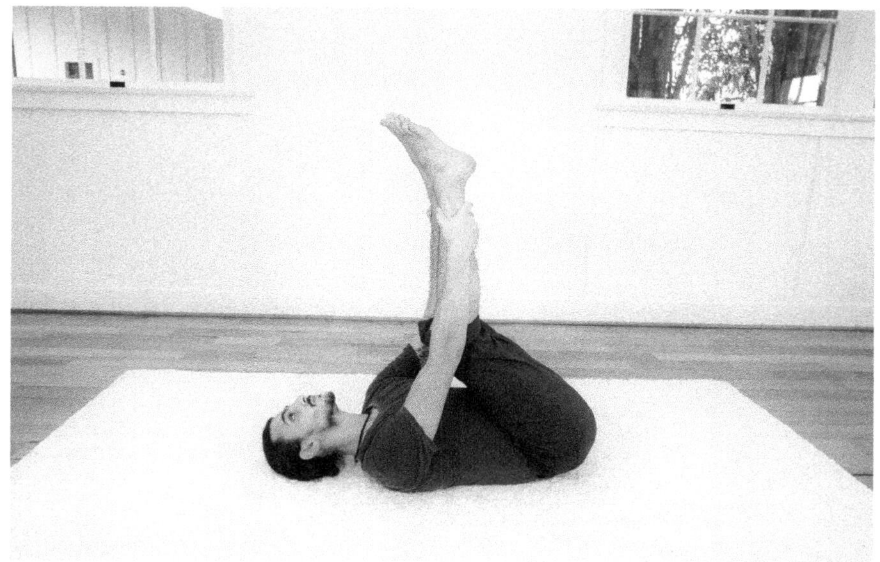

RESISTANCE FLEXIBILITY: Kick your legs away from you, upwards and backwards to resist while your arms pull your legs toward your torso and as you roll back onto your back. Return to the starting position and repeat 10 times.

HELPFUL REMINDERS

1. Reverse movement for strengthening.
2. The Balancing Stretch muscles help you get into the stretch position.
3. The Opposing Stretch muscles help you get the necessary rotation.
4. Your stretch occurs only while you contract and resist.
5. Your breathing is different in every *type* of stretch.
6. Get perspective from others on how each stretch affects you.

#16 ASSISTED (THYMUS)

BENEFITS

Health: Immunity
Body Part: Wrist, Hand
Joint: Wrist, Hand
Movement: Lifting
Good Looks: Radiant, Healthy
Life: Healing, Diet

MUSCLES

Frontalis, Temporalis, Upper Trapezius, Supraspinas, Infraspinatus, Triceps, Wrist and Finger Extensors
Action: Flexion/Abduction/Outward
Stretch: Extension/Adduction/Inward

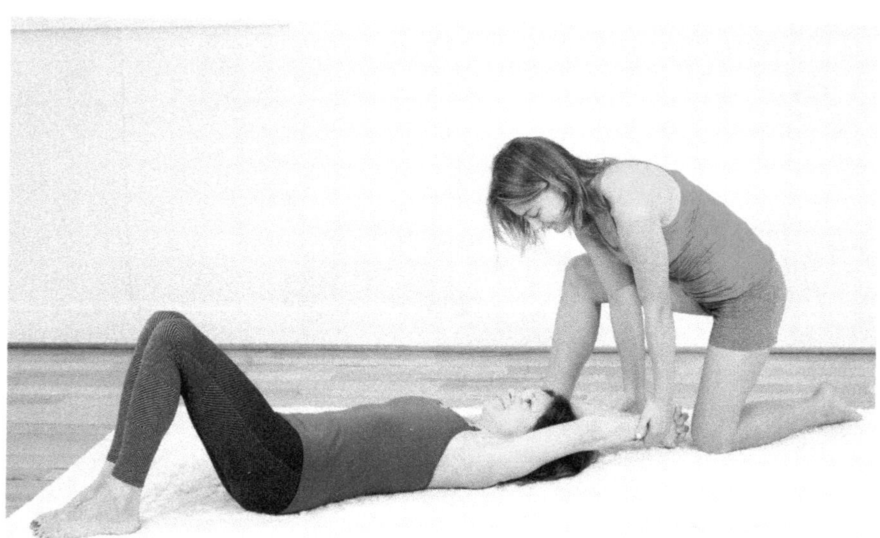

STARTING POSITION: Lie on your back with your arms straight above your head and hands clasped. The assister is behind you and grasps your wrists with their hands.

BALANCING STRETCH

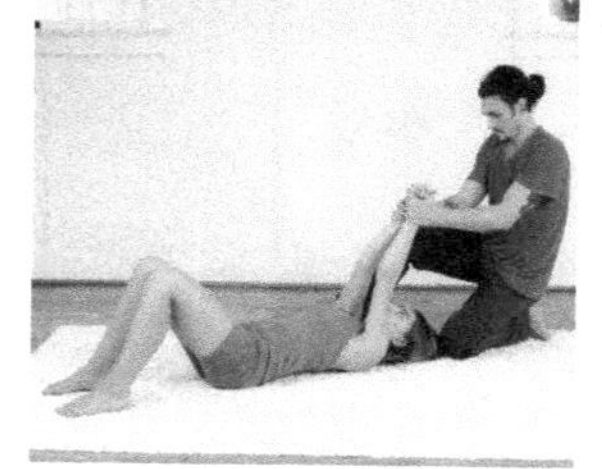

#15 Assisted (Appendix)

OPPOSING STRETCH

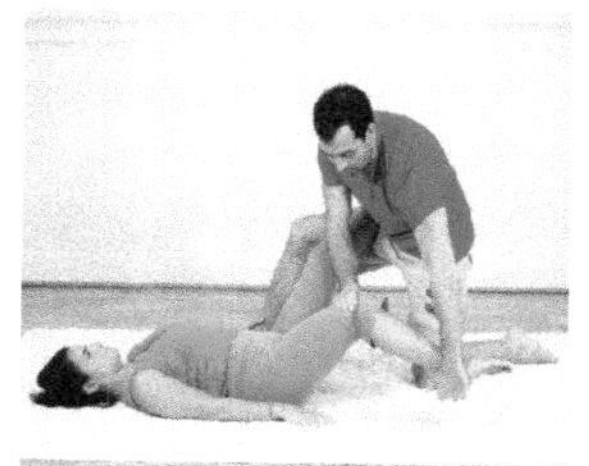

#10 Assisted (Hip Flexor)

ASSISTED HEALING

(TCM)

Organ: Thymus-Tonsils- Spleen
Tissue: Lymph Nodes
Body Part: Arms
System: Internal Immune
Sensory: Exteroceptive
Yin/Yang Element: Yang Sentient Beings

PERSONALITY (GPT)

Group: Physical
Time and Attention: Present and Inside
High Traits: Healing, Diet, Dreams, Flexibility, Forgiveness
Low Traits: Menticidal, Illness
Instinct: Love/ Anger

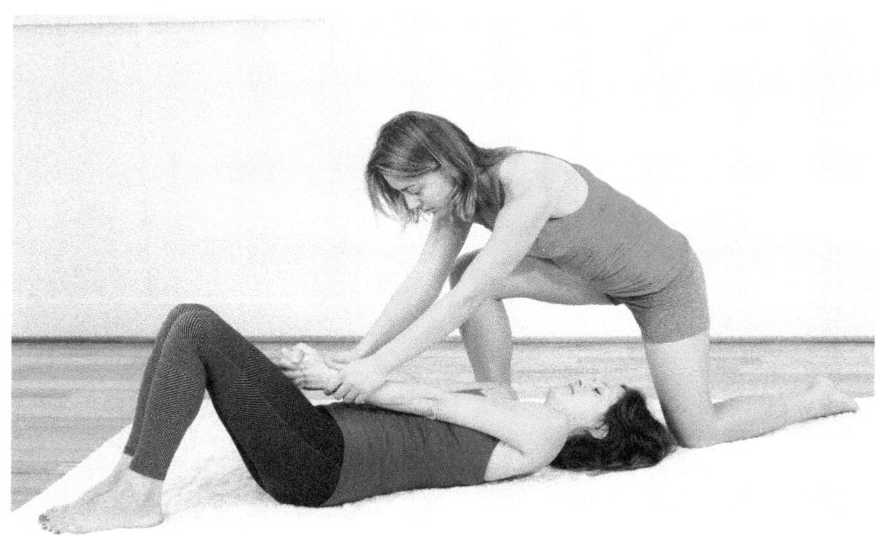

RESISTANCE FLEXIBILITY: Your arms push upwards to resist while the assister lifts your arms over your head down toward your hips. Return to the starting position and repeat 10 times.

HELPFUL REMINDERS

1. Reverse movement for strengthening.
2. The Balancing Stretch muscles help you get into the stretch position.
3. The Opposing Stretch muscles help you get the necessary rotation.
4. Your stretch occurs only while you contract and resist.
5. Your breathing is different in every *type* of stretch.
6. Get perspective from others on how each stretch affects you.

CHAPTER 9
RESISTANCE FLEXIBILITY SERIES
Beginner, Intermediate, Advanced, and Assisted Series

Everyone often does the 16 *types* of stretches in a series. The following are all the Beginner, Intermediate, Assisted and Advanced Resistance Flexibility Stretches in a series for all the 16 types of stretches in each series.

Of course, mix and match to create whatever series of Resistance Flexibility Stretches works best for you.

FREE FIRST MONTH SUBSCRIPTION—

200+ VIDEOS AND EXPLANATIONS

Please check out the 200+ Resistance Flexibility Videos on The Training Archive on our web page:

https://www.thegeniusofflexibility.com/training-archive/join.html

QUESTIONS—> ANSWERS

If you ever have any questions about a stretch, don't hesitate to email us at: https://www.thegeniusofflexibility.com/contact/general.html

...Becoming flexible in all ways *love bob*

Beginner—Starting Position

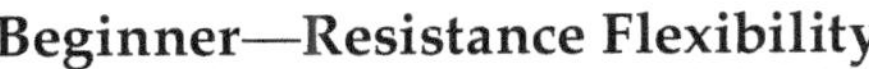

Beginner—Resistance Flexibility

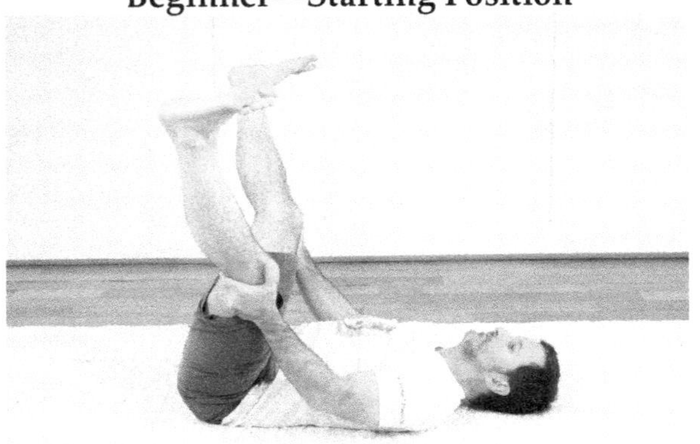

#1 GB

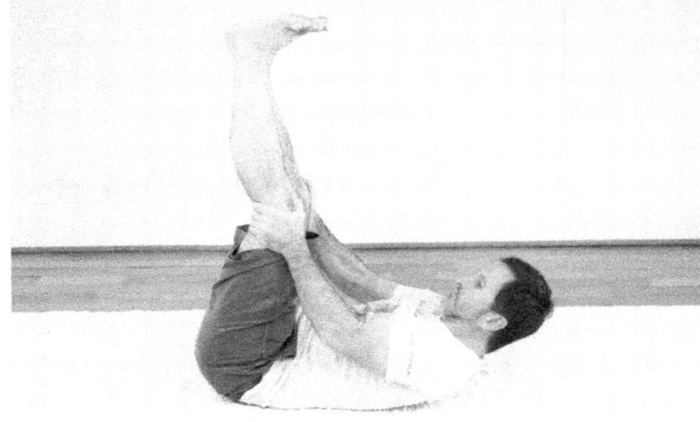

#1 GB

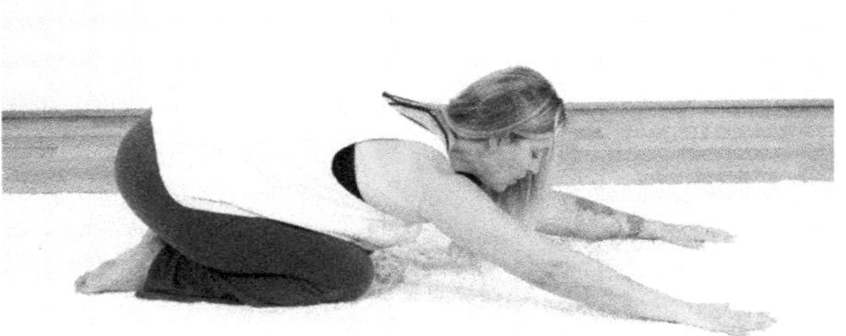

#3 LU

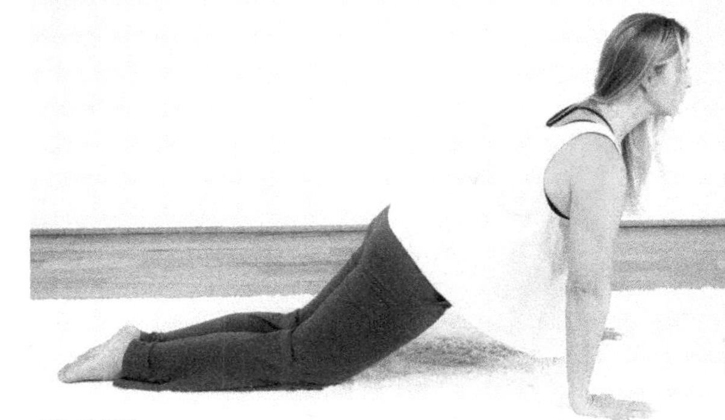

#3 LU

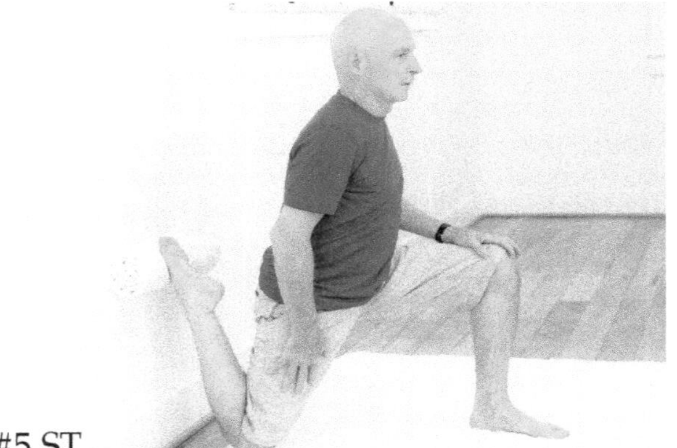

#5 ST

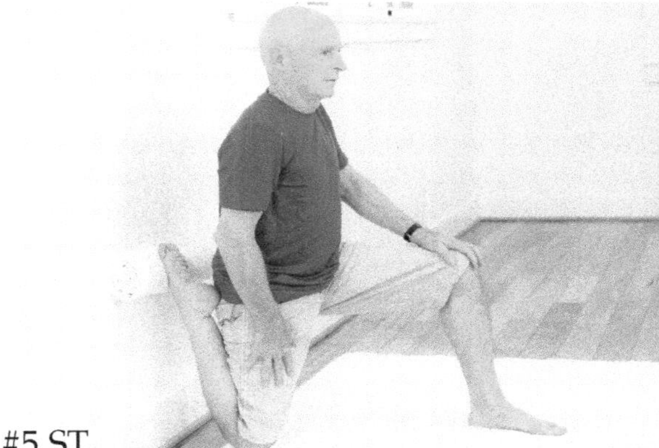

#5 ST

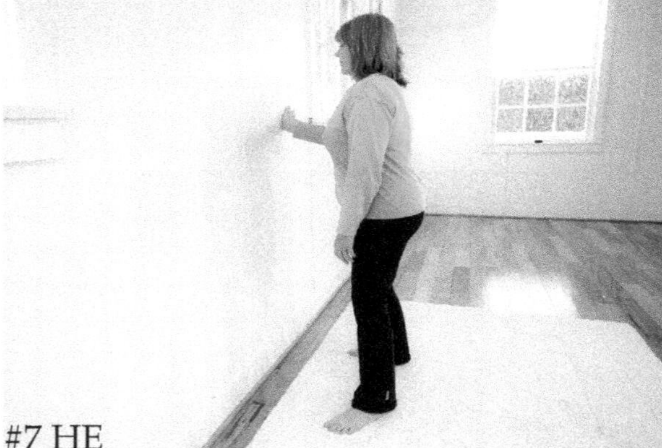

#7 HE

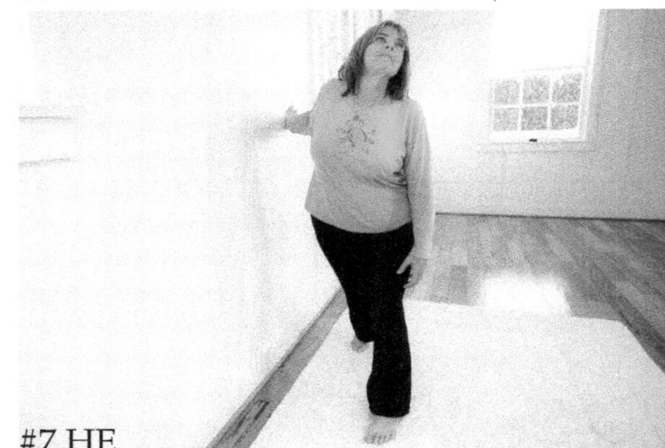

#7 HE

Beginner—Starting Position

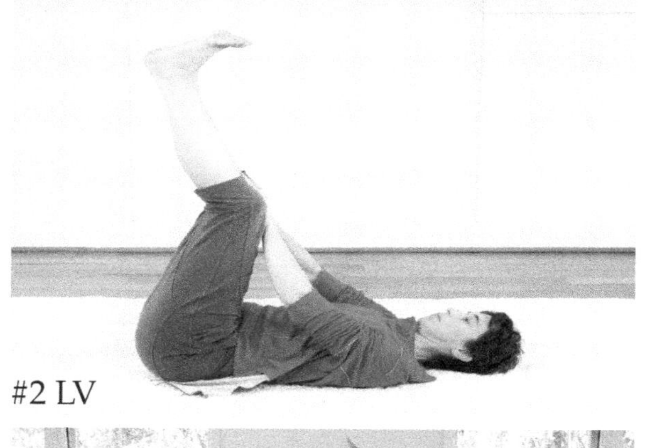
#2 LV

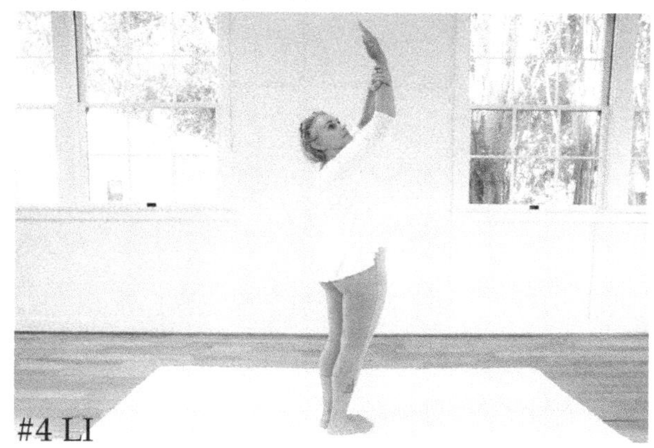
#4 LI

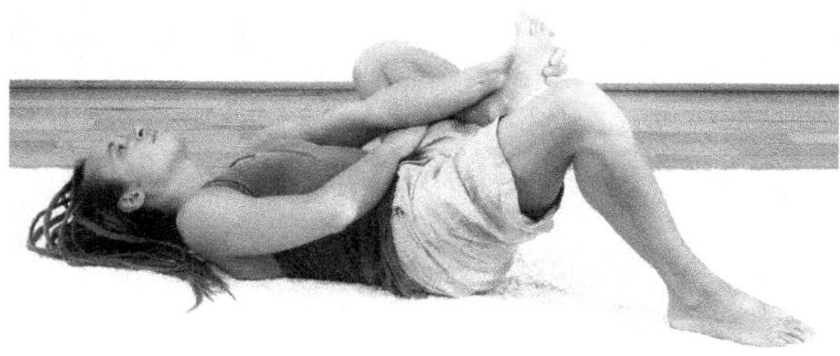
#6 PA

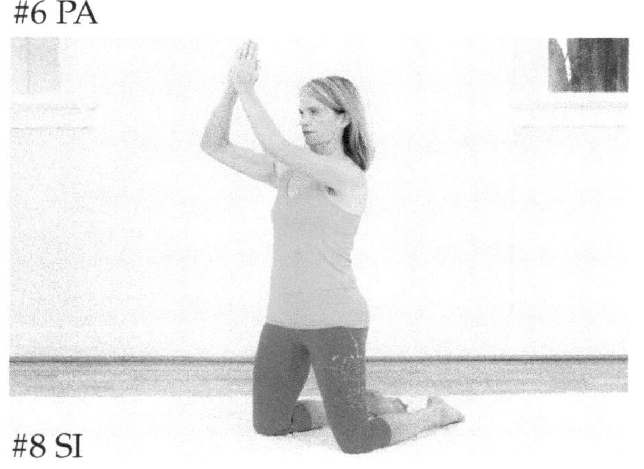
#8 SI

Beginner—Resistance Flexibility

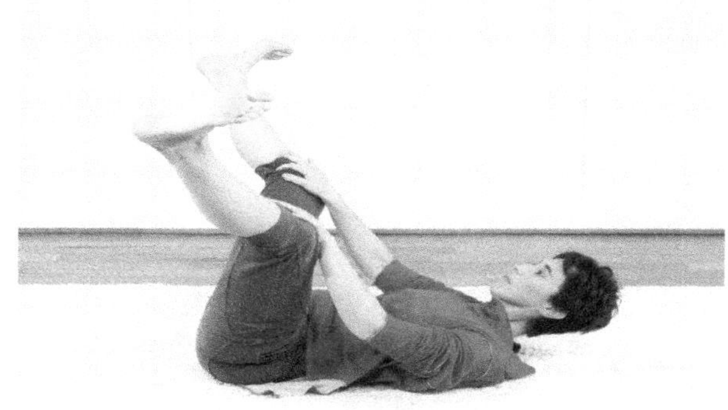
#2 LV

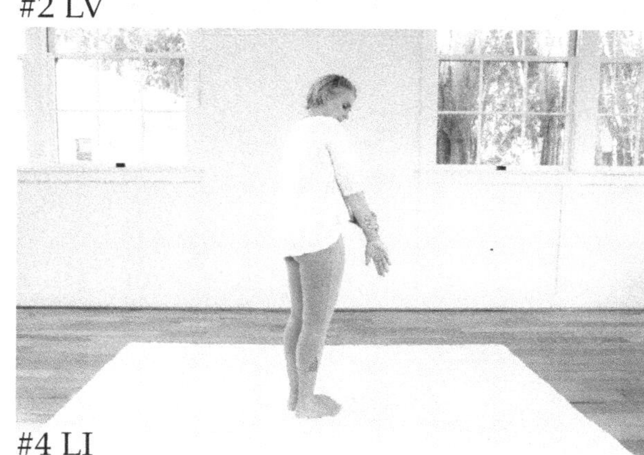
#4 LI

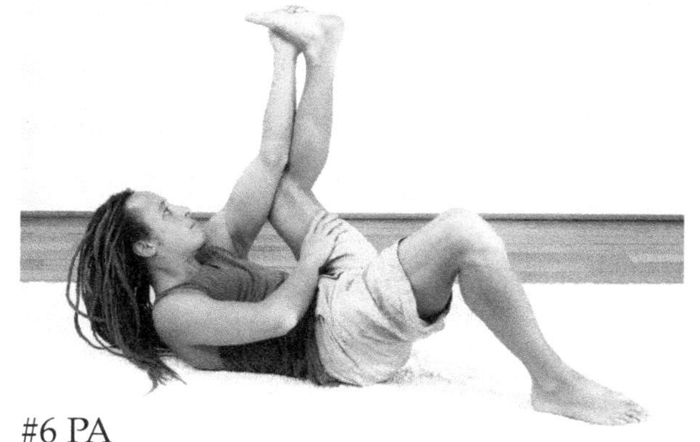
#6 PA

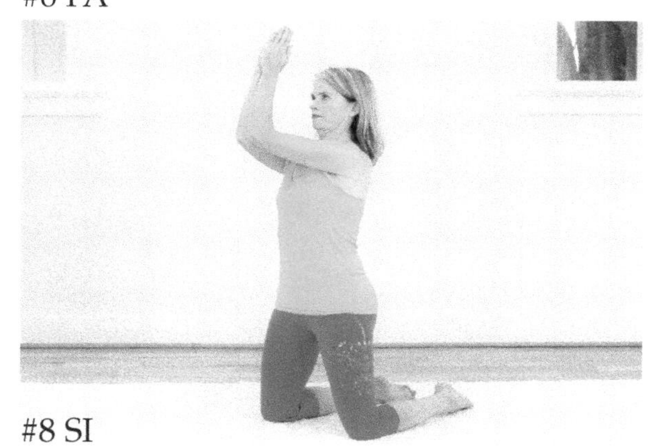
#8 SI

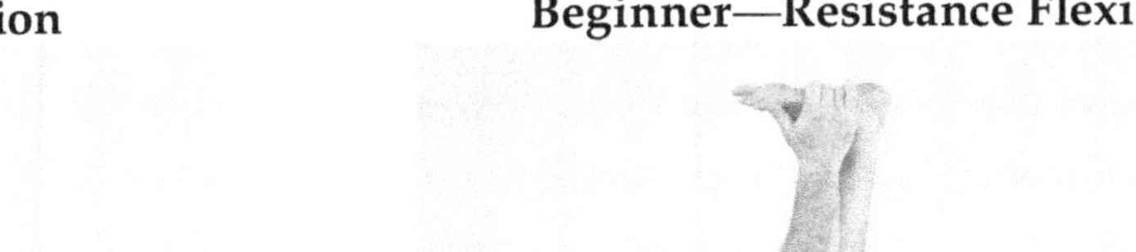

Beginner—Starting Position

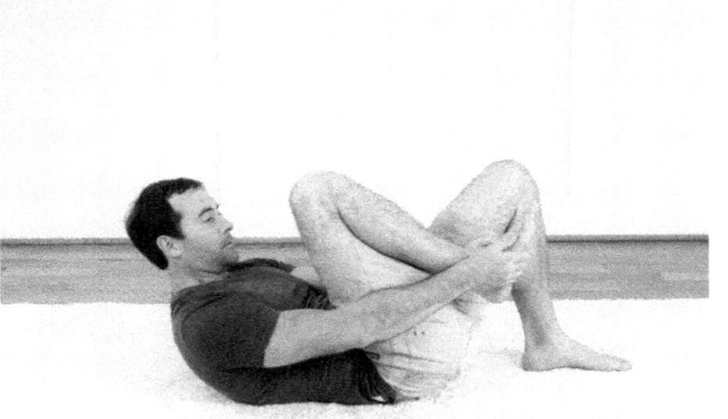

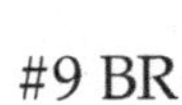

#9 BR

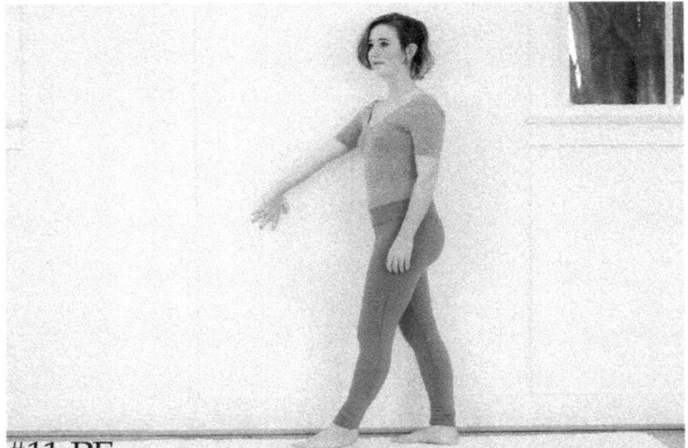

#11 PE

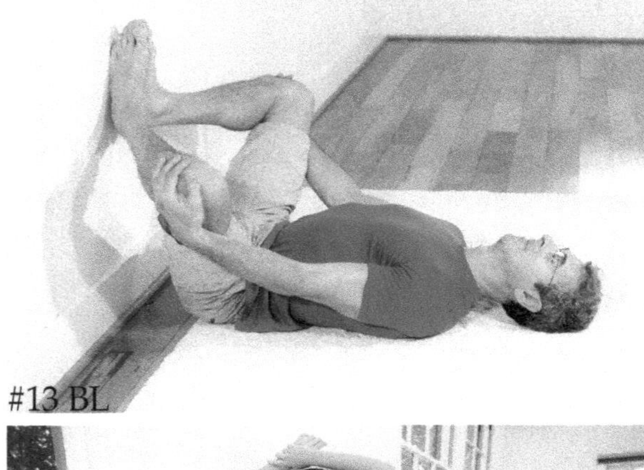

#13 BL

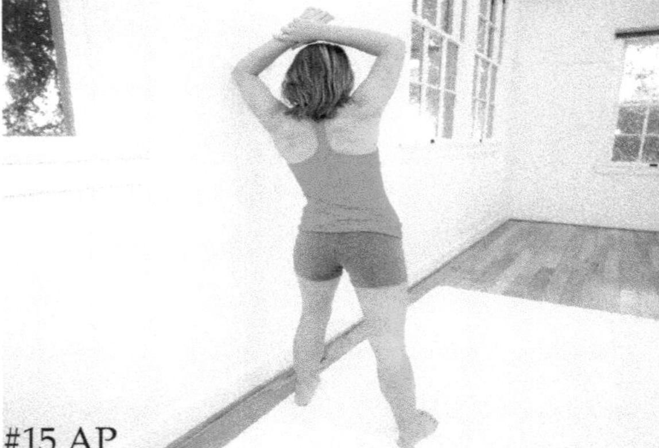

#15 AP

Beginner—Resistance Flexibility

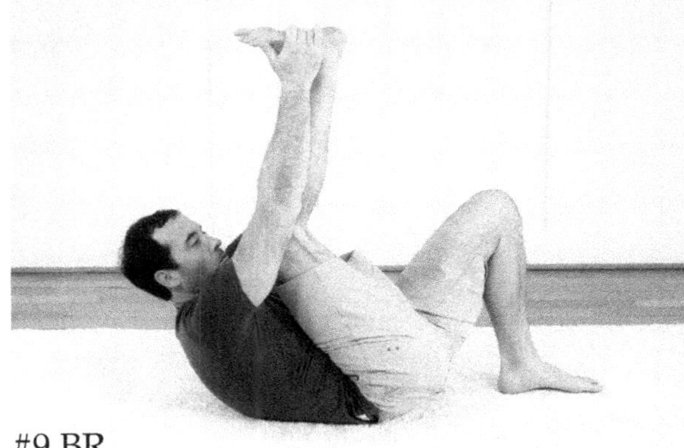

#9 BR

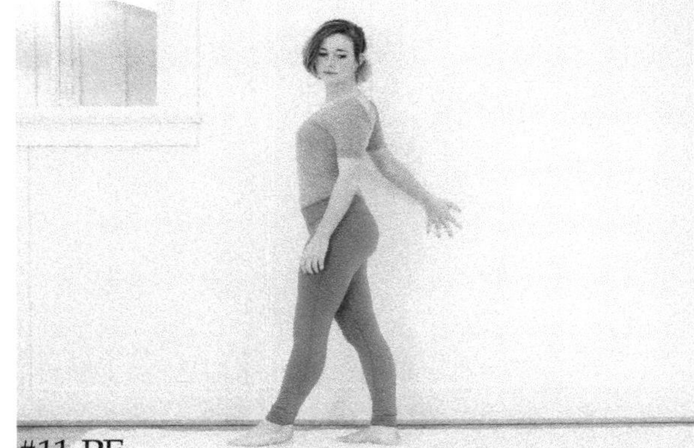

#11 PE

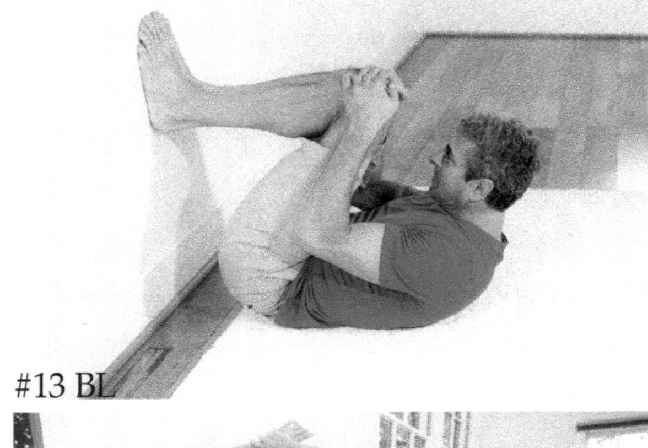

#13 BL

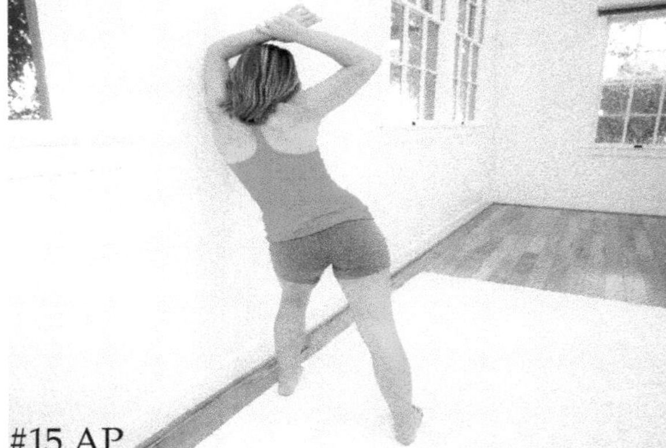

#15 AP

Beginner—Starting Position

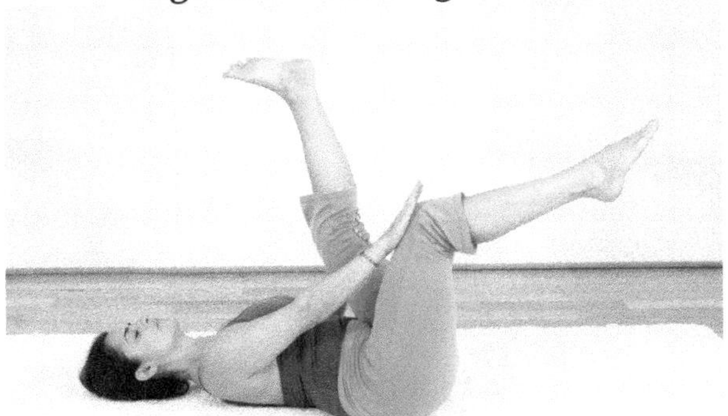

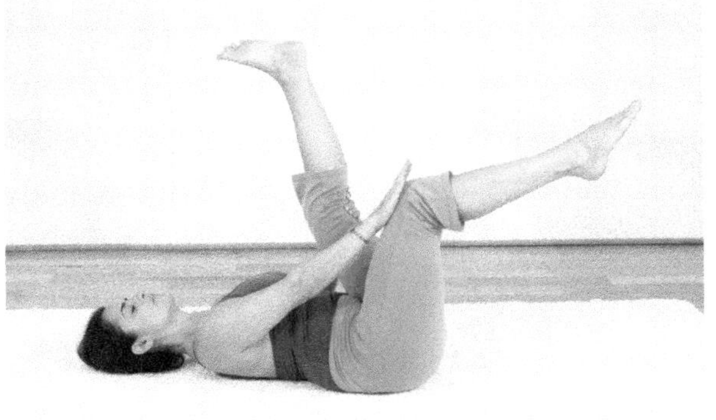

#10 SE

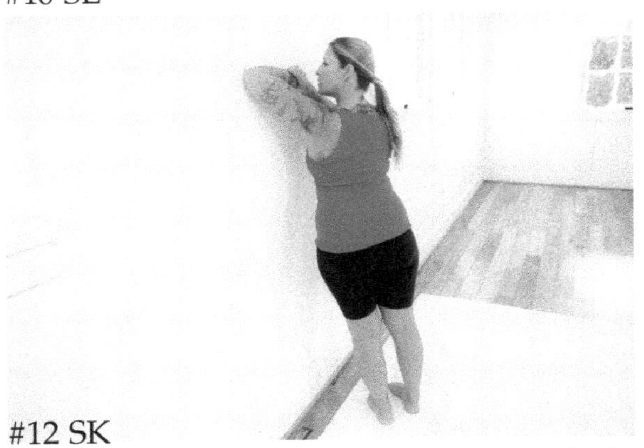

#12 SK

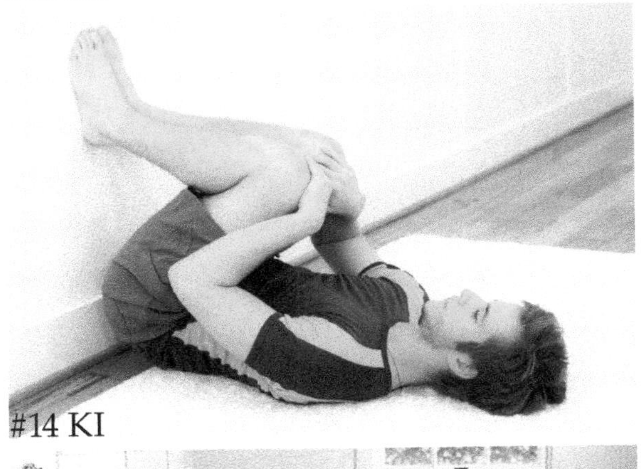

#14 KI

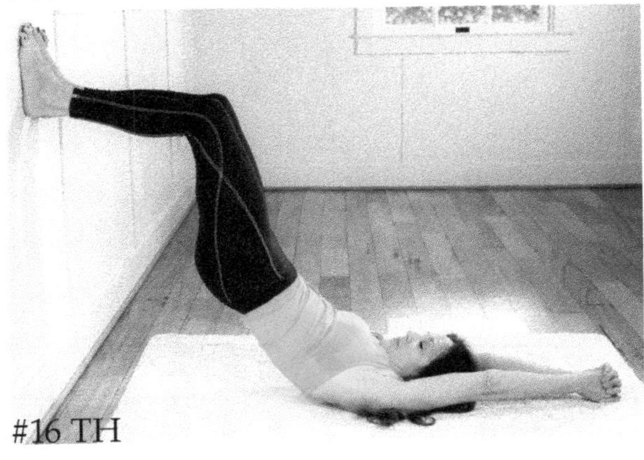

#16 TH

Beginner—Resistance Flexibility

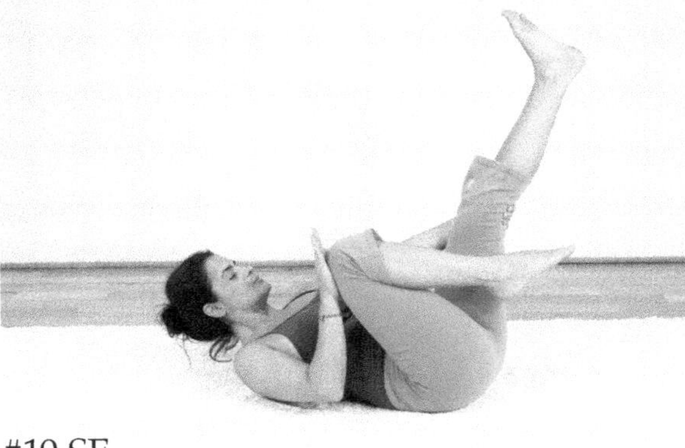

#10 SE

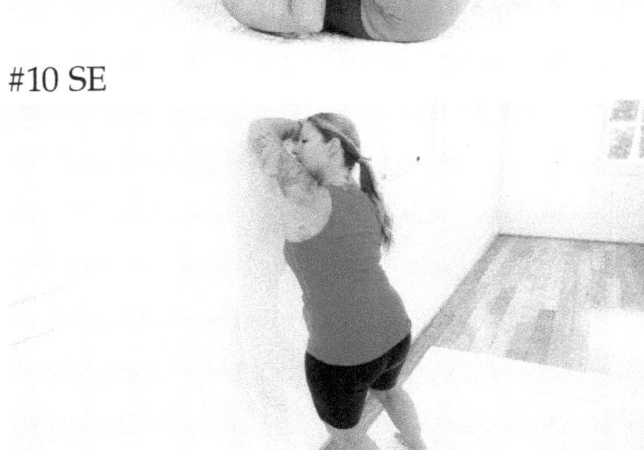

#12 SK

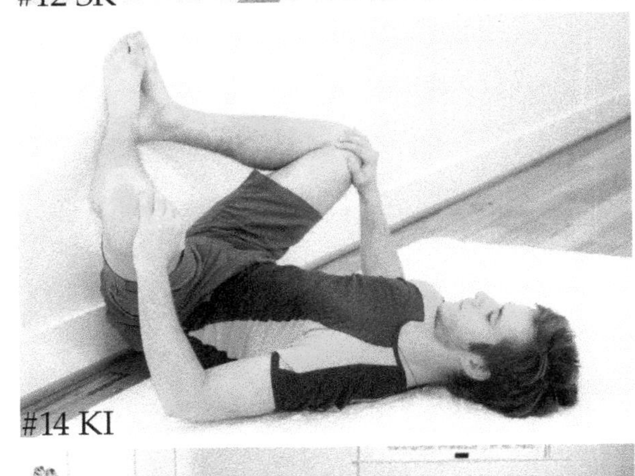

#14 KI

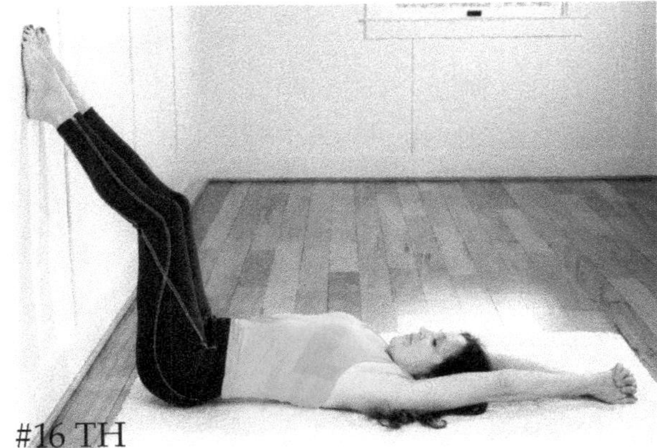

#16 TH

Intermediate—Starting Position

#1 GB

#3 LU

#5 ST

#7 HE

Intermediate—Resistance Flexibility

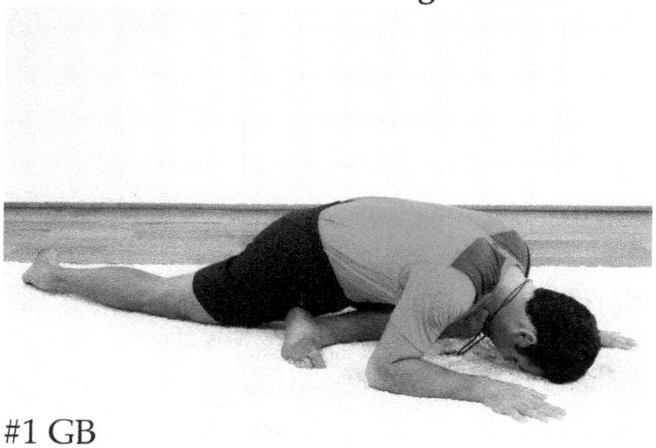

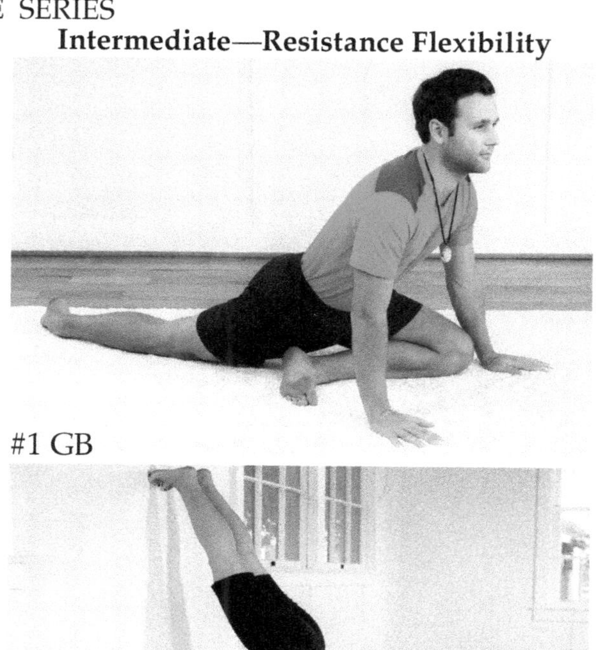

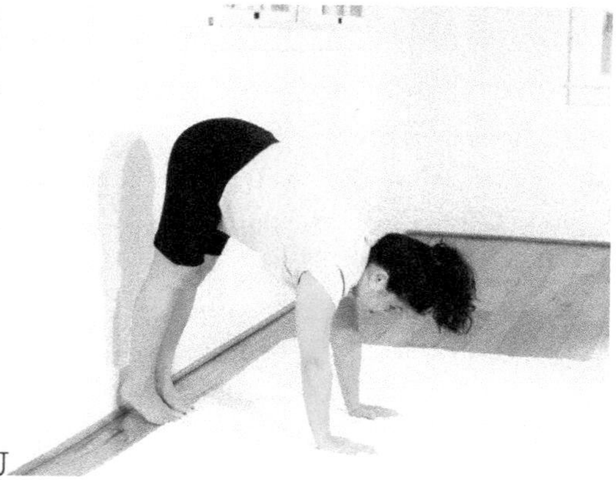

#1 GB

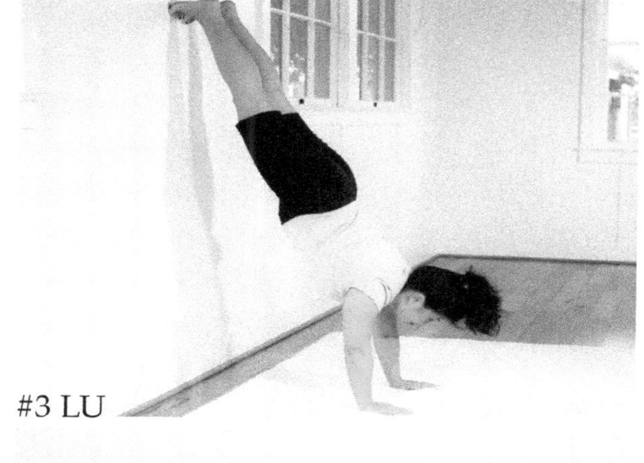

#3 LU

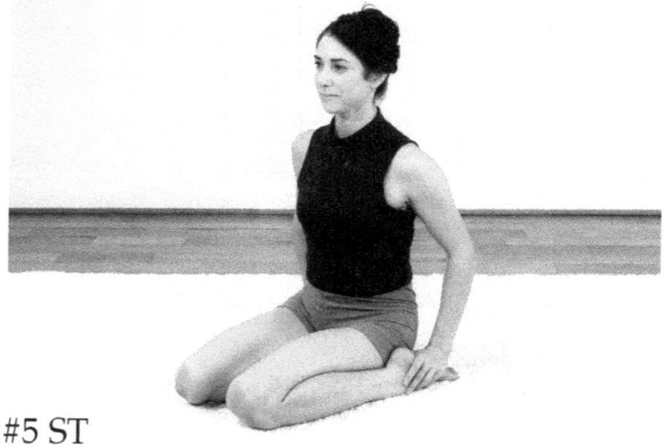

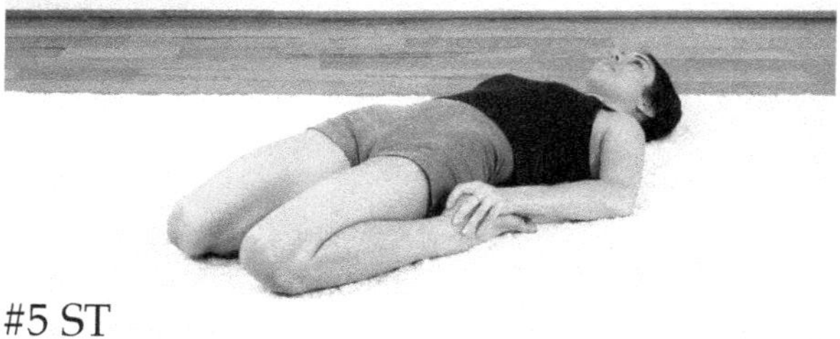

#5 ST

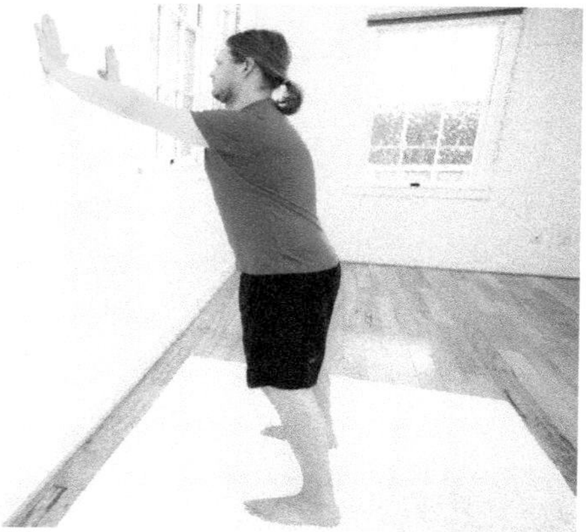

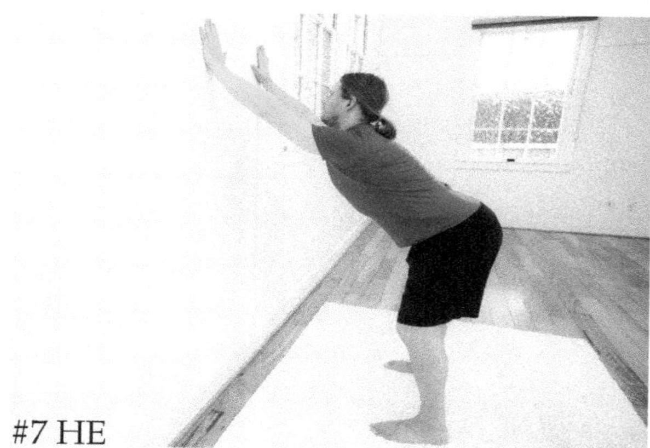

#7 HE

Intermediate—Starting Position

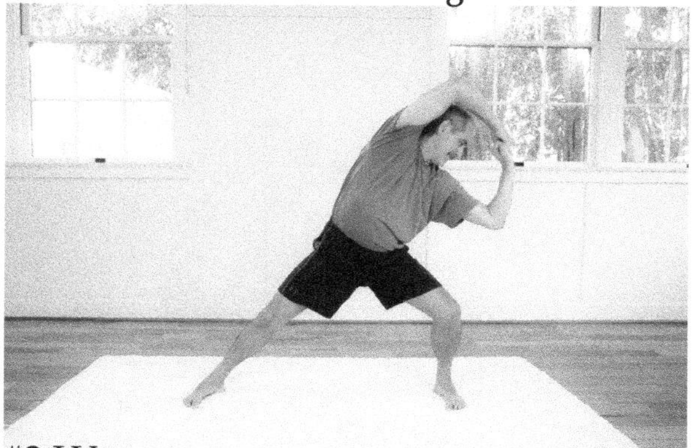

Intermediate—Resistance Flexibility

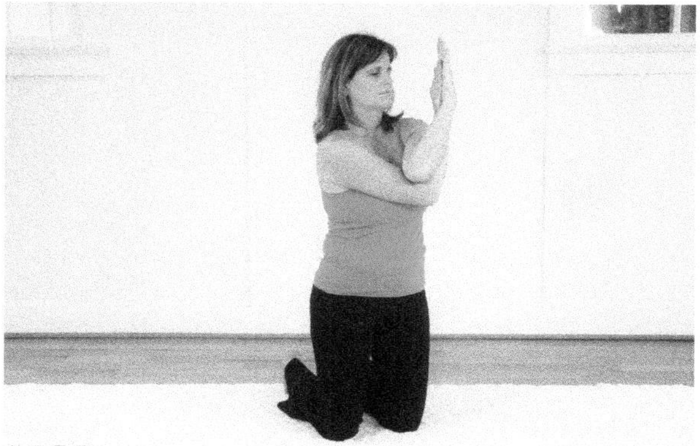

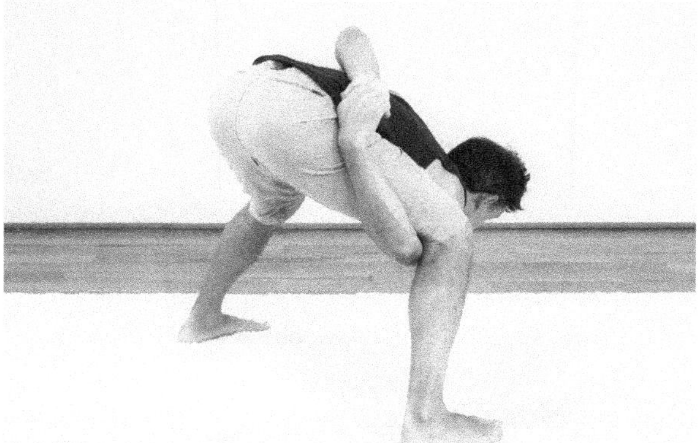

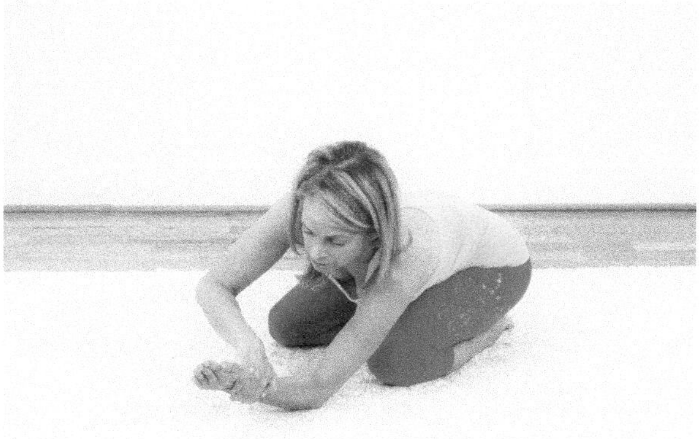

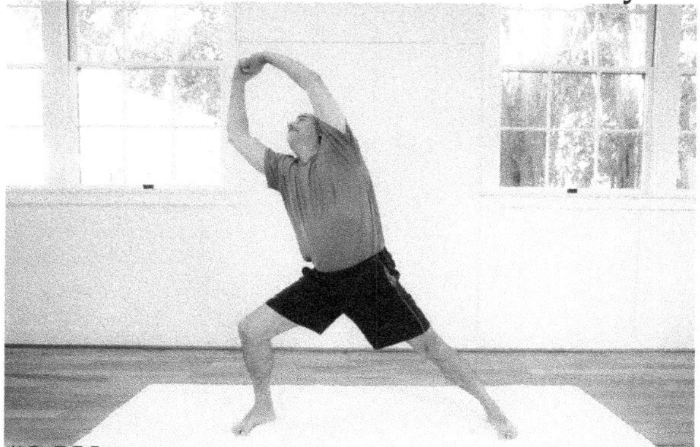

#2 LV

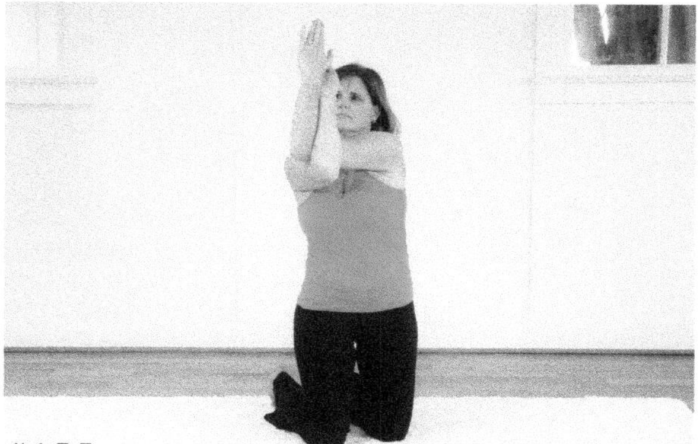

#2 LV

#4 LI

#4 LI

#6 PA

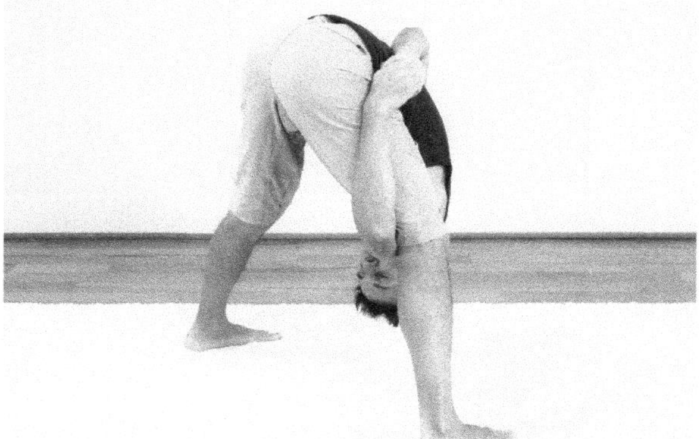

#6 PA

#8 SI

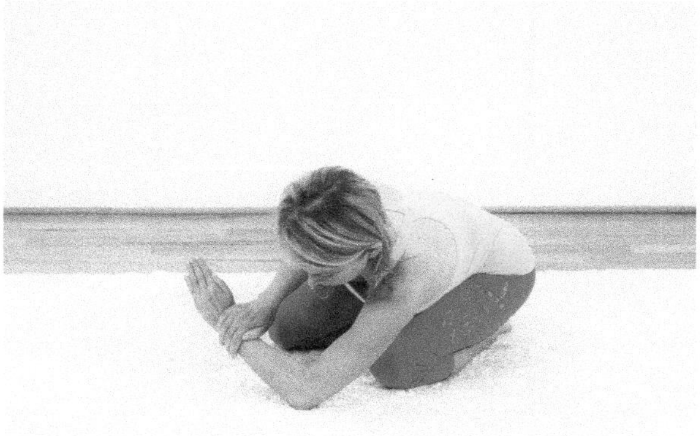

#8 SI

Intermediate—Starting Position

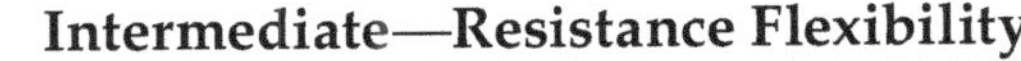

Intermediate—Resistance Flexibility

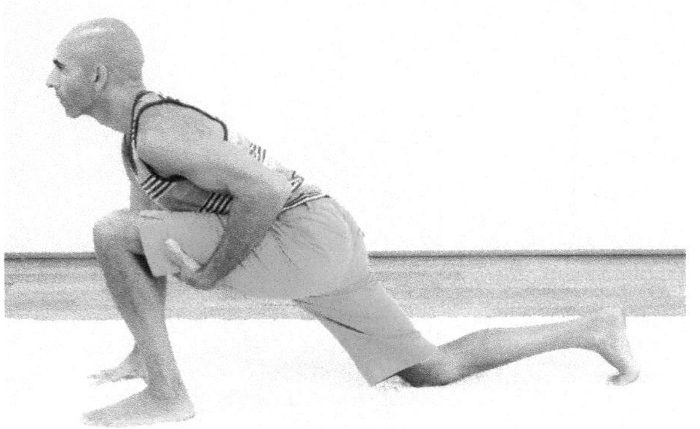
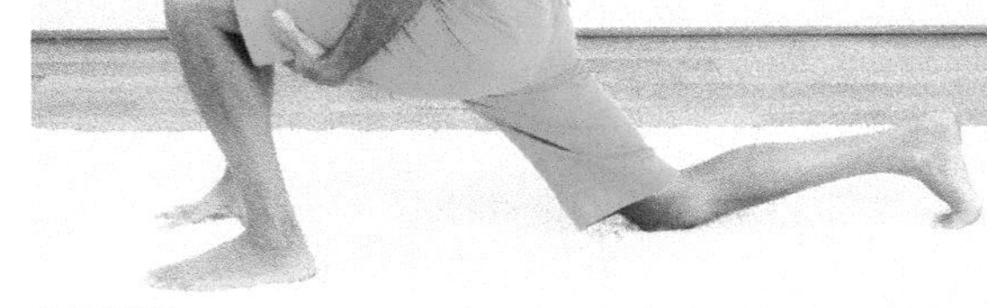

#9 BR

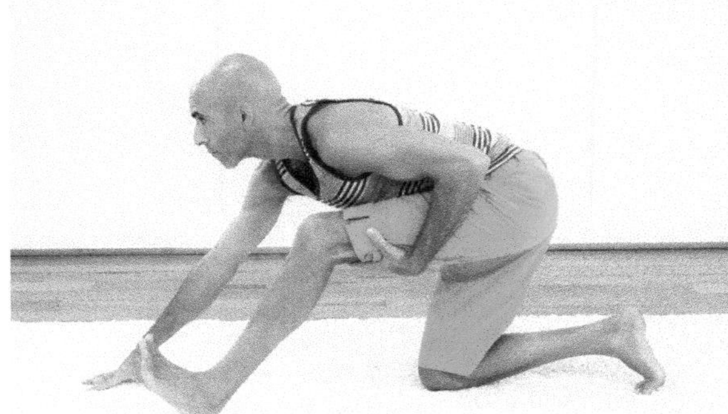

#9 BR

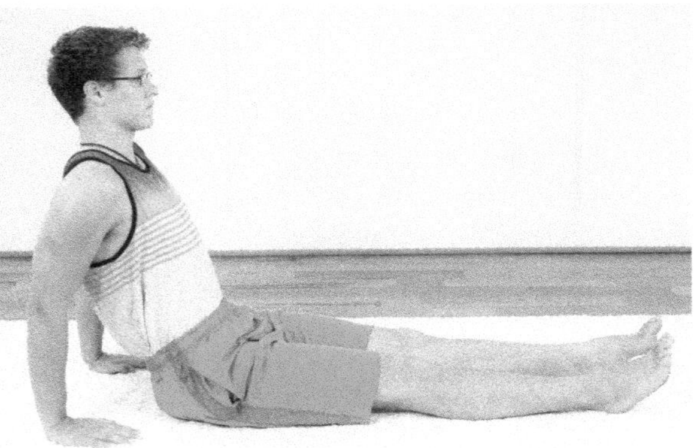
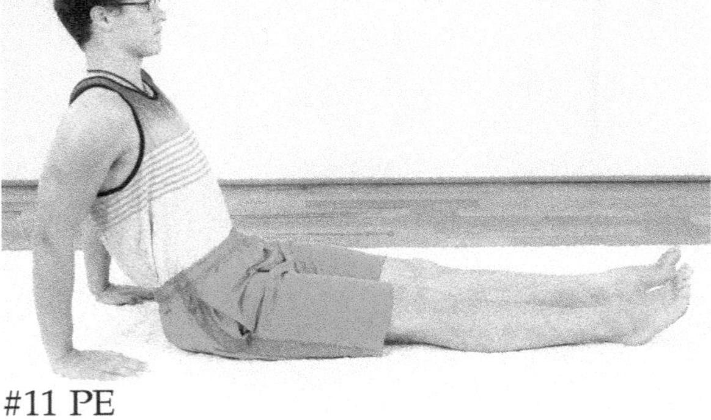

#11 PE

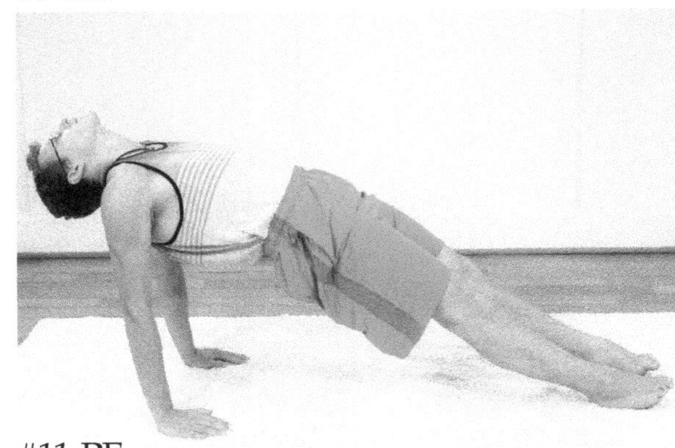

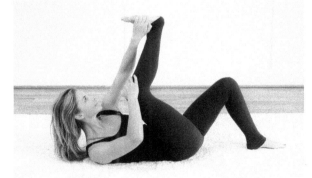

#11 PE

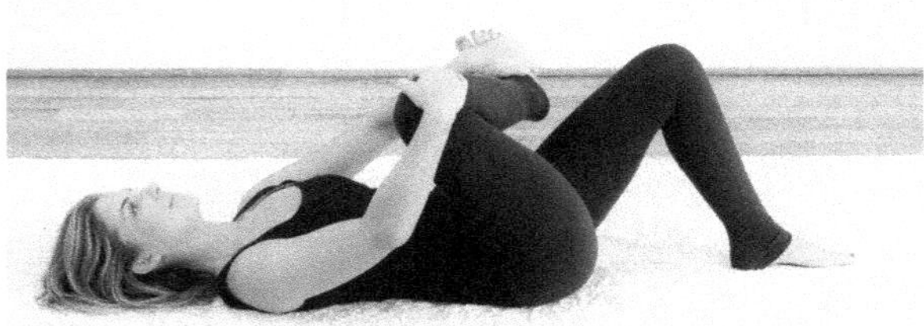
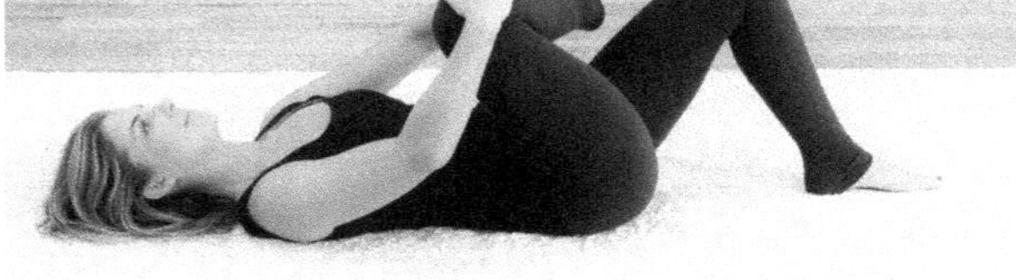

#13 BL

#13 BL

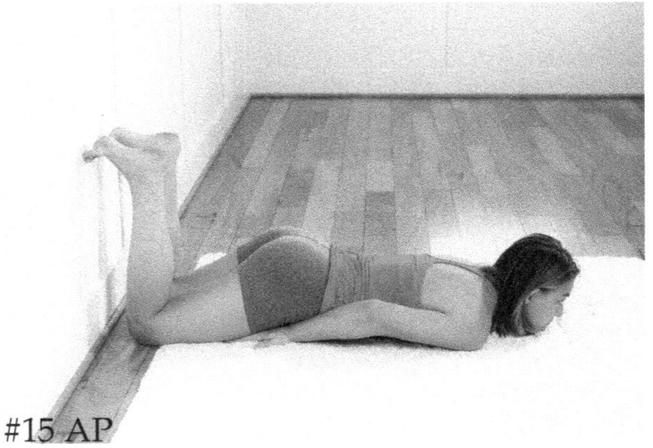

#15 AP

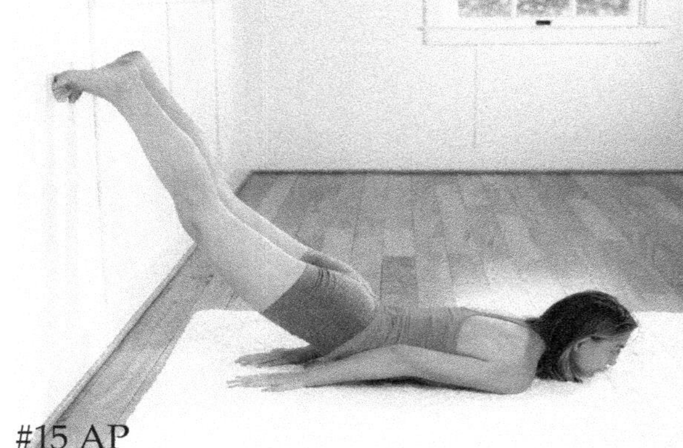

#15 AP

Intermediate—Starting Position

Intermediate—Resistance Flexibility

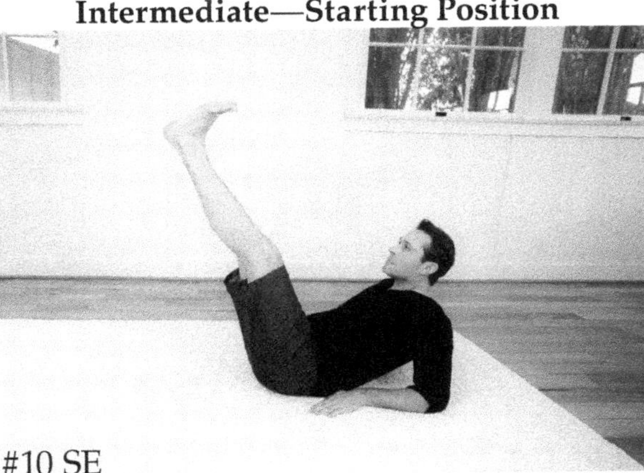

#10 SE

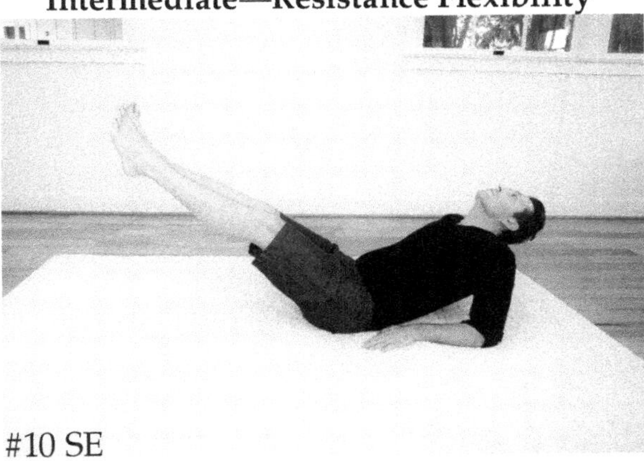

#10 SE

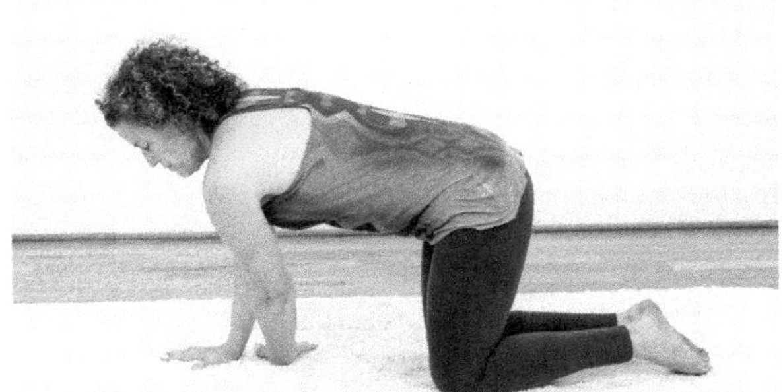

#12 SK

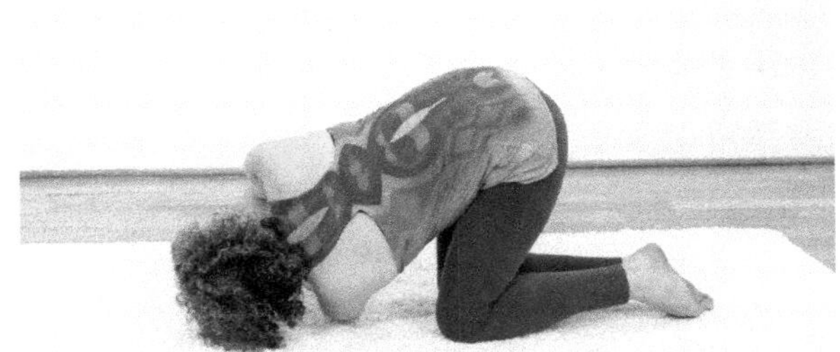

#12 SK

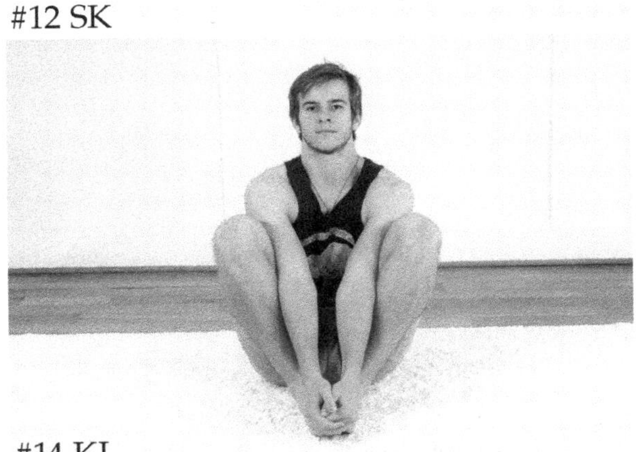

#14 KI

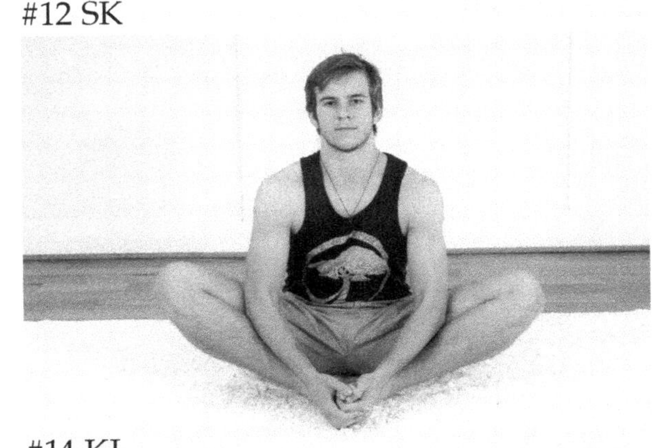

#14 KI

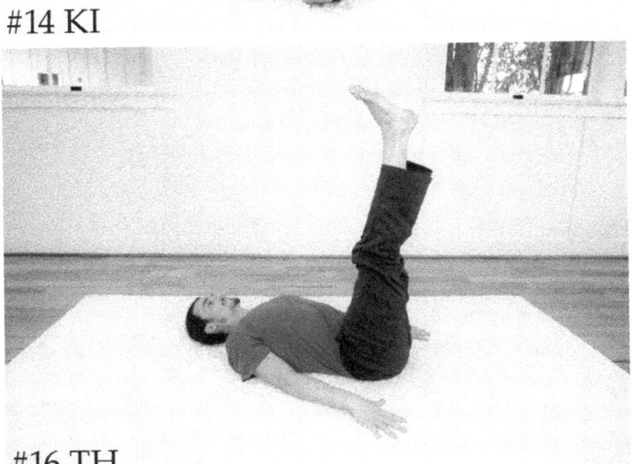

#16 TH

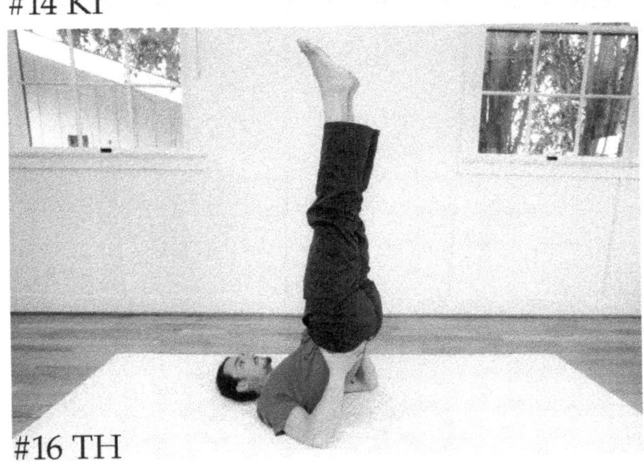

#16 TH

Advanced—Starting Position

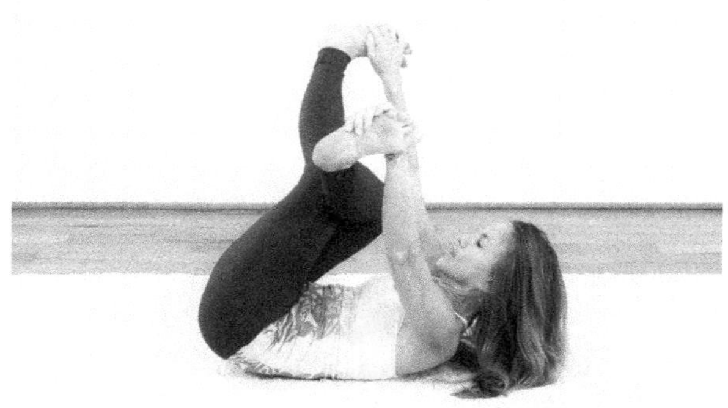

#1 GB

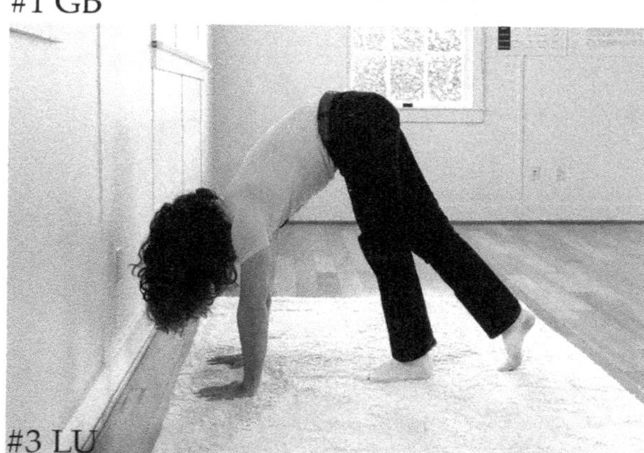

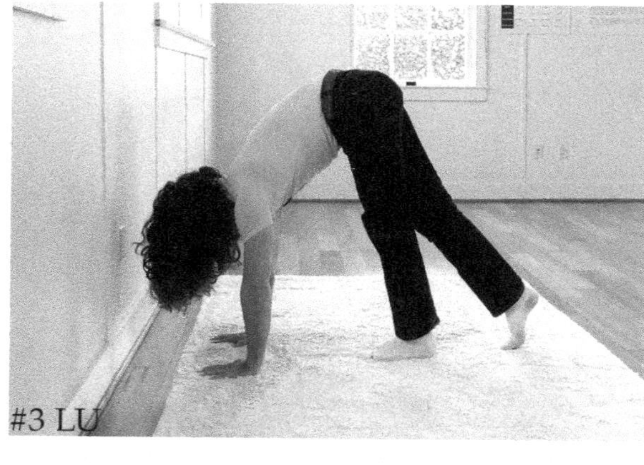

#3 LU

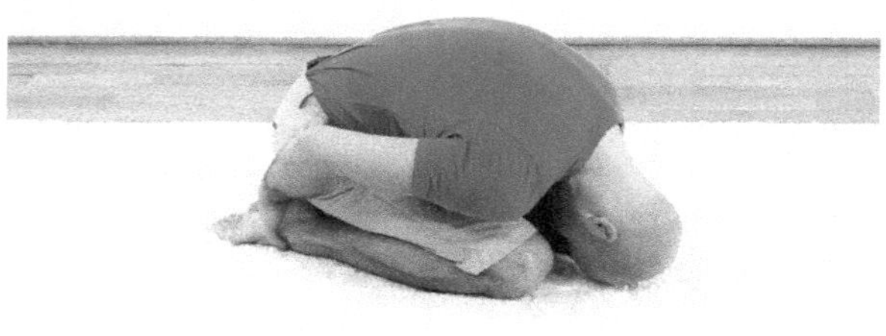

#5 ST

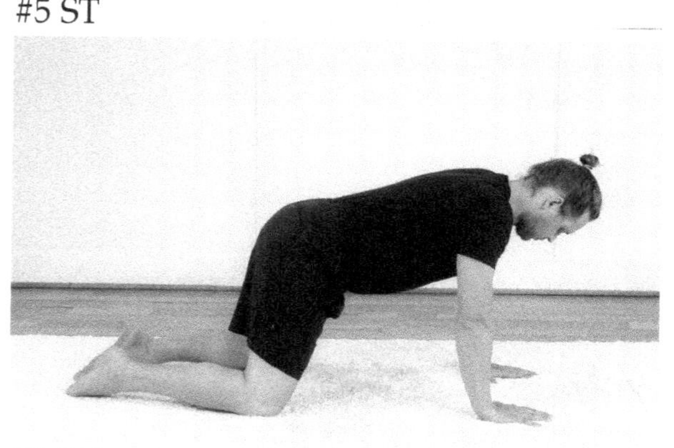

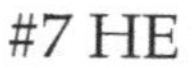

#7 HE

Advanced—Resistance Flexibility

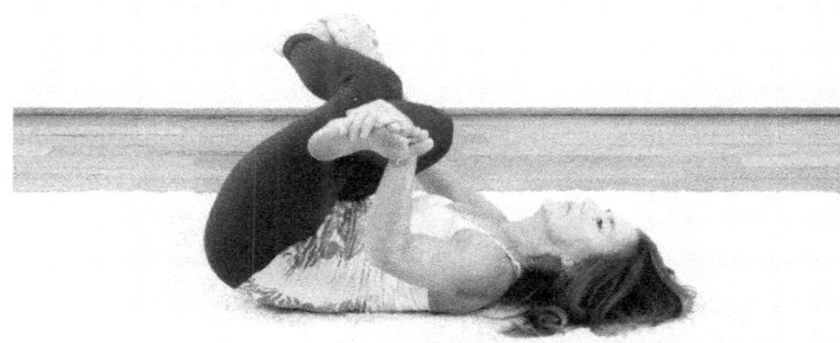

#1 GB

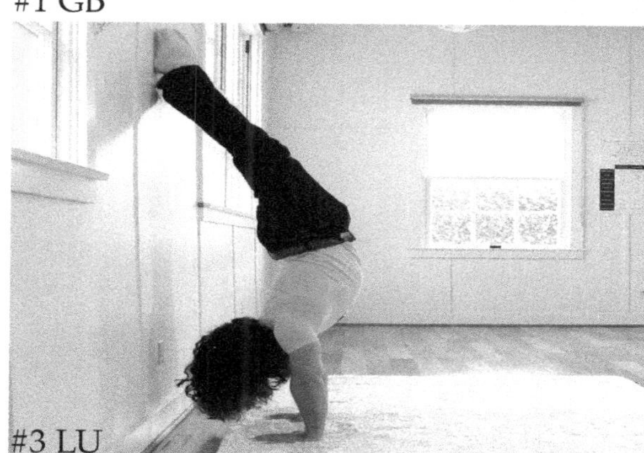

#3 LU

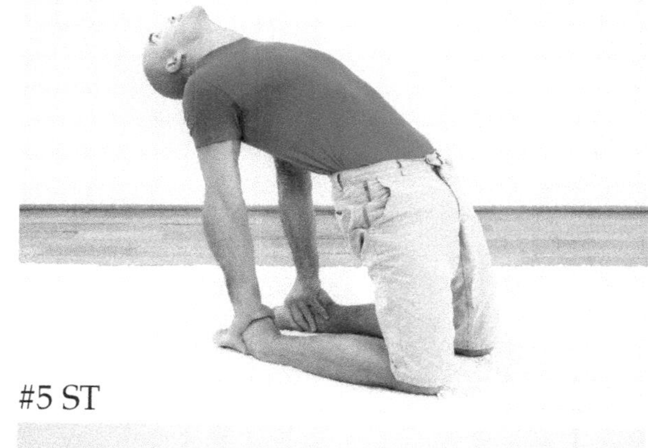

#5 ST

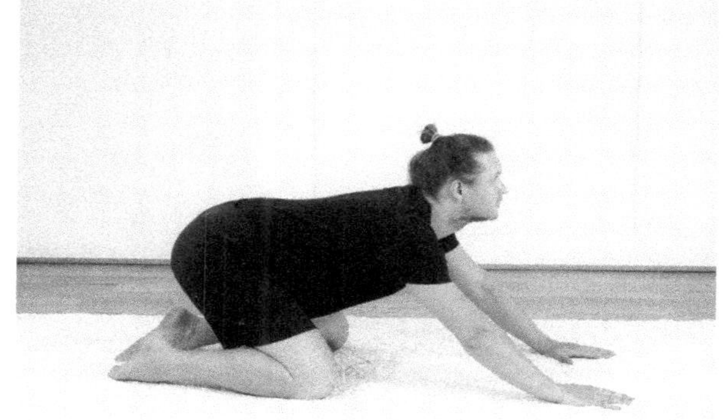

#7 HE

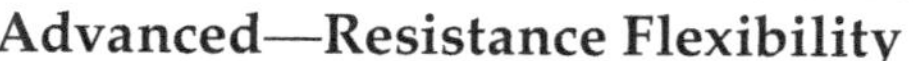

Advanced—Starting Position

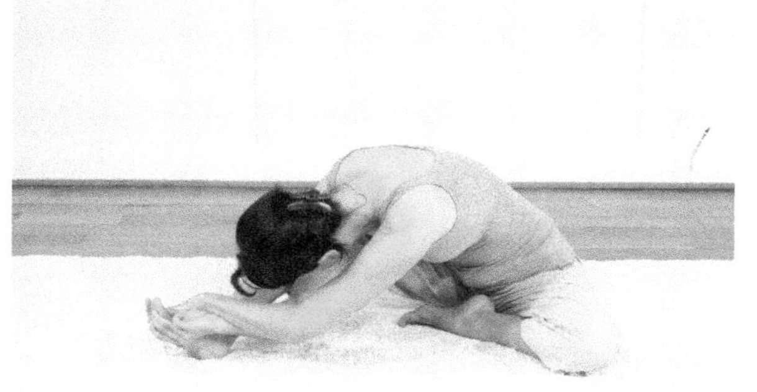

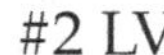

#2 LV

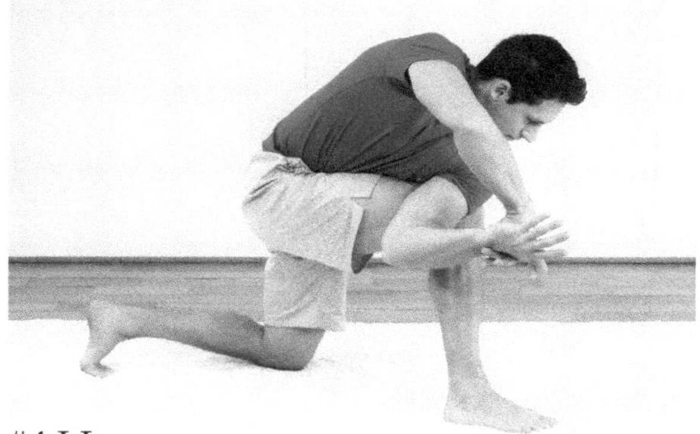

#4 LI

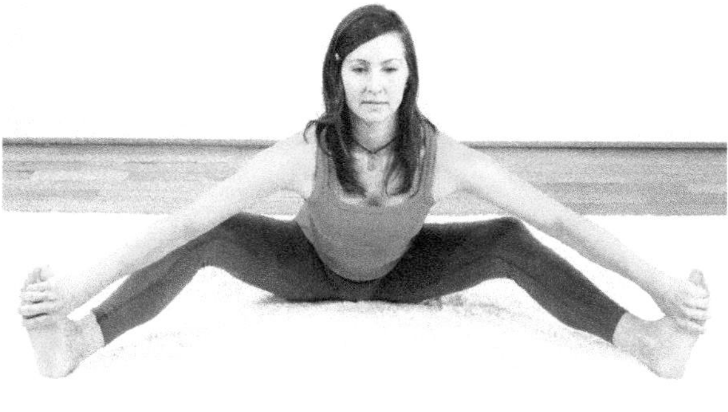

#6 PA

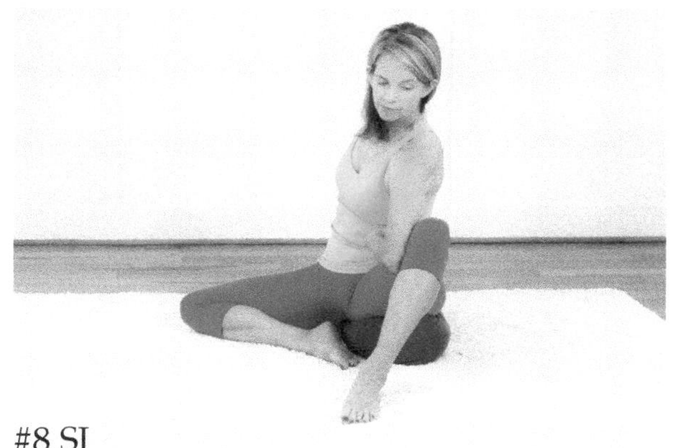

#8 SI

Advanced—Resistance Flexibility

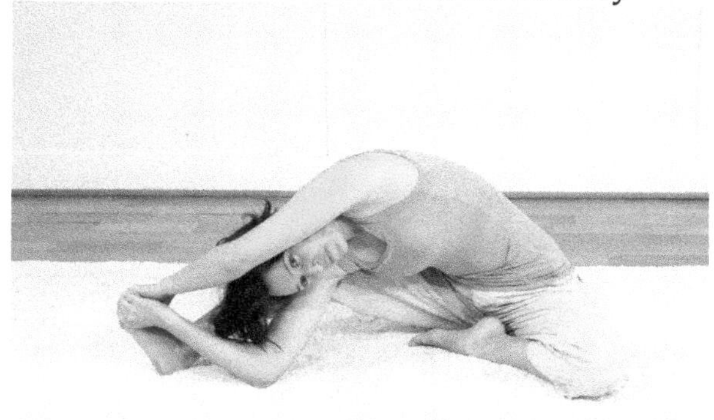

#2 LV

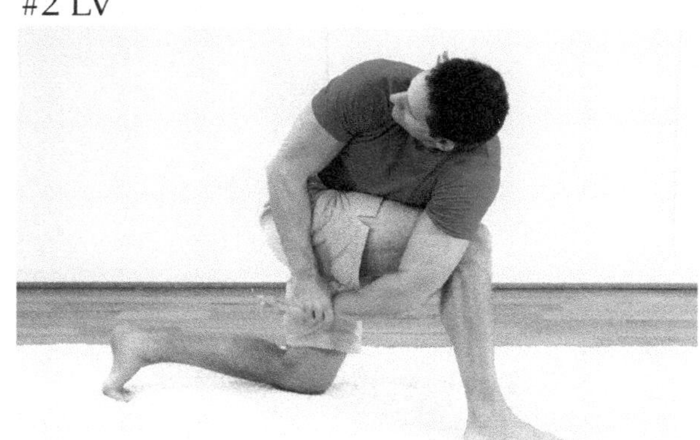

#4 LI

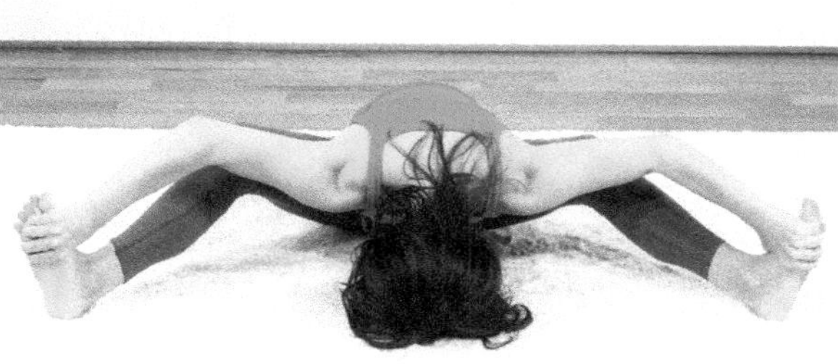

#6 PA

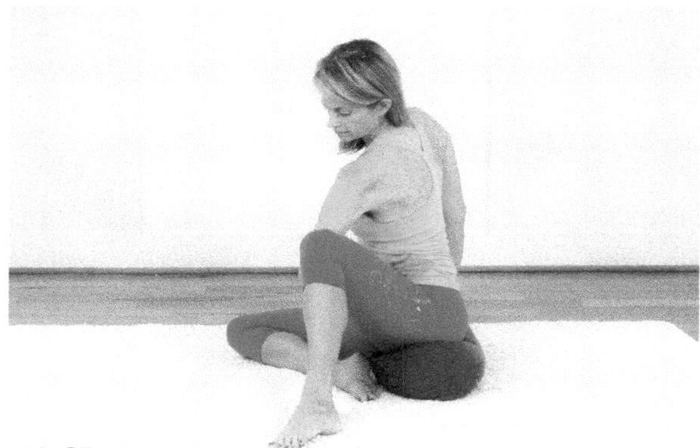

#8 SI

Advanced—Starting Position

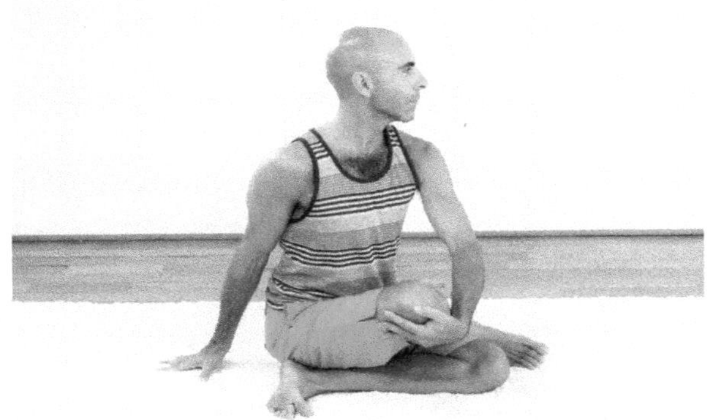

#9 BR

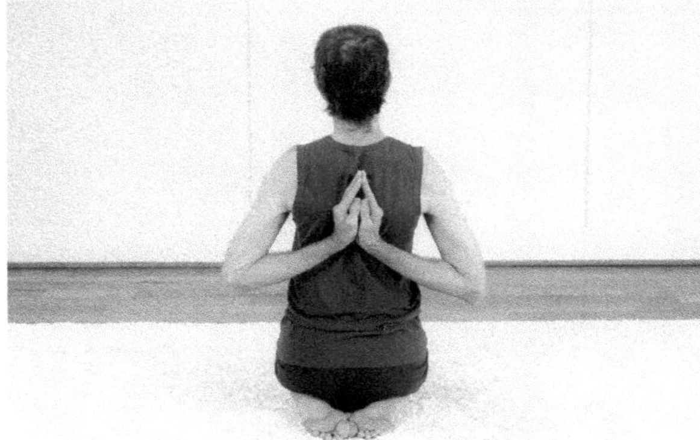

#11 PE

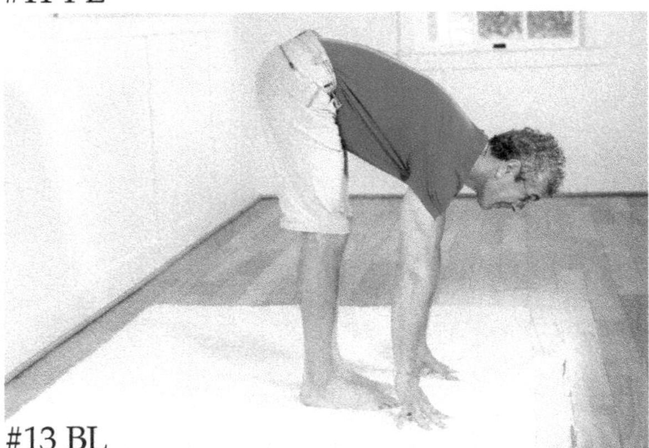

#13 BL

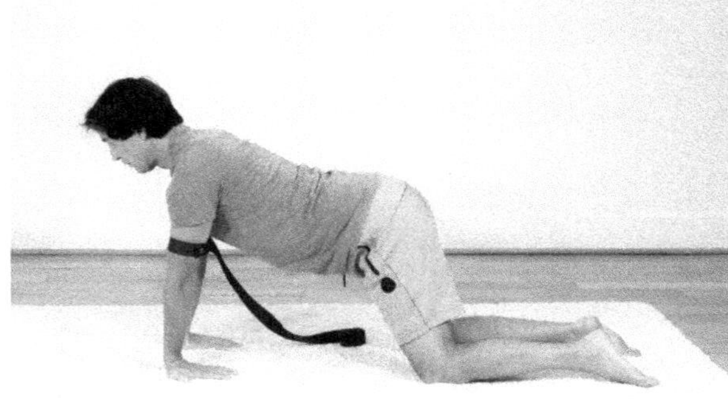

#15 AP

Advanced—Resistance Flexibility

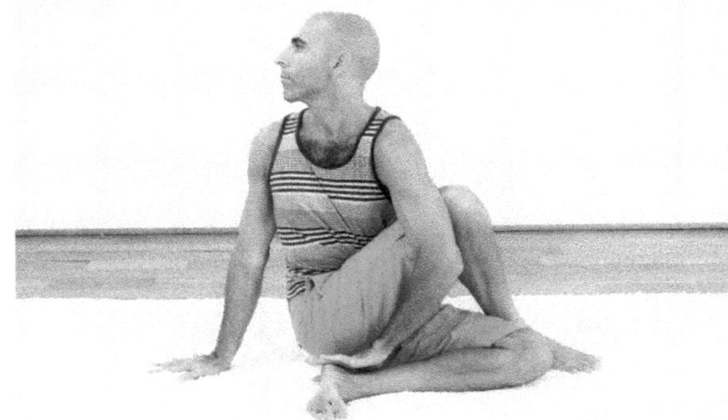

#9 BR

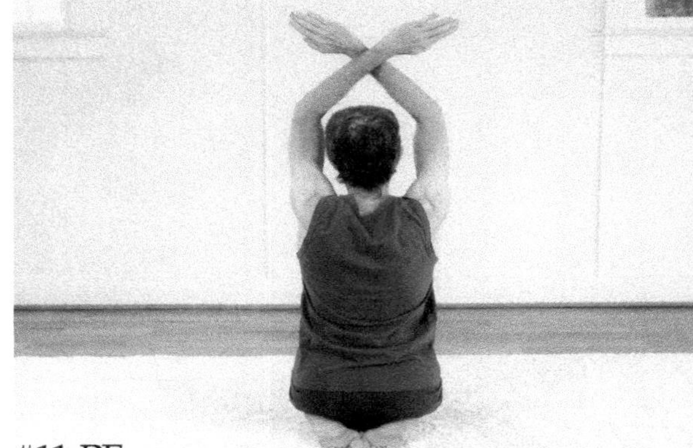

#11 PE

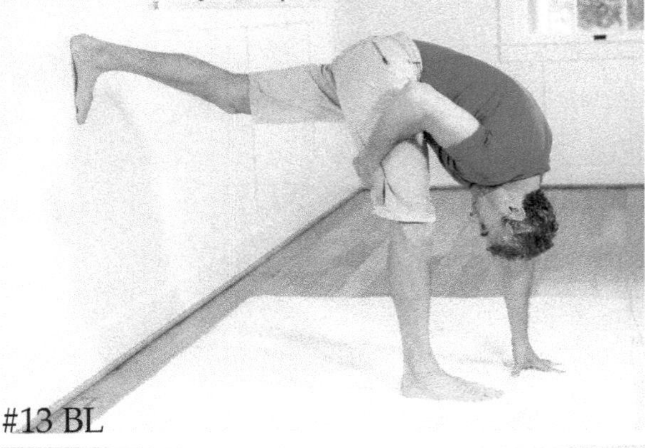

#13 BL

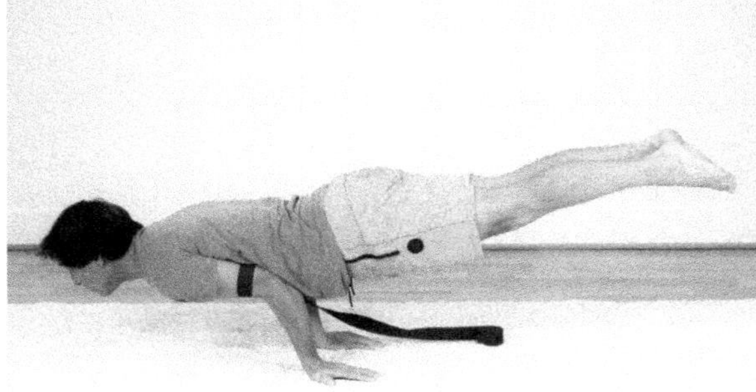

#15 AP

Advanced—Starting Position

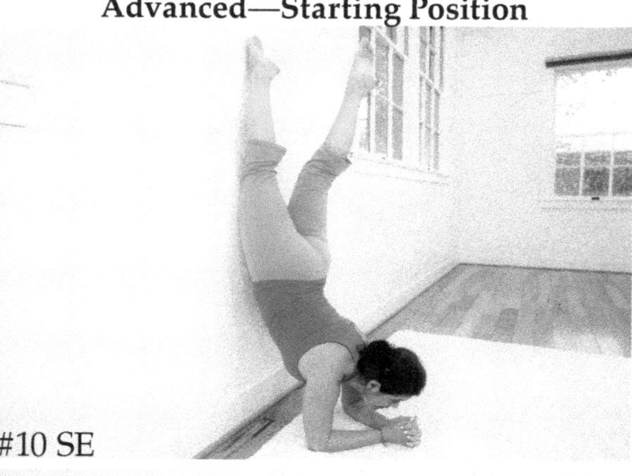
#10 SE

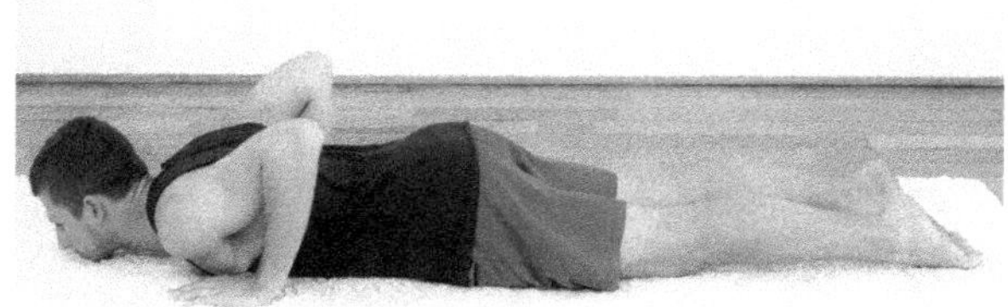

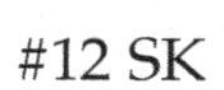
#12 SK

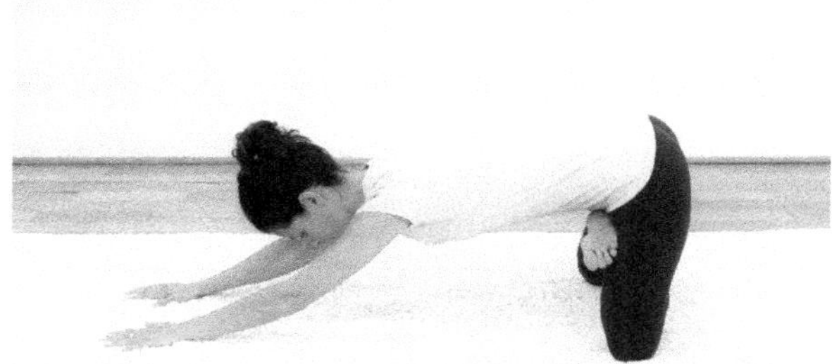
#14 KI

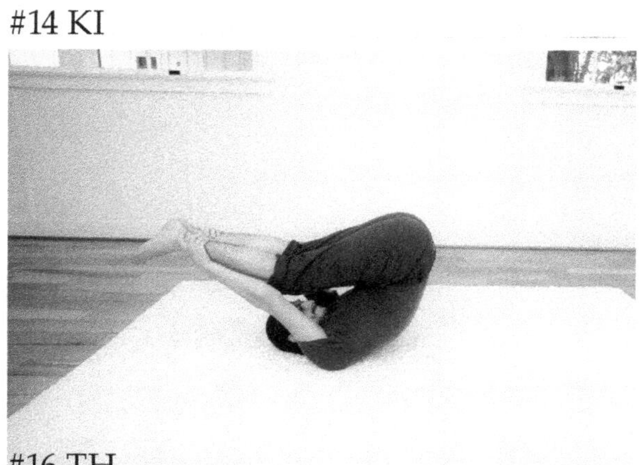
#16 TH

Advanced—Resistance Flexibility

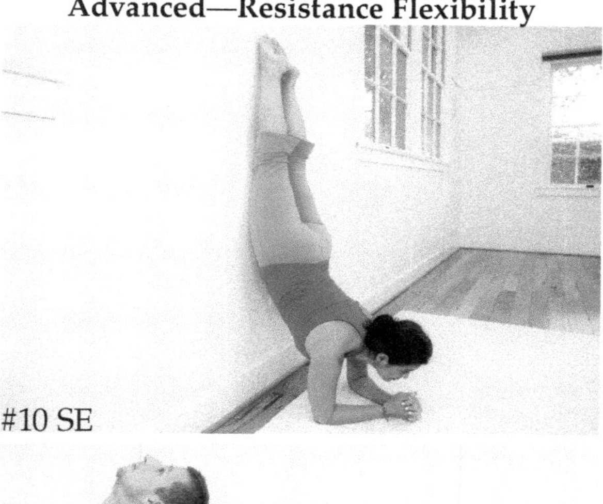
#10 SE

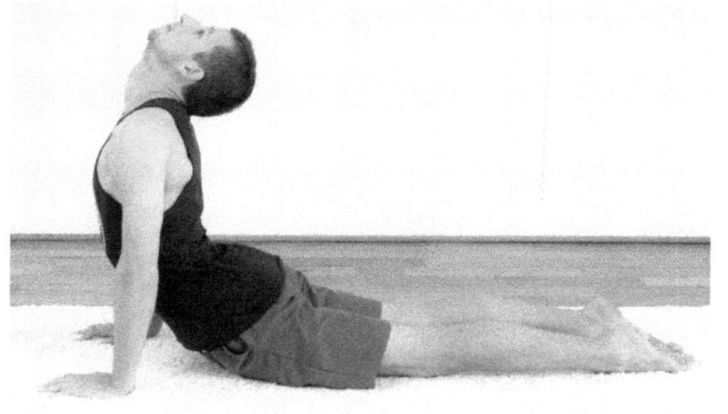
#12 SK

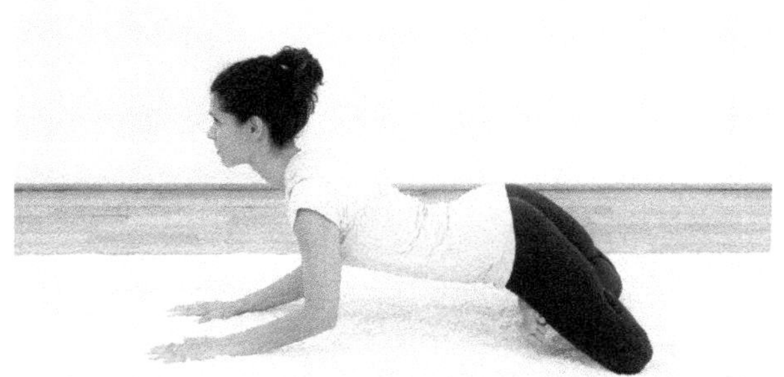
#14 KI

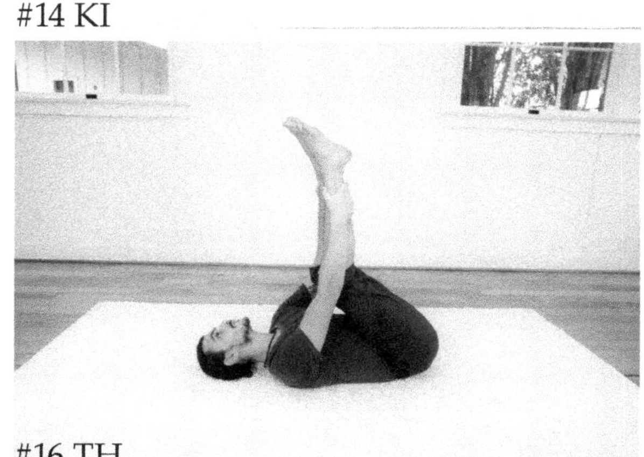
#16 TH

Assisted—Starting Position

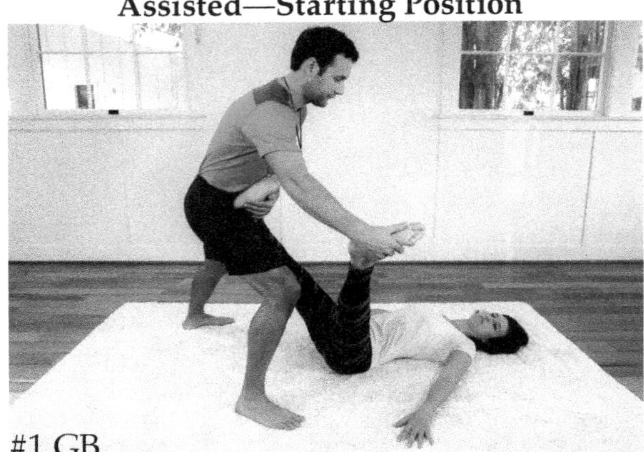

#1 GB

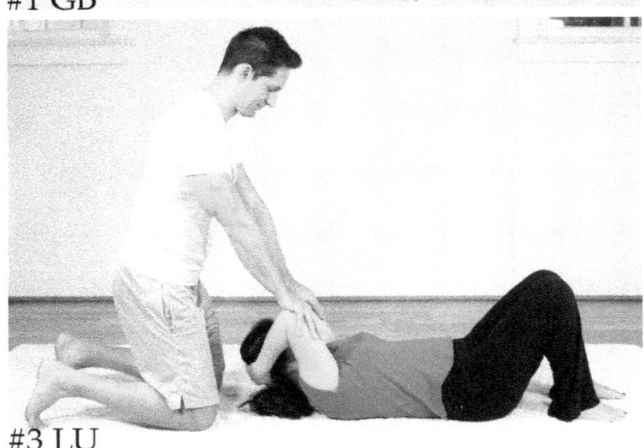

#3 LU

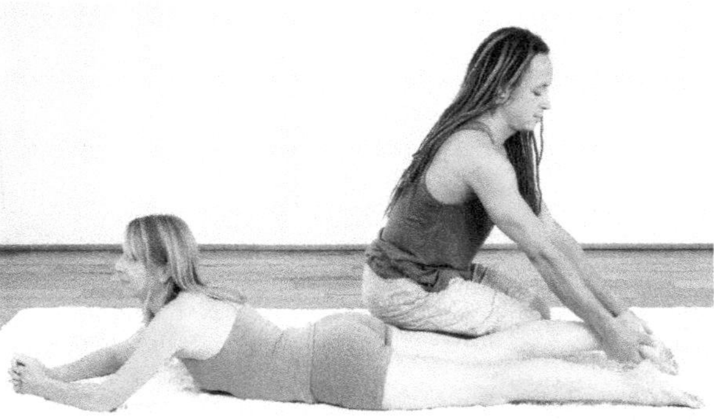

#5 ST

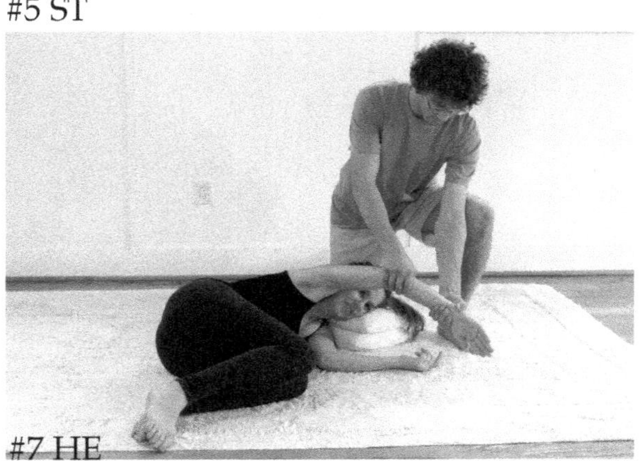

#7 HE

Assisted—Resistance Flexibility

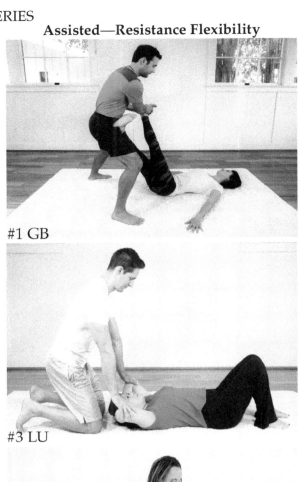

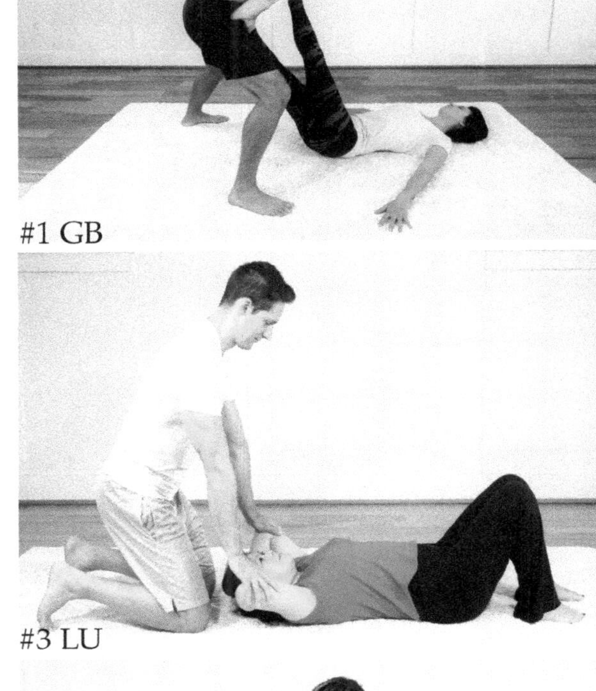

#1 GB

#3 LU

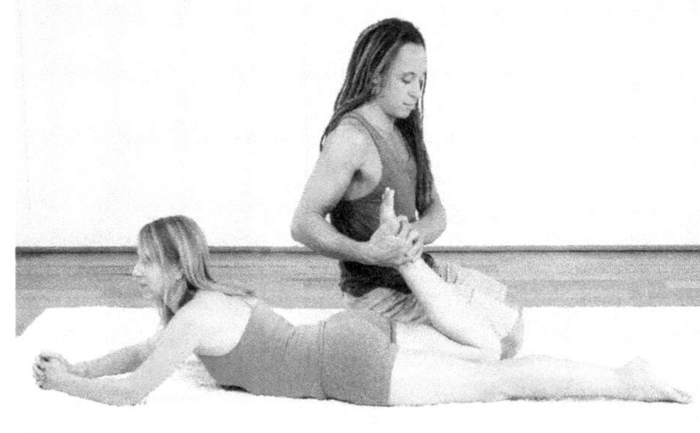

#5 ST

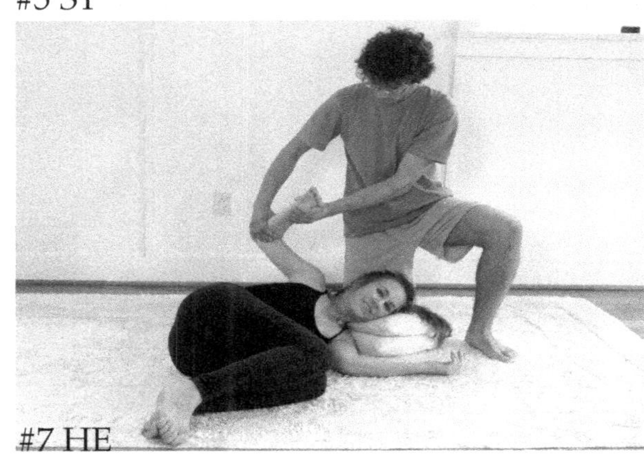

#7 HE

Assisted—Starting Position

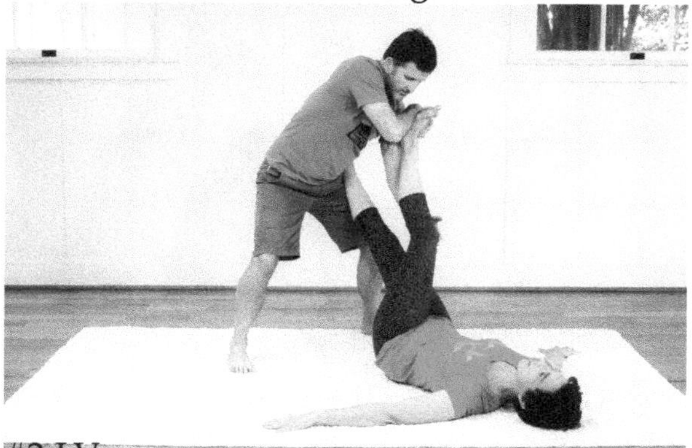

Assisted—Resistance Flexibility

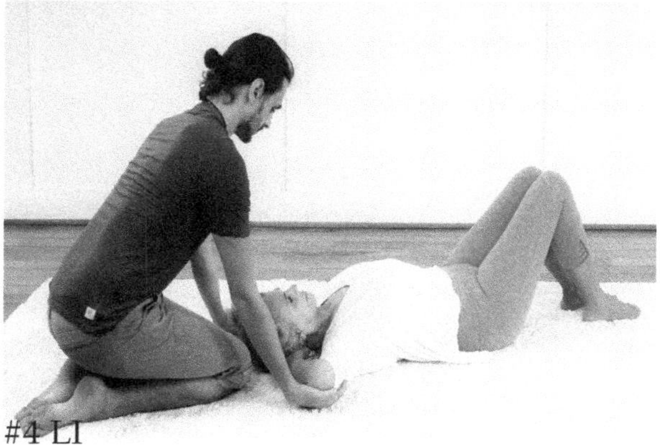

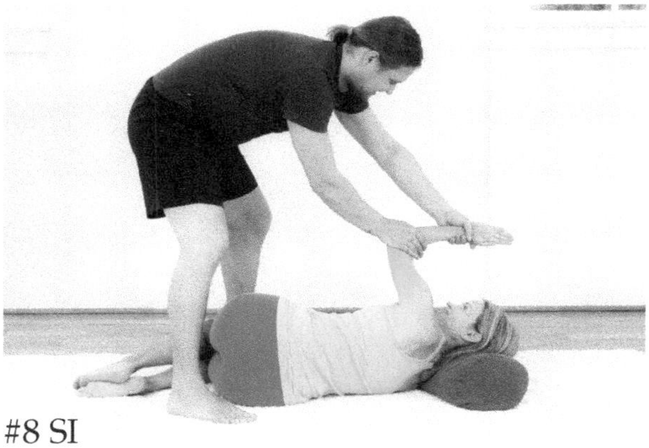

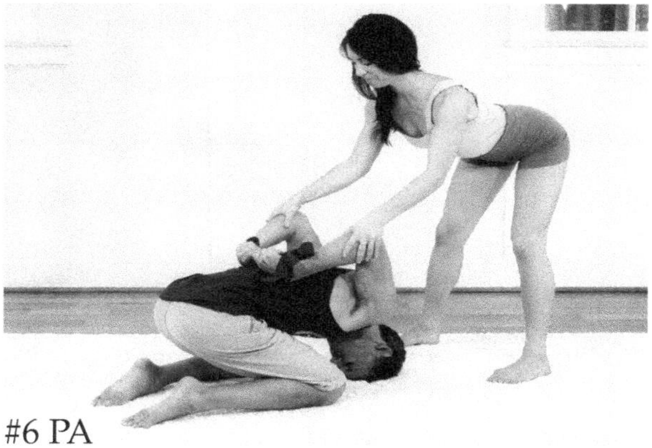

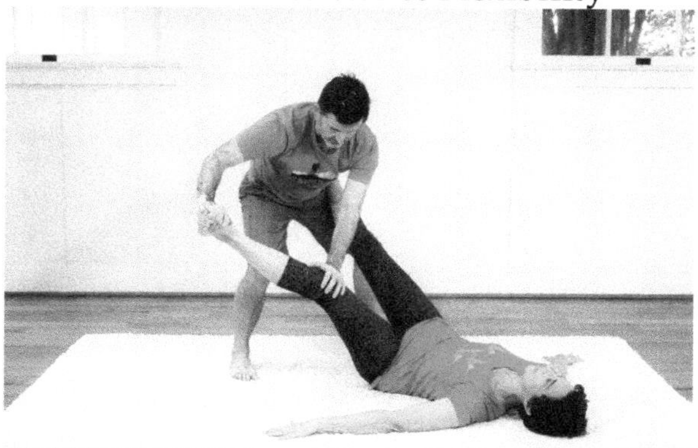

#2 LV

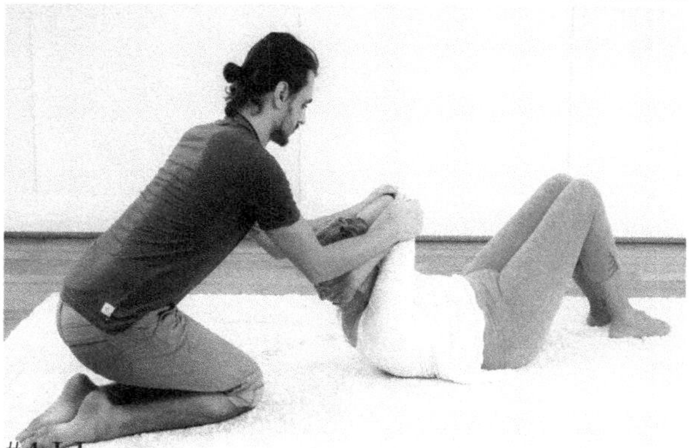

#2 LV

#4 LI

#4 LI

#6 PA

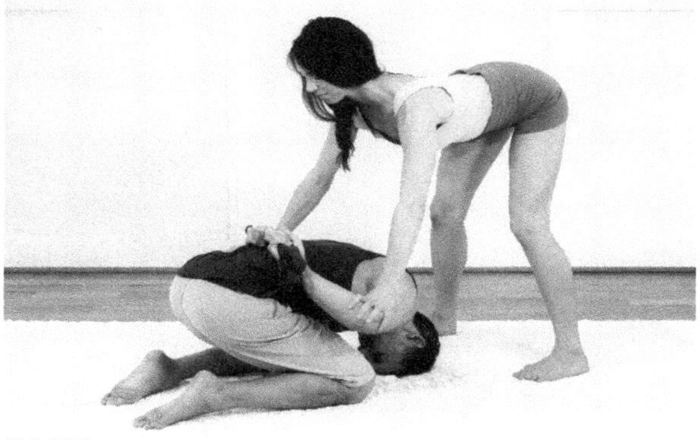

#6 PA

#8 SI

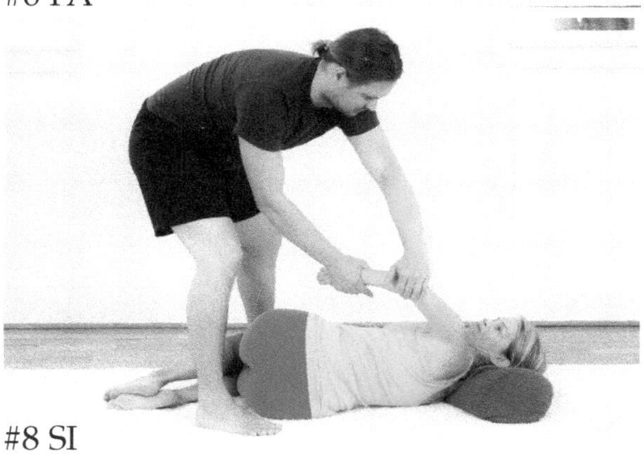

#8 SI

Assisted—Starting Position

Assisted—Resistance Flexibility

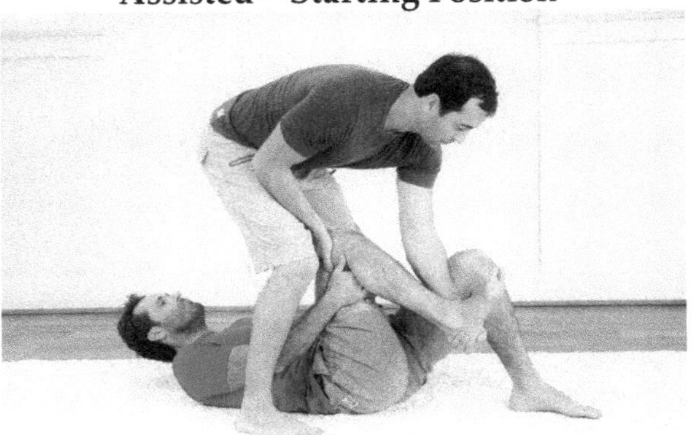

#9 BR

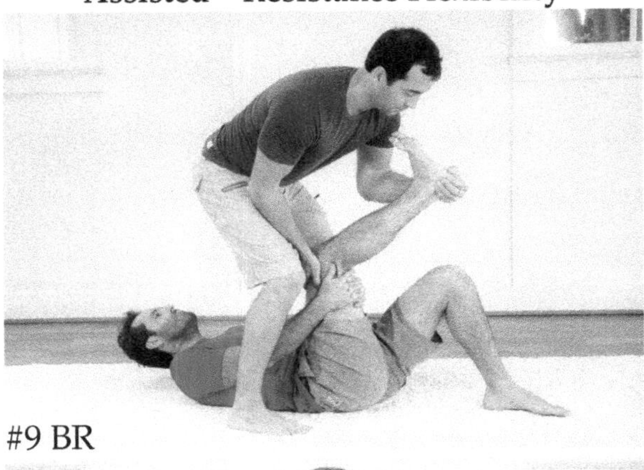

#9 BR

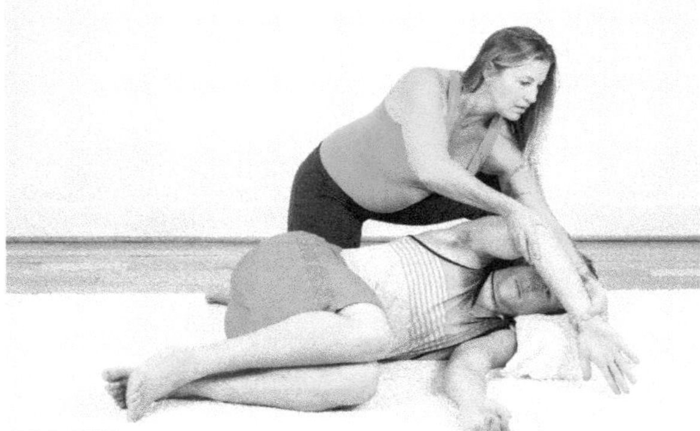

#11 PE

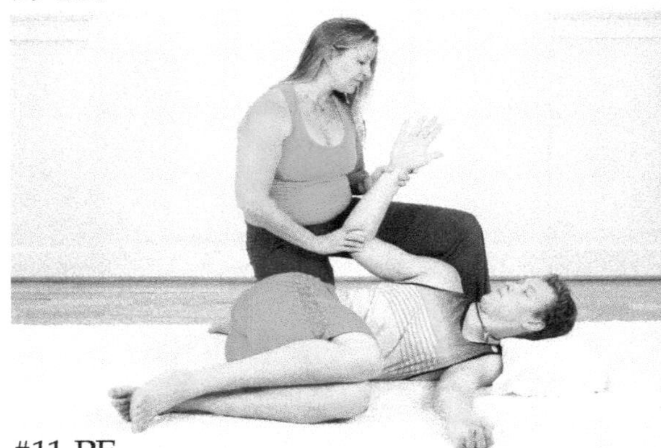

#11 PE

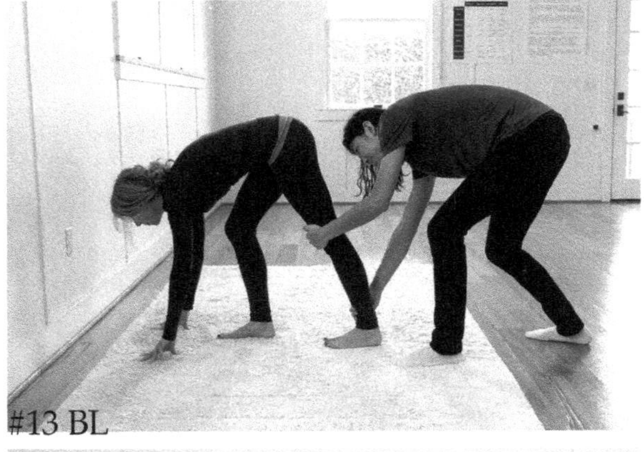

#13 BL

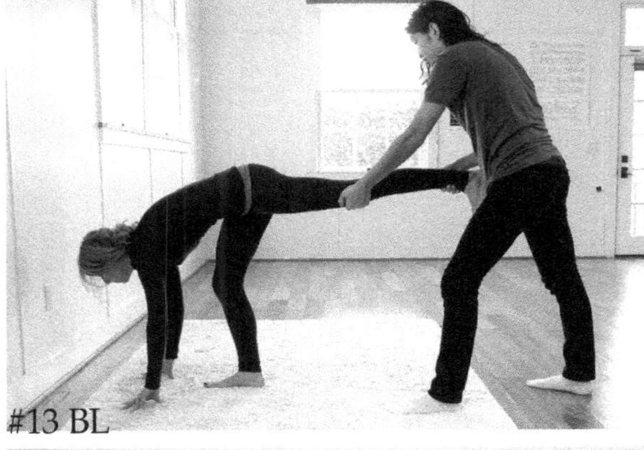

#13 BL

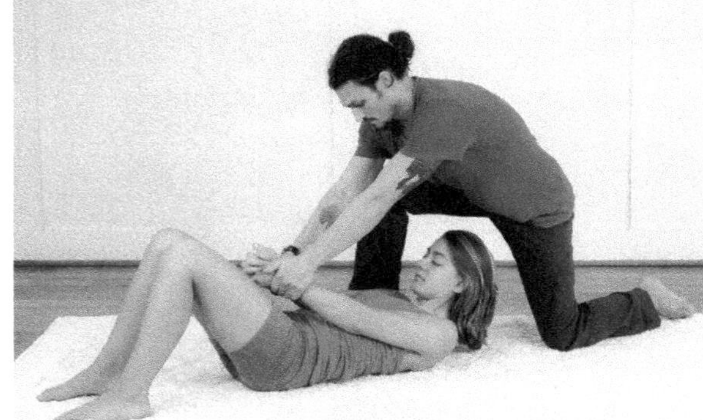

#15 AP

#15 AP

Assisted—Starting Position

Assisted—Resistance Flexibility

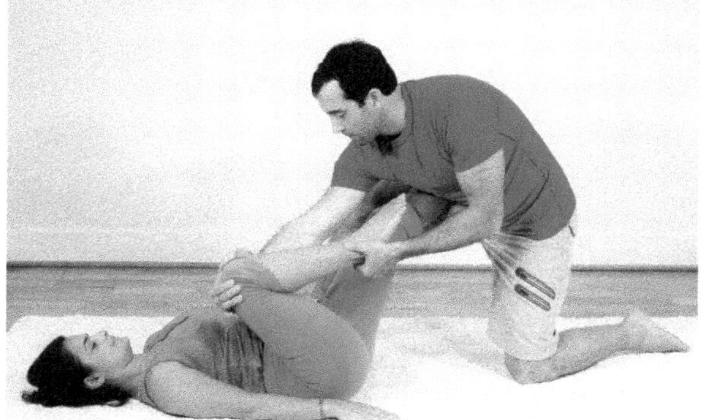

#10 SE

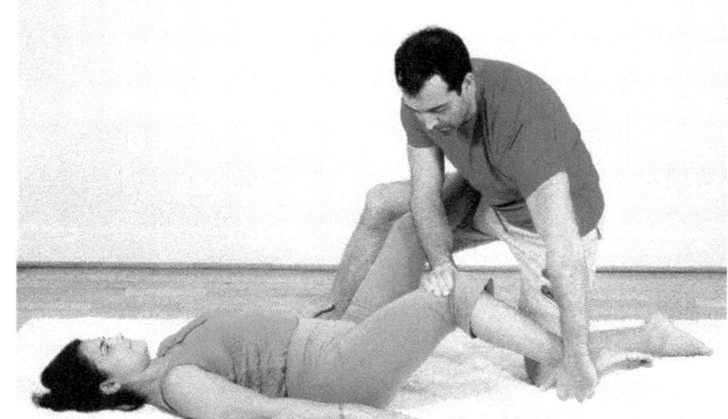

#10 SE

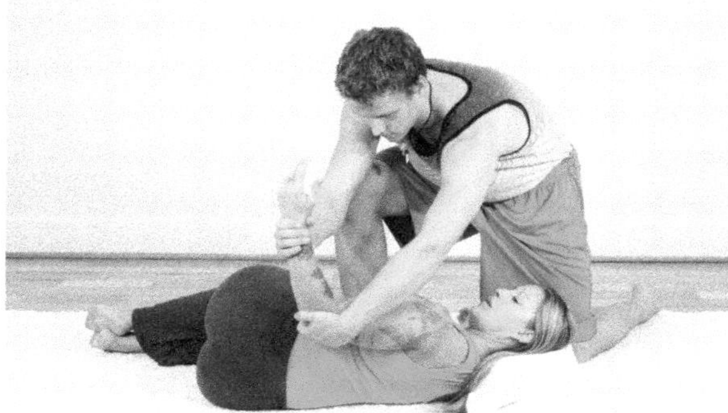

#12 SK

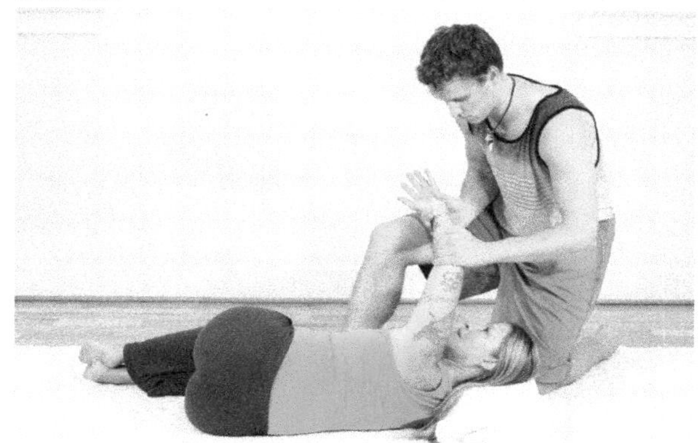

#12 SK

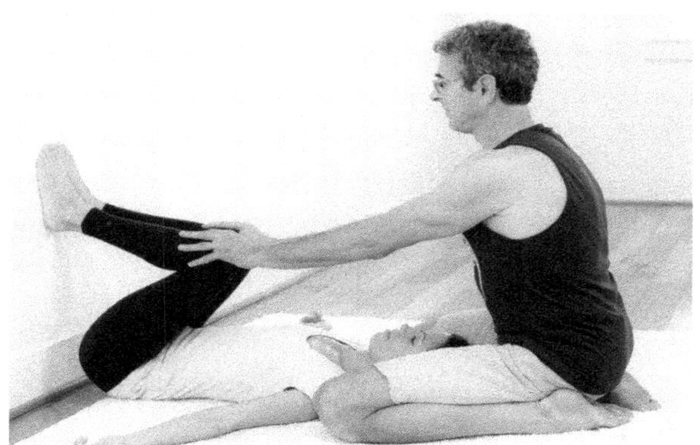

#14 KI

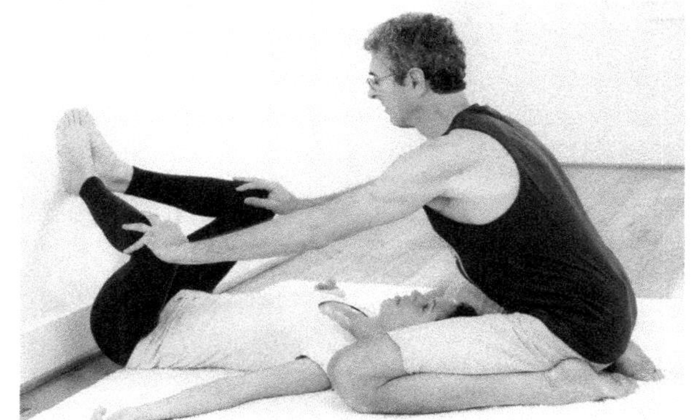

#14 KI

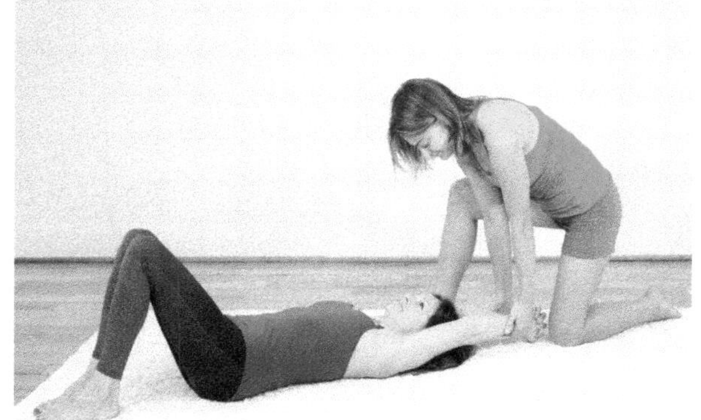

#16 TH

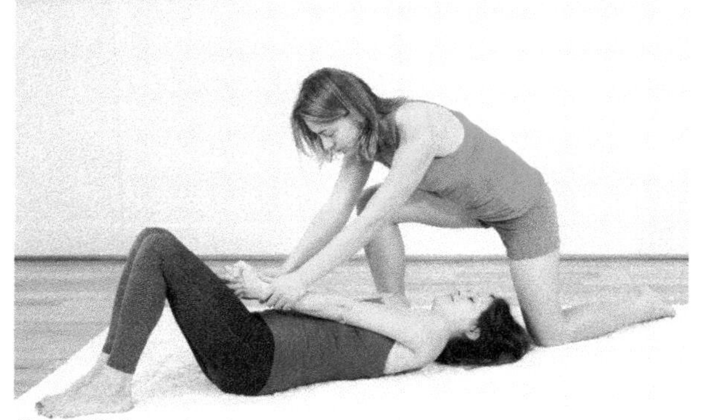

#16 TH

PART III: RESISTANCE FLEXIBITY IN DEPTH

More In Depth Knowledge about Resistance Flexibility

CHAPTER 10

RECOVERY

Enjoying, shortening, and building your recovery capacity

RECOMMENDATIONS FOR RECOVERY

A GOOD SORENESS

Most everyone gets sore from self and assisted Resistance Flexibility. The soreness is not so much produced from using muscles you have never used in a long time; it's more about the dramatic healing that is occurring from the Resistance Flexibility. Not just are you removing from the work of your muscles but everything inside you healing. This includes all your physiological systems, and your psychological, emotional, and spiritual part of yourself. Dare I say you are healing not just yourself but the whole world.

Most strength and aerobic exercise soreness peaks within 24 hours, but soreness from Resistance Flexibility can peak at 48 or 96 hours. Some peopel do not get sore at all, not in the least while others get 'really' sore, but its a good sore,not an injury soreness. Stay calm, and in a couple days you will feel amazing.

PEELING THE ONION

Often when someone is assisted, they uncover that their problem was bigger than they thought and or some people their problems are smaller than they thought or felt. Both of these are common experiences that all of the trainers have witnesses in others and in themselves. As you begin to remove the ADFST, you experience what was causing your problems, and not just the problem itself. Resistance Flexibility is not just getting rid of your problems it is helping your to create those parts of you that were for whatever reason not developed that initially caused you problems. The new you is happening.

Often joint pain is being produced from ADFST in muscles near by the joint. Your joints will be freed once the ADFST is removed.

As you remove the ADFST, you feel much better, better than ever, but you also learn how much work there is to do to get to the bottom of your problem before you get totally out of the problem and live into the solution.

YOUR RECOVERY RATE DEPENDS ON THE HEALTH OF YOUR EXTERNAL IMMUNE SYSTEM

When accumulated dense fascia and scar tissue (ADFST) is freed from your tissue during

Resistance Flexibility, it is absorbed by your blood stream and then cleaned by your lymphatic flow. Depending on the amount of ADFST you remove when doing Resistance Flexibility, as well as how healthy your external immune system operates, will determine the rate you will recover. The frequency of your aerobic health highly correlates with the health of your lymphatic flow and your speed of recovery.

Normal exercise soreness is known to peak about 24 hours after exercising and you return to your normal state within 48 hours. This is not true for Resistance Flexibility. When you do Resistance Flexibility, your soreness peaks within 48 hours and you return to normal within 96 hours.

Some people don't get sore and some get really sore. It all depends on how aerobic they are because a person's aerobic capacity correlates with lymphatic flow 'cleaning'. If you are the type of person that likes to be challenged or take risks regardless of your physical activity, then you will recover fast. If you tend to dislike stress and block irritating sounds instead of letting your mind decide what to block, then you will stiff and sore.

Now it's a bad sore so don't worry. It's not pain. It doesn't feel bad; it's a good sore. Your body is rebuilding and in repair—every part of you.

BE PROACTIVE AND MONITOR THE INTENSITY and REPETITIONS OF YOUR RESISTANCE FLEXIBILITY TRAINING

The more you eat organic nutrient dense food, take in more water than you think you should by keeping a stainless steel or glass container with you, then you are being proactive about the speed of your recovery. Small and more frequent meals are better than big meals.

The greater the intensity of your Resistance Flexibility workout the more you will need to do things to help your body remove the waste products and heal. So learn about what levels of intensity you like and can handle, and notice that your capacity continuously increases over time.

ACCUMULATIVE DENSE FASCIA AND SCAR TISSUE (ADFST)

Everyone has different amounts of accumulated dense fascia and scar tissue (ADFST) in specific areas of their body. Learn where yours is and prioritize those areas and do Resistance Flexibility those areas of concern. The sooner you get scar tissue out of your body, the faster your flexibility and strength will increase.

It is normal to have accumulated dense fascia and scar tissue (ADFST). You can tell how much you have by comparing the resistance in the areas you have ADFST with others. Remember regardless of whom you are or where you come from or how you were raised, the largest amount of ADFST is in everyone's Lateral Hamstrings—Stretch #13.

WHEN TO PRACTICE, HOW OFTEN, SELF OR ASSISTED

Morning Resistance Flexibility sets you up for the whole day. Resistance Flexibility before and after your aerobic exercises prepares your body and helps it recover. The sooner you Resistance Flexibility after exercising the better, as everyone tends to 'glue up' if they don't remove the tenseness and damage to their tissues after exercising.

If you stretch every day like all other animals do, then you will remain flexible as you remove the distresses out of your body from your relationships, your life stresses, etc.

Self-stretching is great but being assisted is ten times better. Pairing up with your friends or hiring an Elite Trainer either ON LINE or in person at one of our four centers in Boston, Los Angles, Santa Barbara, and NYC is wonderful. Being around other people that have prioritized their development and are helping others is a great healing environment.

SLEEP

Not too much could be said for the value of sleep and rest. These two things determine almost more than anything else in how you will recover. Usually after Resistance Flexibility sessions, everyone sleeps better. Sleep rests your body and doing nothing rests your mind.

BENTONITE CLAY

Bentonite clay is benign. I take some anytime I feel like the food at a restaurant is not just right, and when I stretch intensely and I feel a little head achy from the toxicity.

INFRA RED SAUNA OR INFRA RED PAD

Many people that do Resistance Flexibility use infrared saunas or pads. The increase in internal heat facilitates the fascia changes. Fascia is like salt water taffy; the more you heat it, the softer and more pliable it becomes. Heating the body from the outside is not as effective.

Infrared reportedly turns on your internal immune system. That has been my experience. We have Infra Red Saunas in all our Genius of Flexibility Centers.

LYMPHATIC FLOW and AEROBIC CAPACITY

There is a direct correlation between how aerobically rich your muscle tissues are, and how fast they recover. There is also a high correlation between people that like to use stress to develop themselves, and their lymphatic removal of waste material from Resistance Flexibility. Too much stress is obviously not good, but without stress you don't develop.

MASSAGE / SMASHING

We spend a considerable amount of time using our feet to help the lymphatic drainage after Resistance Flexibility. Massage is also helpful but lacks sufficient to weight to significantly help the lymphatic and circulation necessary for the removal of waste material from Resistance Flexibility. So we walk all over the body to help the circulation and lymphatic flows.

HIGH PH WATER

In all of our Genius of Flexibility Centers, we have special water machines that not only filter the water but also transform it into a higher ph. We use a 9-10 ph water as drinking water in our centers. There are various quality machines that do this.

ALKALIZING FOODS

Most people that Resistance Flexibility train eat a lot of high alkaline foods. The fascia is quite acidic when went it being removed from the body. So eating high ph foods is always good.

SOMBRE

Hot/Cold Saves are great for speeding recovery, because the change in temperature helps the lymph nodes to work better and to flush out the waste products.

DIET- SUPPLEMENTS

See Nutrition Chapter 12.

SEX AND RECOVERY

Different *types* have very different responses to having sex and how it affects recovery. For some, it accelerates recovery, and for others it does not. This is something like most things, something each person needs to about themselves and others.

VARITEY OF EXERCISE

Just like it is best to eat a variety of foods, the same is true for exercise. There are of course preferences for everyone, but too much of one type of exercise is not optimal. Vary your aerobic exercise and discover how it helps speeds your recovery. Resistance Flexibility gives the ability to do an ever widening array of exercise.

DAILY RISING AND SLEEPING

Most people that do Resistance Flexibility regularly prefer going early to bed, and getting up early. There are physiological biorhythms that support this way of sleeping. The number of hours you get to bed before midnight is important. The fewer the hours, the more sleep most people need.

FASTING
See Nutrition and Resistance Flexibility Chapter 12

FOOD POISONING AND HEAVY METAL DETOXING
Please consult your professional health care professional for advice on chelation of heavy metals.

PHYSIOLOGICAL HELATH
A person's physiological health has enormous impact on their ability to recover because it determines the health not only of all the tissues of the body but also recovery and rate of healing. You can know more about your physiological health by comparing your flexibility and strengthen in all the 16 types of stretches.

BREATHING
There are four stages of breathing: Inhaling, holding the inhale, exhaling, and retention of the exhale. Each type of stretch involved a person in two of these more than the other. Discover how your body wants you to breathe in stretching and in everything else you do.

PSYCHOLOGICAL HEALTH
Like physiological health, psychological health highly determines recovery. How you handle your love/anger, fear/fearlessness, excitement/anxiety, and calm/fright all have huge impacts on your recovery. The different types of stretches specifically help to develop all 16 high/low personality traits.

SPIRITUAL VALUES
Perhaps less known is how a person's spiritual values affect them in all aspects of themselves and others. This is the largest single factor affecting recovery. Your life is reflected in your body. As you become more flexible in all ways, your life will also reflect your health and connect you to healthy things in your life.

Diaries

"I love being stretched before I go to dance class or before I perform, assisted RF is great, and self stretches work too...makes such a difference in movement and the ecstasy part of the experience. Of course, post-stretching makes recovery happen, so that the next day I am moving forward instead of having to start from square one."
BonnieCrotzer@TheGeniusofFlexibility.com Elite Resistance Flexibility Trainer

"Being stretched is the BEST! I used to wonder how many sessions it would take to get rid of the ADFST, but now I am focused on the instant improvements I feel and the upgrades to my looks, personality, and over all well- being...and I want MORE!"
MimiAmrit@TheGeniusofFlexibility.com Resistance Flexibility Intern

"My motto when it comes to Resistance Flexibility: stretch, get stretched, and stretch others. I find that practicing all three of these yields the best results. Self-stretching provides me with enormous insight into myself, but self stretching alone leaves me feeling frustrated with being unable to take myself where I know that others can take me. Assisted stretching gives me a much faster and more thorough change when compared to self stretching, but assisted stretching alone makes me entirely dependent on others instead of being empowered with a practice that I can use by myself if need be. Assisting others allows me to learn from the person I'm assisting how to get a better stretch for myself by seeing what they are doing while getting stretched that I don't do. It's also great strength training. But, assisted stretching alone would only leave me feeling bound up, tight, and over extended. I've found that a combination of stretching, getting stretched, and stretching others hits my sweet spot."
LutherCowden@TheGeniusofFlexibility.com Elite Resistance Flexibility Trainer

"There's nothing quite like the 'good sore' that can happen after an intense RF session. The soreness after my first few times being assisted was intense, and now I only rarely get sore. I've learned to enjoy the soreness when it occurs. It feels like a teacher to me, as it prevents me from substituting and compensating in my movements, and makes me aware of the parts of my body that were otherwise sensationless. I make sure to keep moving when my body is sore, so that I can take advantage of this heighted state to learn how to defer to my body, and to recover at a faster rate."
LutherCowden@TheGeniusofFlexibility.com Elite Resistance Flexibility Trainer

"I remember the morning after I was assisted in RF for the first time, I felt more mobile in so many ways, like my bones got to settle in a new and better place. But I was so sore; I could barely sit my ass down on the toilet, nor get up! I was much assured that I got some major changes! It was great. I have heard many folks share about the toilet problem too post first stretch, very funny."
BonnieCrotzer@TheGeniusofFlexibility.com Elite Resistance Flexibility Trainer

"Some people tell us after their first time getting assisted resistance flexibility trained that they were surprisingly not sore at all. More often most people says that they have never been as sore even from their most intense workout as they are from their resistance flexibility session. It's a good sore not a bad sore you get when you do something wrong. At first it can be surprising because you don't feel the

dramatic fascia change during the stretch session...but afterward you know that a lot happened! I find that once the soreness dissipates in my own body after stretching, the new physical real estate that is available in my body is phenomenal. I feel like a super human sometimes. I have power, movement, and strength at a whole new level. I feel invigorated and more alive than ever before. You discover that it is going to take some work to solve your problems at the root...but you also feel like 'what is the other option?" A partial or non-solution, solution. This doesn't really make sense and just prolongs the process. It is much more efficient to chip away at it and marvel at the changes."
BerylHagenburg@TheGeniusofFlexibility.com Resistance Flexibility Intern

"What can be revealed as the layers of ADFST are removedcan be frightening, because you realize how many licks it might take to get to the center of the tootsie pop! But its also so exciting because its fun to solve problems; problems will always be around to get solved, and in the process, we get to help and be helped."
BonnieCrotzer@TheGeniusofFlexibility.com Elite Resistance Flexibility Trainer

"When I first started Resistance Flexibility, one of my primary motivations for practicing was that the movements made me feel really good. It was that simple. But, as I progressed, I became more psychological in my analysis of myself and instead of settling for just feeling good; I demanded optimal functioning of my body and myself in all ways. Through this I have learned how much work it takes to resolve areas of chronic stress and tenseness in the body."
LutherCowden@TheGeniusofFlexibility.com Elite Resistance Flexibility Trainer

"The quality of food and water that I consume are a great support for my stretching practice. The 2 play off of one another. The more I stretch the more healthy I want to eat and the more water my body and tissue can absorb...and the healthier I eat and the more I hydrate, the greater my capacity to stretch. Resistance flexibility is a movement. People can change who they are in a community where everyone is supportive and in the same boat. Your very presence and participation is giving to others while you receive. GOF centers are designed with one thing in mind- development and expression of the greatest technology on the planet- the human being."
BerylHagenburg@TheGeniusofFlexibility.com Resistance Flexibility Intern

"Following a session of being stretched by another trainer, I've experienced different degrees of soreness, occurring later than my usual exercise. I'm also extremely thirsty for water, as I can feel my tissues instantly re hydrating! So I make certain to drink copious amounts of purified water. Within the 24 – 48 hrs, I've also experienced exhaustion to the point of requiring immediate sleep. Upon recovery, I feel great!"
MimiAmrit@TheGeniusofFlexibility.com Resistance Flexibility Intern

"I consider myself an experiment. I eat certain types of food and see how they affect my functioning. The same goes for my physical exercise. I've tried spending many hours a day self-stretching, or self stretching a bit each day. I've tried getting assisted occasionally, daily, and once for 10 continuous hours in one day. All of these different ways of training myself have yielded different types of results. I'm continuously refining my training in this way and find the entire process to be quite fun."
LutherCowden@TheGeniusofFlexibility.com Elite Resistance Flexibility Trainer

"Removing dense fascia and scar tissue from my body is like removing the parts of myself that are dead to life. These are the parts of myself that I have misidentified as my true self. This is the tissue that prevents me from living my life to the fullest. Dealing with dense fascia and scar tissue is challenging, but rewarding, in that it gives me a physical outlet for dealing with the equivalent psychological and emotional parts of myself that would otherwise be too far away for me to problem solve."
LutherCowden@TheGeniusofFlexibility.com Elite Resistance Flexibility Trainer

"A good sleep schedule is crucial. I feel like I waste so much of what I gain when I don't go to bed early and wake up early. As my body gets healthier, I am able to let go of social and other obligations and prioritize my own health. When I do this I become so much more present and aware in all of my interactions and activities."
BerylHagenburg@TheGeniusofFlexibility.com Resistance Flexibility Intern

"I always travel with bentonite clay, activated charcoal, and oil of oregano. These help my digestive system in case I eat food that makes me sick. Oil of oregano boosts my immune system. And I love sitting in an infrared sauna and sweating until I'm drenched."
LutherCowden@TheGeniusofFlexibility.com Elite Resistance Flexibility Trainer

"Getting smashed after getting stretched is like the cherry on top. It allows me to lie down and be passive while someone walks up and down my hamstrings and other areas to facilitate the removal of waste products from my body. I gain valuable feedback from the person smashing me as to where I'm tense and/or have dense fascia. The sensation that arises from the physical pressure allows my brain to know where I'm tense and then my body naturally begins to relax."
LutherCowden@TheGeniusofFlexibility.com Elite Resistance Flexibility Trainer

"I have been happily self employed for the last twenty seven years as a very successful and sought after Licensed Massage Therapist. Soon after my first year in the field, I was fortunate enough to meet Bob Cooley, who's RFST has enabled me to release fascia throughout my own body, increase my flexibility and core strength, improve my posture, avoid repetitive injuries and free me from worries and stress; my conditioning after 25 plus years in a very physically punishing career is remarkable and would have been impossible without Bob Cooley and RFST. I feel youthful and healthy, I can totally focus on my clients' needs and, without question, and Resistance Flexibility will always be a very important part of my life."
Joanna DiRice LMT

"Fasting. I get RF stretched when I am fasting, and it accelerates the change in my ADFST and has high impact of the health of my organs, truly clearing out. Recovery gets faster too."
BonnieCrotzer@TheGeniusofFlexibility.com Elite Resistance Flexibility Trainer

"In being an athlete playing up to the levels of professional, I have always been into the getting the most amazing nutrients in my body for recovery, however also to have the edge to achieve the up most performance. While playing college and pro hockey with intense schedules of up to 82 games and with rigorous preparation of becoming a pro natural bodybuilder, I have taken almost everything you could

try for superfoods, protein powders, creatine, glutamine, Chinese tonic herbs etc. What I found out is if the organs meridians are blocked off from the fascia to receive energy, oxygen and blood flow then how could all these amazing nutrients be absorbed efficiently? With the stretching have noticed much more ability to actually reap the full benefits of these supplements and superfoods. As my body and spleen/ pancreas can produce enzymes more efficiently by doing the stretches getting a much different result by taking the same supplement, getting more energy and experience of what I'm paying for. Makes the resistance flexibility a perfect combination with nutrition and supplementation, with my clients as being a nutritionist has been life changing for them to get the results they always wanted to get with eating healthy and trying to lead that lifestyle, however the organs are the key to receive this."
ScottBottoroff@TheGeniusofFlexibility.com Elite Resistance Flexibility Trainer

"I had spend an enormous number of hours doing aerobic exercise, loving every second of it. So when I began to do Resistance Flexibility I rarely became sore. But when being assisted by many people to help remove my ADFST, I can get sore but with this soreness is a much better ease of movement and health. Like most people, I like a good sore."
Anonymous

CHAPTER 11

COMMON CONCERNS SOLVED

Low Back Pain No More

Proactive and Preventative Health Strategies

COMMON CONCERNS

Many, many commons problems can be solved with Resistance Flexibility. This includes concerns with posture, movement, physiological, psychological, emotional maturation, and spiritual development. The following are stretch for some of these most common *types* of wellness concerns.

PHYSICAL

LOW BACK PAIN

There are world conferences on Low Back Pain, but never did I see a study that simply told people that most low back pain may be coming from inflexible hamstring or muscles on the sides of your legs. So try these Resistance Flexibility stretches for your hamstrings: #13 (BL) and for your hips: #1 (GB).

POSTURE

Most people have tried their whole lives to have good posture, endlessly trying to remind themselves to sit up straight or pull their shoulders back. But bad posture is not a memory problem; it is simply insufficiency in flexibility and strength. The following list can help you to practice specific stretches for each of the most common posture problems.

1. PELVIS TOO FLEXED FORWARD WITH A HYPEREXTENDED LOWER BACK

Most people think that their pelvis is too anteriorly flexed with a resulting sway in their lower back is because the muscles on the front of their body are too short, but it is rarely true. Instead it is the hamstrings that are not flexible enough to shorten to extend your pelvis. Try these for your three hamstrings: #6 (PA), #9 (BR), and #13(BL)

2. KYPHOTIC CURVES IN YOUR THORACIC SPINE

Often some people have increased backward curves in the mid section of their spine, these are called kyphotic curves. They can come from either muscles on the back of the torso not being flexible enough to shorten to erect you, and/or from muscles on the front of your torso are too short to allow you to straighten up. Try these Resistance Flexibility stretches for both the front and back of the middle of your torso: #15(AP) and #16 (TH).

JOINTS

One way to understand how to target distress in the major 8 joints of the body comes from TCM. The following list can help you to practice the specific stretches for each of these major joints.

Lower Body:

Hip Girdle	#1 (GB) and #2 (LV)
Hip Joint	#5 (ST) and #6 (PA)
Knees	#9 (BR) and #10 (SE)
Ankle and Feet	#13 (BL) and #14 (KI)

Upper Body:

Shoulder Girdle	#3 (LU) and #4 (LI)
Shoulder Joint	#7 (HE) and #8 (SI)
Elbows	#11 (PE) and #12 (SK)
Wrist and Hands	#15 (AP) and #16 (TH)

PHYSIOLOGICAL

All of the 16 *types* Resistance Flexibility exercises have concomitant potential health benefits for all the organ systems in the body based on Traditional Chinese Medicine (TCM) Theory. Review this chart on which RF exercises to practice to help you evaluate and affect the wellness of all your physiological systems.

	Organ—Tissue—Systems
#1	GB—Ligaments—Digestive System (Fat Metabolism)
#2	LV—Tendons—Detoxification
#3	LU—Oxygenation—Air Elimination System
#4	LI—Venous Blood Flow—Waste Elimination System
#5	ST—Muscles—Muscular System
#6	PS— ascia—Digestive System (Enzyme Catalysts)
#7	HE—Blood Volume—Arterial Circulation
#8	SI— Cerebral Spinal Fluid—Cranial Sacral System

<u>Organ</u>—<u>Tissue</u>—<u>Systems</u>

#9 BR—Nerves—Nervous System

#10 SE—Hormones—Endocrine and Reproduction System

#11 PE—Arterial Blood Flow—Arterial Circulation

#12 SK—Skin—External Immune System (Integumentary)

#13 BL—Bones—Skeleton System

#14 KI—Joints—Urinary System

#15 AP—Cartilage—Elimination of Toxins

#16 TH—Lymph Nodes—Internal Immune System

SPECIAL CONCERNS

There are many special concerns people about their health. Viruses reek havoc with one's health. Concussions can also be helped. Try the following stretches for these special concerns.

Viruses #16 (TH)

Concussions #8 (SI, #11(PE), and #16 (TH)

PSYCHOLOGICAL

According to Genetic Personality *Type* (GPT) Theory, each of the sixteen different types of Resistance Flexibility exercises are concomitant with helping to developing high personality traits while dismantling their opposite low traits. Try the Resistance Flexibility stretches that you would like help in developing those specific high personality traits or dismantle their opposite low traits.

#1 GB—Devotion/Dependency

#2 LV—Freedom/Codependency

#3 LU—Empowerment/Suppression

#4 LI—Ambition/Obsession

#5 ST—Sobriety/Addiction

#6 PS—Peaceful/Martyrdom

#7 HE—Right Action/Avoidance

#8 SI—Creativity/Depression

#9 BR—Trust/Paranoid

#10 SE—Intimacy/Mood Disorder

#11 PE—Transparency/Self Defeating

#12 SK—Community/Antisocial

#13 BL—Diversity/Narcissism

#14 KI—Understanding/Splitting

#15 AP—Integrity/Depersonalization

#16 TH—Forgiveness/Menticidal

EMOTIONAL

Emotional maturation is something that everyone can build regardless of the holes in their upbringing. Try the four types of Resistance Flexibility stretches to develop these types of emotional qualities.

#8 (SI) Self Affirmation

#10 (SE) Self Worth

#13 (BL) Self Esteem

#2 (LV) Self Liking

GOOD LOOKS

It is not well understood that a person's looks are a reflection of how they are being with others and not simply their physical endowment. The sixteen different types of stretches can dramatically positively affect your looks. Try these different Resistance Flexibility stretches to help you develop those specific *types* of looks. (Possible famous people may represent these *types* of looks.)

#1 (GB) = Sensual, Pleasing, Appealing, Devine,

Lady Gaga, Matthew McConaughey

#2 (LV) = Pretty, Handsome, Decorative, Ravishing,

Fan Bingbing, Bill Clinton

#3 (LU) = Powerful, Commanding, Remarkable,

Shohreh Aghdashloo, Chris Hemsworth

#4(LI) = Elegant, Perfection, Friendly, Splendid, Charming,

Daniel Radcliff, Naomi Scott

#5 (ST) = Cute, Distinguished, Twinkle in the eyes, Unconventional

Leona Lewis, Bruce Lee

#6 (PA) = Bedazzling, Astonishing, Angelic,

Cheryl Cole, Enrique Iglesias

#7 (HE) = Lovely, Joyful, Inner Beauty

Hugh Grant, Oprah Winfrey

#8 (SI) = Beautiful, High Fashion, Dramatic, Fabulous, Classy

Whitney Houston, Bruno Mars

#9 (BR) = Alluring, Aristocratic, Sophisticated, Superb, Rich

George Vanderbilt, Deviprana (Vedanta Temple Santa Barbara)

#10 (SE) = Sexy, Star, Persona, Good Looking, Gorgeous, Spectacular

Beyonce, Elvis Presley

#11 (PE) = Transparent, Precious, Jewel, Rare, Magnificent,

Bryan Brothers, Pardis Sabeti

#12 (SK)= Stylish, Ravishing, Delightful, Reverence, Striking, Stunning,

Jennifer Lopez, Brad Pitt

#13 (BL)= Image, Reflective, Iconic, Luminescent, Statuesque,

Mariah Carey, Kevin Costner

#14 (KI) = Vast, Deep, Echoing, Absorbing, Illuminated from within

Halle Berry, Will Smith

#15 (AP) = Iridescent, Lustrous, Pleasant,

Meryl Streep, Kevin Spacey

#16 (TH) = Radiant, Glowing, Healthy, Bewitching, Wholesome

Jodi Foster, Mickey Rouke

SPIRITUAL

The Reflection Principle of the Types

The magnificent association of things inside yourself and things outside yourself becomes a principle behind understanding life. Because *types* is such an associatively based system, this inner and outer connection is experienced frequently. For example, one of the *types* is associated with the functioning of the sexual organs, and this *type* also characteristically presents themselves like a peacock in their social behavior. Curiously enough, the traditional Hatha Yoga stretch for the exact muscles associated with this *type* is called peacock! On a more global scale, Gandhi said "Be the change you wish to see in the world." What *types* of things in the world reflect what you are like?

Is it possible, that the *types 16* highest personality traits form the basis for all the different *types* of religions? Perhaps each spiritual tradition is a magnificent pillar that supports spirituality, each providing their high traits as paths to spiritual enlightening. All of these different pathways must be equal in value, none better than any other, yet each offering a different way to the top.

16 Types of Enlightenment—

Joy, Delight, Health, Empowerment,

Sobriety, Devotion, Trust, Understanding,

Equanimity, Bliss, Ecstasy, Freedom, and

Peace, Harmony, Integrity, and Benevolence.

CHAPTER 12

NUTRITION AND RESISTANCE FLEXIBILITY

www.HealthSafari.com

INTRODUCTION

As you Resistance Flexibility train your body, you will experience significant upgrades in the health of all your tissues. Optimizing your nutrition greatly accelerates these upgrades and helps increase flexibility. As you would expect, we find that people who eat a diet rich in organic vegetables and low in sugar and processed foods have tissue that is more elastic and easier to change. The purpose of this section is to give you an overview of the most cutting-edge ways to optimize your nutrition. For healthy, organic product reviews and recommendations related to this overview, visit the Health Hunts section of HealthSafari.com at www.healthsafari.com/health-hunts.

FIRST IMPROVE YOUR DIGESTION

Eating high quality food is only as beneficial as your ability to digest it and assimilate nutrients. Resistance Flexibility training the muscle groups associated with digestive organs (Stomach, Gall Bladder, Liver, Pancreas, Small Intestine and Large Intestine) can dramatically improve your ability to break down, process and eliminate food. For example, preliminary thermographic studies demonstrate that people who have been Resistance Flexibility trained on a regular basis for more than six months enjoy stress-free digestion. They tend not to experience issues such as acid reflux, gall bladder stress, liver stagnation and constipation that typically show up on a thermogram. Furthermore, many individuals with severe, genetically based digestive issues have fully resolved them with Resistance Flexibility.

HYDRATE

The foundation for optimal nutrition begins with proper hydration. *More than 80%* of people live in a chronically dehydrated state. Drinking plenty of water in the morning and afternoon is best. Allow your organs time to rest at night by not drinking or eating three hours before bedtime.

Drink high quality spring water, mineral water or filtered tap water. Do not drink unfiltered tap water as it is typically contaminated with fluoride, chlorine, volatile organic chemicals (VOCs) and endocrine disrupting chemicals from prescription medication residues. The most effective filtration technologies include granular activated carbon (GAC), kinetic degradation fluxion (KDF), capillary membrane, carbon block, fibredyne block, deionization, ion exchange, ceramic and reverse osmosis (RO). The best filters use a combination of these technologies. If you have a reverse osmosis (RO) filtration system, be sure to remineralize your water with a remineralization cartridge; RO strips water of its beneficial minerals. RO also wastes a lot of water.

WAYS OF EATING

Follow your instincts to find what foods work for your body. Doing the Thymus Roll Down (*page 238*) is an excellent way to discern what foods truly nourish you. Developing flexibility in the Thymus meridian helps people crave foods that are healthy for them, eliminating the need for an overly restrictive eating regimen. There are *many* healthy ways of eating. Consider eating the plants associated with your ethnic home—the foods of your ancestors. Be aware that foods that nourish you might be harmful to your friends or family members.

We have found that knowing your Genetic Personality Type (GPT) is extremely useful for optimizing your diet. People of the same GPT tend to like the same foods and have the same nutritional needs and deficiencies. This is an active area of research that will be included in the forthcoming book *Diet and the Types.* Other useful methods of dietary typing include *Eat Right 4 Your Blood Type* by Dr. Peter D'Adamo and *The Metabolic Typing Diet* by Bill Wolcott. *Healing with Whole Foods* by Paul Pitchford is an excellent book that identifies foods to help you heal particular organ systems.

You may find the concept of 90/10 or 95/5 useful. Eating very healthy 90%-95% of the time and then allowing yourself to eat things that you normally would not 5-10% of the time works well for many people. While nutritional needs are highly individual, below are some guidelines and suggestions.

VARIETY IS KEY

Eat a variety of organic, non-GMO vegetables and fruits. Support your local farmer's market whenever possible. You'll get to know the amazing people that produce organic food. Food from your local market is fresher and more nutritious than anything you can buy in a grocery store. If you are interested in growing your own vegetables, *The Vegetable Gardener's Bible, 2nd Edition* by Edward Smith is an excellent resource.

Your diet will naturally evolve as you do. Excessive consumption of any food can produce a negative immune response over time, so it's important to listen to your body's needs and let your diet change with the seasons. For example, many people who eat cooked eggs on a daily basis develop an egg protein allergy.

Healthy vegetables include: spinach, arugula, asparagus, lettuces, endive, broccoli, celery, kale, chard, collard greens, beet tops, turnip tops, snap peas, green beans, cabbage, brussels sprouts, artichokes, okra, bok choy, spring onions, chives, leeks, cilantro, fennel, turnip greens, parsley, microgreens, watercress, sprouts, and cucumbers. These vegetables taste great in a salad, steamed, stir-fried, juiced or blended in a smoothie. Don't boil your vegetables! Boiling destroys nutrients. It's important to eat some *raw* green vegetables every day. Microgreens or arugula can easily be tossed on top of most any dish.

Root vegetables such as beets, radishes, turnips, celeriac, yams, yuca, parsnip, rutabaga, jicama, water chestnut, and yacon are delicious. Steam them or cook them in a soup. Pickled vegetables like kimchi and sauerkraut are rich in probiotics and make excellent side dishes.

For more information on fermented foods, read *The Art of Fermentation* by Sandor Ellix Katz. Don't forget about onions, rhubarb, peppers, tomatoes, mushrooms, garlic and the many other healthy plants not mentioned here!

Chlorella and spirulina, species of algae, are powerful additions to a healthy diet. Drinking a shake with the Vitamineral Greens made by Health Force Nutritionals or the Super Food made by Boku is a great way to start your day. These dehydrated powders are packed with healthy green vegetables from the land and the sea—they help detoxify your body. Green vegetables are both alkalizing and immune boosting; they create the foundation for any truly healthy diet. For more information on green foods, see *The Green Foods Bible* by David Sandoval.

Eat fruits in smaller amounts (no more than 2 servings per day on average) and try to have them separate from other foods (by at least 30 minutes) to improve digestion. Choices: blueberries, blackberries, raspberries, cherries, currants, cranberries, goji berries, mango, grapes, grapefruits, guavas, coconuts, figs, kiwi, orange, banana, apple, mangosteen, pineapple, papaya, peach, passionfruit, pear, persimmon, pomegranate, pomelo, pumpkin, raspberry, strawberry, dragonfruit, lemons, limes, cantaloupe, mulberries, nectarines, honeydew, rambutans, squash, watermelon and avocado.

Fresh fruit makes an excellent dessert! Lower sugar fruits like avocado are easily digested in combination with other foods. Starting your day by drinking a cup of hot water with fresh squeezed organic lemon juice is a great way to hydrate, oxygenate, balance your pH and boost your immune system.

PROTEINS

Healthy sources of animal protein include cage-free, organic eggs, grass-fed beef, grass-fed bison and wild seafood. In addition to being cleaner, grass-fed meat contains more beneficial omega-3 fatty acids than meat from grain-fed animals. Wild salmon, sardines, flounder and haddock tend to contain less mercury than other fish. Eating mackerel, sea bass, tuna and other species can be highly toxic to your body due to their high mercury levels.

When eaten in small amounts, sprouted quinoa and germinated brown rice are decent sources of protein (look for TruRoots brand). These can be cooked and ready to eat within 15 minutes. Quinoa has the advantage of being a complete protein. Unfortunately, quinoa and brown rice register relatively high on the glycemic index and can cause elevations in blood sugar. If you are trying to improve your insulin sensitivity, these foods are not the best choice. When eaten on a regular basis, beans are also not an optimal source of protein. They contain complex carbohydrates that can disrupt your blood sugar levels. Buckwheat and amaranth can be consumed occasionally, but are also relatively high carbohydrate foods.

As a rule of thumb, most people can handle eating roughly 15g of carbohydrate per meal without experiencing spikes in blood sugar. (This varies considerably between individuals, due to genetic and epigenetic factors). A quarter cup of dry quinoa contains 30g of carbohydrate and 5g of protein. A quarter cup of dry brown rice contains 40g of carbohydrate and 4g of protein. For this reason, consuming brown rice or quinoa protein powder is better for many people than eating cooked versions of these foods. Boku Super Protein is a clean, brown rice based protein powder. One scoop of Super Protein contains 10g of carbohydrate and 18g of protein. Garden of Life's Organic Raw Protein, which contains both brown rice and quinoa, offers 3g of carbohydrate and 17g of protein per scoop.

Non-grain, plant-based sources of protein include nuts and seeds, organic pumpkin seed powder, hemp seed powder, pea protein powder and sacha inchi seed powder. One scoop of organic pumpkin seed powder contains about 3g of carbohydrate and 19g of protein.

RAW DAIRY

Grass-fed, raw dairy, when eaten in small amounts, is healthy for many people. Raw dairy in the form of milk, cheese, kefir and butter is a living food that is rich in beneficial bacteria, food enzymes and natural vitamins (especially vitamin A, vitamin K and vitamin E). Pasteurized dairy, on the other hand, is a dead food that should be avoided at all costs. Pasteurization destroys raw milk's nutrients, enzymes and healthy bacteria and promotes the growth of pathogens in milk. Pasteurized milk, cheese and yogurt are highly toxic.

Some people do not respond beneficially to grass-fed, raw dairy. In many cases, this is due to them consuming dairy products from A-1 cattle, which produce milk that has a mutated amino acid in its beta-casein protein. This mutation can lead to negative health effects including upper respiratory congestion, increased phlegm production and digestive distress. Unfortunately, most cattle raised in the United States and Europe are A-1. In many cases, switching to an A-2 breed of cattle makes all the difference. Jersey's, Guernsey, Asian and African are the healthier, A-2 cattle breeds to seek out. Goats and sheep are naturally A-2. To learn more about the importance of A-2 vs. A-1 dairy, read *Devil in the Milk: Illness, Health and Politics of A1 and A2 Milk* by Keith Woodford.

Some people cannot tolerate any raw dairy due to their genetics or epigenetics. Experiment and find out what works for your body. To locate raw dairy producers in your area, visit the Weston A. Price Foundation's campaign for real, raw, grass-fed milk: www.realmilk.com.

Superfoods and Healthy Snacks.

Most green vegetables are considered superfoods due to their high nutrient density and anti-inflammatory properties. Other superfoods include acai, chia seeds, black sesame seeds, reishi mushroom powder, dried cordyceps mushrooms, chaga mushroom powder, sun-dried botija olives, sea buckthorn seed oil, pine nuts, longan fruit, blue-green algae from Klamath Lake, chlorella, spirulina, hydrilla, moringa, ashitaba, dandelion root, chicory root, manuka honey, organic noni juice and raw cacao. For more information on superfoods, read *Superfoods: The Food and Medicine of the Future* by David Wolfe.

For a healthy snack, try trail mixes with raw, sprouted nuts and seeds like almonds, pistachios, pumpkin seeds, walnuts, pecans and brazil nuts. These nuts and seeds are also available as raw nut butters, which are more processed, but still make a great occasional snack when spread on a stick of celery, an apple or a pear.

Other trail mixes include macambo seeds, sacha inchi seeds, tiger nuts, jujube dates and goldenberries. Tiger nuts are an excellent source of resistant starch and help promote the growth of healthy bacteria in your guts. Instead of potato chips, try sweet potato chips cooked in coconut oil or gluten-free almond crackers. Grass-fed beef jerky, bison jerky and wild salmon jerky also make great snacks. Eat coconut butter and try naturally sweetened coconut macaroons for dessert.

ADATOGENIC HERBS AND HERBAL TEAS

Most every modern prescription drug is a synthetic derivative of a compound that was first identified in an herb. When you consume the whole herb, you ingest hundreds (or thousands) of natural phytonutrients that work in unison to help heal your body. Herbs are not normal foods—they are powerful healing plants. Therefore, you'll have to experiment to find out which ones work for you. Beware of overly complex herb combinations. You could consult a Chinese medicine doctor, acupuncturist, herbalist or naturopath to assist you. The Jing Herbs Optimal Health Analysis is a free online tool that can help identify herbs that will work for you: www.JingHerbsAnalysis.com.

While some herbs are used clinically and only for short periods of time, others are ingested regularly as part of a healthy diet. In particular, the class of mild herbs called adaptogens is especially useful. Adaptogens can help you perform better under stressful conditions by facilitating balance and homeostasis in the body. If you are not currently consuming adaptogenic herbs, then now is the time to start. Adaptogens are an easy and delicious way to take your tissue health and performance to the next level.

Adaptogenic herbs come as superfood powders or herbal teas (check out Ron Teeguarden's Dragon Herbs and Jing Herbs). Perhaps the best place to start is to brew a cup of gynostemma tea. Gynostemma has been shown to increase strength, stamina and longevity. Next, you could add some eleuthero or reishi mushroom powder to your cup of tea. Before you'll know it, you'll have a mini tonic bar in your home!

Other healthy adaptogenic herbs include ashwaganda, astragalus, holy basil, hawthorn, elderberry, eucommia, ginger, ginseng, guyusa, he shou wu, schisandra, licorice root, green tea, nettle, rhodiola, rooibos, rose hips, rosemary and turmeric. For more information on the health benefits and uses of adaptogenic herbs, see *Adaptogens in Medical Herbalism* by Donald Yance.

INTERMITTENT FASTING

Intermittent fasting is a powerful technique that can help you balance your blood sugar, lose weight and reduce inflammation. Intermittent fasting increases your sensitivity to insulin and leptin and helps you become fat adapted. This means you'll be able to efficiently burn body fat as fuel when you don't eat for a few hours, instead of feeling starved. Getting fat adapted is one of the most beneficial things you can do for your overall health; you will be less likely to develop diabetes and other chronic diseases.

Here is a sample intermittent fasting protocol. While intermittent fasting, it is important to eat healthy fats and avoid high carbohydrate and sugary foods.

06:00am – 10:00am : Fast

10:00am – 10:45am: High Intensity Aerobic Workout

10:45am – 11:30am: Resistance Flexibility Training

11:30am – 06:00pm : Eat

06:00pm – 10:30pm : Fast

10:30pm – 06:00am : Sleep

Following this kind of fasting protocol for just two or three weeks can result in permanent improvements to your physiology. Many people have no problem intermittent fasting and choose to make it part of their lifestyle. For others, intermittent fasting doesn't work at all. Read *The 8 Hour Diet* by David Zinczenko and Peter Moore for more information about intermittent fasting.

JUICE FASTING

Many people benefit from an annual or bi-annual fresh green vegetable juice cleanse that lasts between three and ten days. Other people enjoy shorter one-day or three-day juice fasts throughout the year. We have seen that juice fasting can accelerate the fascial upgrades caused by Resistance Flexibility training. This could be due to the fact that after your body burns through its fat reserves, it begins to break down excess fascia and scar tissue. Juice fasting can cause your body to generate large quantities of metabolic enzymes, because you do not need to produce nearly as many digestive enzymes while you fast. It is thought that these metabolic enzymes assist with breaking down excess fascia and scar tissue. We have not seen juice fasting cause a complete elimination of dense fascia or scar tissue in the deep muscles of the body. However, improvements do occur and when combined with Resistance Flexibility training, the results are impressive.

Use a slow masticating juicer to squeeze your juice. Masticating juicers do not destroy valuable food enzymes. The pre-squeezed juice sold in stores is not at all suitable for a juice cleanse, because it's not fresh, nutritious or enzymatically rich. Focus on juicing green vegetables and herbs like kale, celery, lettuces, arugula, chard, collard greens, spinach, cabbage, beet greens, cilantro, basil, and mint. Use beets, carrots, apple, lemon and lime sparingly to flavor your creations. If you plan to drink fruit juice as part of your cleanse (pineapple, orange, apple, etc.), then limit it to one small serving each day. Otherwise, you will not cleanse your body but flood it with sugar.

Drinking a high potassium vegetable broth at least two times per day is essential while juice fasting. Potassium broth helps balance your electrolyte levels. Even when you are not juice fasting, you can serve this broth as an appetizer:

Add the following chopped vegetables to a very large pot: One beet, beet tops, three carrots, carrot tops, one yam, three sticks of celery, celery tops, three leaves of kale, one half cabbage, one turnip, ginger, garlic, two teaspoons Himalayan salt. Then, add enough clean water to submerge the vegetables. Simmer for 45 minutes. (Do not let the water boil.) Next, strain away the solids and toss them out. Enjoy! Potassium broth keeps for 24-48 hours if refrigerated. Reheat before serving.

You have to be careful while juice fasting. Toxins are released into your body during this time. Drink plenty of clean water and get a lot of rest. Do not try to participate in high intensity or stressful activities. Juice fasting is traditionally carried out in a relaxing spa environment. Try to create something like this for yourself, especially if you choose to do an extended juice fast. For more information on juice fasting, read *How to Keep Slim, Healthy, and Young with Juice Fasting* by Paavo Airola.

SUGAR: HEALTHY TISSUE'S WORST ENEMY

While everyone likes a good dessert once in awhile, the body has an extremely low tolerance for all forms of processed sugar. Cut these out of your diet to immediately improve your tissue health and overall health. As you would expect, we find that people who eat processed sugars suffer an increase in accumulated dense fascia throughout the body and especially in the medial hamstrings (Pancreas meridian). Resistance Flexibility training the Pancreas meridian (page 158) can help you eliminate sugar cravings by improving your digestion. Sugar consumption is associated with energy highs and lows. Increasing the health of the Pancreas meridian leads to good, sustained energy levels throughout the day.

Recent research demonstrates that the systemic inflammation caused by eating processed sugar damages almost every system in the body and incapacitates the immune system. Processed sugar is poison. Some of the worst sugars are high fructose corn syrup, brown sugar, sucrose, glucose, fructose, cane sugar, cane juice and turbinado. Agave, once touted as a healthy alternative, is also very damaging to the liver due to its high fructose content. Artificial sweeteners such as aspartame and other sugar alcohols are, generally speaking, even worse than processed sugars. Read *Sugar Crush* by Dr. Richard Jacoby to learn more about how sugar impacts the body.

There are some sweeteners that, when used in moderation, are much better for you than others. These include coconut sugar, coconut flakes, dates, date sugar, maple syrup and raw honey. These alternatives affect individuals differently, but when eaten occasionally, in small amounts, one of these sugars will likely agree with your body.

Stevia and lo han guo (monkfruit) are healthy alternatives to processed sugars, assuming that you get the pure versions without any additives or fillers.

EAT HEALTHY FATS

To get healthy, most people need to eat more healthy fats, less sugar and less carbohydrate. Healthy fats are unrefined fats from plants or animal sources that are highly saturated or monounsaturated, or higher in omega-3 fatty acids. To improve your ability to digest fats, try the gall bladder stretch (page 118).

Healthy fats are part of the solution to sugar cravings. The ability of your cells to use ketones (derived from fat) when glucose is low in the bloodstream indicates that the mitochondria of your cells are healthy and functioning properly. However, if you eat a diet high in sugar or carbohydrates, then you will always feel starved when you haven't eaten for a few hours. This indicates that the mitochondria of your cells are not functioning very well, ketones can't be used as fuel and your energy production system needs some work. Along with the Pancreas exercises (page 158), eating more healthy fats, less sugar and less carbohydrates is the easiest way to increase energy production in the body. Healthy fats help improve your insulin sensitivity, curb sugar cravings and are satisfying to eat. Coconut oil has been shown to be the most satisfying.

Healthy fats can also reduce inflammation, balance your metabolism, support weight loss and improve the health of your skin. For athletes, eating healthy fats is essential to the recovery process because it helps balance your hormones. To enjoy the full benefits of eating healthy fats, limit your sugar intake to less than 20g per day.

Sources of healthy fats include avocados, unrefined extra virgin olive oil, coconut oil, coconut butter, unheated organic nut oils, raw nuts (almonds, pecans, seeds, macademia), organic cage-free eggs, grass-fed meats, wild salmon, ghee and raw organic butter. Saturated fats found in coconut oil contain fatty acids that are highly effective destroyers of viruses, bacteria and parasites. For more information on healthy fats, read *Know Your Fats* by Dr. Mary G. Enig.

When cooking, be careful not to burn your oils. If you see smoke rising from the pan, then you have turned the oil rancid. Burning the oil causes dangerous free radicals to be released into your food. Due to its relatively low smoke point, olive oil is not a good option for cooking. Coconut oil is a great option because it is an almost completely saturated fat. Other options include grass-fed butter and ghee, almond oil and avocado oil.

Unhealthy fats include soy oil, peanut oil, corn oil, safflower oil, sunflower oil and canola oil because they contain a high Omega 6: Omega 3 ratio and tend to be oxidized during processing. Read the label and cut oils out of your diet to improve your health.

Although it is touted as healthy and used to cook most of the prepared food at Whole Foods Market, canola oil is damaging to your health! It increases Omega-6 levels, is usually genetically modified and contains a toxic chemical called erucic acid. For more information on the negative health effects of GMO foods, see Jeffrey Smith's awesome film *Genetic Roulette.*

FOOD ALLERGIES AND SENSITIVITIES

It's estimated that 70% of people have developed some form of a food allergy. Most people are not aware of their allergy. Practicing the Stomach exercises (page 150) can help decrease food sensitivities.

The following nine foods account for 90% of food allergies: peanuts, tree nuts, dairy, eggs, wheat, soy, fish, shellfish and sesame. Identifying food allergies does not necessarily require an advanced blood test. In fact, an elimination diet is often a more effective approach, due to the inaccuracies associated with blood testing. Holistic physician Dr. Stephan Rechtschaffen, cofounder of the Omega Institute, advocates the following protocol, which has helped many people identify their food allergies:

If you want to know if you are allergic to gluten, for example, you could completely eliminate gluten from your diet for 7 days. See how you feel. Many people feel worse for the first 4-5 days and then notice a significant improvement on days 6-7. Then, on the 8th day, consume a significant amount of gluten. This approach should produce a magnified negative response on day 8 or day 9 if you are allergic to gluten.

THE TROUBLE WITH GLUTEN, GRAINS, AND GLUTEN-FREE FOODS.

Gluten and other grains like soybeans, oats, sorghum, barley, rice and corn all contain proteins that are generally difficult for our bodies to digest. This stems from the fact that we did not evolve to eat grains of any kind. For many people, reducing or eliminating wheat and other grains from your diet can cause dramatic improvements to your health and cognitive function. Other people are not so negatively affected by eating grains and can get healthy eating a diet that is composed of up to 15% grains. The hybridized, high-gluten forms of wheat grown in America today are certainly less healthy than heirloom European varieties. Non-organic corn and soy, prevalent in the processed food supply, have been shown to contain significant amounts of glyphosate, the active ingredient in RoundUp, and should be treated strictly as poison.

Many individuals that have tested negative for Celiac's disease believe they are not allergic to gluten, but this is not necessarily the case. The symptoms of non-celiac gluten sensitivity, for example, are almost identical to those of Celiac disease. It's a useful exercise to completely eliminate *all* grains from your diet for a week or two and see how you feel. Foods labeled gluten-free are not necessarily healthy; they often contain other grains, processed sugars, binders and fillers. *Wheat Belly* by Dr. William Davis and *Grain Brain* by Dr. David Perlmutter are outstanding books on the science of eating wheat and other grains.

HEAL YOUR GUTS!

Leaky gut syndrome is a hidden epidemic that causes many secondary health problems. It is estimated that *over 80% of people* experience some degree of leaky gut, which is associated with chronic inflammation in the body. Over 11,000 studies about leaky gut have been published in the scientific literature. Still, the medical profession largely denies the condition has no protocol to diagnose it. Practice the Small Intestine exercises (page 174) to help heal your guts.

Leaky gut can cause the following symptoms: chronic diarrhea, constipation, gas, bloating, nutritional deficiencies, and suppression of the immune system. Leaky gut is also linked to impaired cognitive function and can cause headaches, brain fog, memory loss and overall fatigue. You can dramatically improve your brain functioning by healing your guts.

The small intestine acts like a net. Normally, only nutrients are allowed to pass through this highly selective net and enter your blood. However, if the net has holes ripped in it, then large particles escape into your blood. The immune system may see these particles as foreign objects and attack them.

Eating processed foods such as hydrogenated vegetable oils, gluten and pasteurized dairy typically causes the initial tearing of the small intestine. Eliminating these foods from your diet, along with fried foods and canned foods, can help you heal your gut. Other causes of leaky gut include exposure to toxic chemicals, mold, prescription medications and toxic skin care products.

Organic, grass-fed bone broth has been shown to help heal leaky gut, as well as probiotics, aloe vera juice, fish oil and the supplements proline, glycine, l-glutamine and collagen. For more information on this topic, see the *Healing Leaky Gut Program Course* by Dr. Josh Axe.

GET A NUTRITIONAL BLOOD TEST

The most important nutrient for you today is the nutrient that you are low in. Advanced micronutrient blood testing can help you identify vitamin, mineral and amino acid deficiencies, as well as determine your heavy metal levels. In most states, you will simply need to coordinate with your physician to receive these tests. Call in advance and arrange for them to order you the test and draw your blood. Pricing varies depending on your location and practitioner. Genova Diagnostics, SpectraCell Laboratories and Cyrex Laboratories are leaders in nutritional testing.

The Genova Ion Nutritional Test is excellent. This test measures vitamins, minerals, antioxidants, amino acids, essential fatty acids, minerals and heavy metals in your blood. Genova also offers advanced food allergy testing.

SpectraCell Labs offers a nutritional test that measures 35 nutritional components, including vitamins, minerals, antioxidants and amino acids.

Cyrex Labs offers nutritional testing for specific concerns such as gluten sensitivity and food allergies.

SUPPLEMENT TO BALANCE OMEGA 6: OMEGA 3

We have found that Resistance Flexibility helps people achieve excellent health without taking a lot of supplements. However, there are some nutritional needs that you'll only get by supplementation. Taking an animal-based Omega-3 fatty acid supplement each day is essential.

For millennia, humans evolved and lived with an Omega-6 to Omega-3 fatty acid ratio of 1:1 in the bloodstream. However, due to eating processed foods and unhealthy oils, the average person in the Western world now has a ratio of about 15:1 or 20:1 (depending on the study). High Omega-6 levels are linked to inflammation and can cause many preventable diseases, including heart disease. This means we need to avoid high Omega-6 fats, eat high Omega-3 fats and take an Omega-3 supplement.

The best Omega-3 supplements come from an animal source such as fish or krill, because they contain eicosapentaenoic acid (EPA) and docosahexaenoic acid (DHA), which are the most beneficial Omega-3 fatty acids. EPA and DHA are linked to reduced inflammation and improvements in heart health. Plant-based Omega-3 sources, such as hemp, chia seeds and flaxseeds, contain alpha-linoleic acid (ALA), which does not provide the same health benefits as EPA and DHA. If you are vegetarian, consider taking an algae-based Omega-3 supplement—these are 100% vegetarian but contain EPA and DHA.

THE BEST SUPPLEMENTS

If you eat a healthy, whole-food based diet, then you won't need to take a lot of supplements. However, some nutrients are very difficult or impossible to obtain through diet. For many people, a basic supplement regimen includes:

Vitamin D-3, suspended in olive oil or coconut oil: It is estimated that 85% of people are Vitamin D deficient. While daily sun exposure is part of a healthy lifestyle and provides some Vitamin D, taking a D-3 supplement is essential. Vitamin D has been shown to increase bone health, fight infection, stop abnormal cell growth and prevent most every disease.

Whole Food Multivitamin: Consider taking a high quality, whole food multivitamin, like those produced by Garden of Life and MegaFood to get a broad spectrum of essential vitamins and minerals. While conventional multivitamins contain isolated or synthetic vitamins and minerals, whole food multivitamins are sourced from real food and contain valuable co-factors and phytonutrients.

Animal based Omega-3s: As previously discussed, taking an animal-based Omega-3 supplement is essential for good health.

Probiotics: Taking a probiotic supplement, such as those produced by Garden of Life and MegaFood, is a great way to help heal your guts. Probiotic capsules are best taken at bedtime. You could also eat fermented foods like kimchi or sauerkraut (with lunch or dinner) to increase the growth of healthy bacteria in your guts.

Digestive Enzymes: If you have trouble digesting food, consider taking plant-based digestive enzymes prior to each major meal. Digestive enzymes dramatically help many people lose excess weight. Options include Swedish Bitters and plant-based digestive enzyme capsules. In the long term, you will want to heal your digestive organs so that you do not become dependent on enzymes. In the short term, enzymes can help your digestive organs heal by giving them a break from overworking. For more information on the importance of enzymes, read *Enzyme Nutrition* by Dr. Edward Howell.

Other useful supplements include Co-Q10, astaxanthin (BioAstin) and minerals. To discover the specific supplements you need, you could take one of the nutritional blood tests mentioned above or hire someone that helps people optimize their nutrition. Consult *Disease Prevention and Treatment* by the Life Extension Foundation to learn how herbs and supplements can be used to treat virtually any disease or health condition.

DETOXIFICATION

In the modern world, we are constantly ingesting toxins through the air we breathe, the water we drink and the food we eat. Reduce your exposure by eating organic food, filtering your air and water and using only non-toxic skin care products and cleaning supplies. The Appendix exercises (page 230) can help you eliminate toxins.

Toxins such as lead, mercury and aluminum tend to get stored in fat tissue. In fact, the presence of heavy metals in your bloodstream encourages your body to increase fat storage. Many people become less healthy after losing weight, because toxins flood the body as excess fat is eliminated. Along these lines, Resistance Flexibility training can cause toxins to be released into the body. After stretching, be sure to drink plenty of clean water and choose easy to digest foods such as juices, superfood powders, hot soups and green salads.

To determine the levels of heavy metals and other toxins in your body, visit a holistic physician and receive a heavy metal chelation challenge and urinalysis test. If you currently take prescription drugs, ask your physician before trying any of the following detox methods. (Prescription drugs are generally toxic and can be eliminated by foods and supplements that detoxify the body.)

Eating plenty of raw green vegetables and drinking raw green vegetable juice on a regular basis is a good place to start. Other mild detox methods include chlorella, spirulina, cilantro, garlic, plant-based MSM, bentonite clay, coconut charcoal and dehydrated seaweed. Of these options, many people find that liquid bentonite clay (look for Sonne's or Great Plains) works the best. When people begin to Resistance Flexibility train, they often experience headaches during or directly after stretching. We have found that drinking a couple teaspoons of bentonite clay dissolved in a large glass of water is highly effective at eliminating these headaches.

Dr. Schulze produces many outstanding herbal products for periodic detoxification including colon cleanses, liver/gallbladder cleanses and kidney/bladder cleanses. Visit www.herbdoc.com to learn more. For more medically intensive detox needs, find a holistic physician that offers DMPS injections.

Going in an infrared sauna is another useful way to detoxify. Infrared saunas heat your body from the inside out and have been shown to help dislodge heavy metals and other toxins from deep tissues. For detox purposes, infrared saunas are more effective than electric saunas or steam rooms.

Mercury amalgam fillings cause significant toxicity to the body and can impair many physiological systems. No level of mercury is safe. Only let a trained holistic dentist remove mercury amalgams from your mouth. If not performed properly, removal of mercury amalgams can cause large quantities of mercury to enter your body. For more information on this topic, read *Holistic Dental Care: The Complete Guide to Healthy Teeth and Gums* by Nadine Artemis and Victor Zeines D.D.S. To locate a holistic dentist, visit the Holistic Dental Association at holisticdental.org.

BUILDING YOUR NATURAL MEDICINE CABINET

Keeping a supply of natural medicines on hand is key to staying healthy. The moment you feel a cold virus, flu or infection coming on, try the Thymus exercises (page 238) to help boost your immune system, open your natural medicine cabinet and start treating yourself.

Essential immune boosting products include food-based Vitamin C powder, ginger tea, ginger extract, elderberry extract, turmeric extract, echinacea extract and goldenseal extract. Oregano oil has powerful anti-bacterial properties. Boku Super Immune Tonic and California Naturals Immunity Shots are great combination products to keep on hand. For colds, try mucus dissolving enzymes, black elderberry syrup, manuka honey lozenges or a neti pot with neti salts. Homeopathic medicines such as Umcka, Boiron Coldcalm and Boiron Sinusalia also help. For flu concerns, try Boiron Oscillococcinum. Wormwood and black walnut are useful for dealing with intestinal parasites.

For millennia, essential oils have been used to create health and longevity and to treat disease. These oils are powerful medicines that can be rubbed on your skin or taken orally in small amounts. Ty Bollinger's outstanding documentary series *The Truth About Cancer* examines how essential oils are being used to effectively treat brain cancer and other forms of cancer.

You can supercharge a cup of herbal tea by adding a few drops of food grade, organic essential oil. Here are some of the most beneficial essential oils: frankincense, myrrh, oregano, peppermint, rose, rosemary, tea tree, lavender, clove, eucalyptus, lemon, cinnamon, cypress, grapefruit, peppermint, ginger, cedarwood, bergamot and melaleuca. With a bit of research, you can use essential oils to improve your health. Read Dr. Josh Axe's *Essential Oils Guide* to learn more.

CONCLUSION

Getting healthy should be simple and fun! Your body instinctively knows the foods that you need to heal and become your healthiest self. Resistance Flexibility helps connect you to these instincts. You will likely undergo significant dietary changes when you begin to stretch. Listen to your body. Try new ways of eating.

Hiring a Holistic Health Coach is a great way to get on the fast track to excellent health. Holistic Health Coaches are trained to coach you in ways that are compatible with your lifestyle, helping you achieve optimal health and success in all areas and never recommending overly restrictive, impossible to follow eating guidelines.

For healthy, organic product reviews and recommendations related to the foods mentioned in this chapter, visit the Health Hunts section of HealthSafari.com at www.healthsafari.com/health-hunts.

CHAPTER 13

THE GENIUS OF FLEXIBILITY CENTERS

Sustainable Trainers and Eco-Sustainable Centers

ACTIVITIES IN ALL CENTERS

There are ongoing Resistance Flexibility private sessions, classes, Affiliate Certification Trainings, and workshops in all centers. See TheGeniusofFlexibility.com for contact and information.

"We have worked with all types of people from all socio-economic, racial, and spiritual backgrounds. The way we help them is to develop those parts of them that for whatever reason were not yet developed-we develop them in all ways physically, psychologically, emotionally, and spiritually. We concentrate on helping everyone to simply become better them.
BobCooley@TheGeniusofFlexibility.com

WELCOME TO THE GENIUS OF FLEXIBILITY CENTERS

The Genius of Flexibility Centers creates a traditional healing environment that includes group participation, transparency, group perspective, and where the healing of the healers is a priority.

It is important for people participating at the center to understand how classes and private sessions are conducted. Often the activities involved in healing are in stark contrast to the current corporate health practices where the medical practitioner isolates the client in a closed room, and only they treat the person.

During both classes and private sessions:

1. Other people in the room are asked to give their perspective, feelings and knowledge on the changes that have occurred for someone who has been assisted or after their self-stretch. The perspective of others honors and acknowledges the genius of others knowledge.

2. Everyone can be asked to participate to help assist another person. Resistance Flexibility training often requires many people to help generate the movement necessary to help someone.

3. All four aspects of a person are discussed which is essential to creating those parts of a person that have yet to be developed and which are the root causes of their health concerns.

4. Though time slots are arranged, often both the beginning and ending times are somewhat flexible in order to allow both the participants and the practitioners to accomplish the work that has been attempted to help everyone.

5. Everyone needs to embrace the valuable opportunity to learn from others experiences. Often other people are assisted during a private session or discussions occur that are of significant value to everyone.

THE GENIUS OF FLEXIBILITY SANTA BARBARA

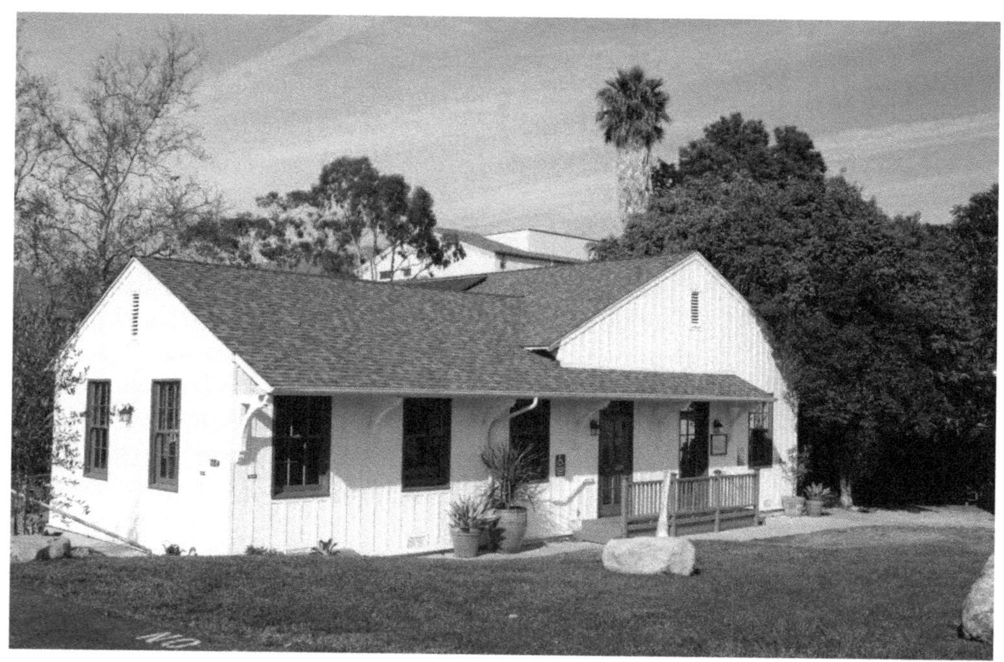

914 A Santa Barbara St. Santa Barbara, CA 93101
Contact:
www.TheGeniusofFlexibility.com/contact/
Owner:
BobCooley@TheGeniusofFlexibility.com

SB Elite Resistance Flexibility Trainers:

LutherCowden@TheGeniusofFlexibility.com

NickWare@TheGeniusofFlexibility.com

ChrisRenfrom@TheGeniusofFlexibility.com

BonnieCrotzer@TheGeniusofFlexibility.com

SB Resistance Flexibility Interns:

NoelChristensen@TheGeniusofFlexibility.com

KajHoffman@TheGeniusofFlexibility.com

SamuelCamburn@TheGeniusofFlexibility.com

KatConnorsLongo@TheGeniusofFlexibility.com

KarenMason@TheGeniusofFlexibility.com

PatrickGregston@TheGeniusofFlexibility.com

JohnBagasarian@TheGeniusofFlexibility.com

ChrisPearsall@TheGeniusofFlexibility.com

AlexNolte@TheGeniusofFlexibility.com

EthanDupris@TheGeniusofFlexibility.com

RichardGregston@TheGeniusofFlexibility.com

BrianMay@TheGeniusofFlexibility.com

PeterDonovan@TheGeniusofFlexibility.com

THE GENIUS OF FLEXIBILITY LOS ANGELES

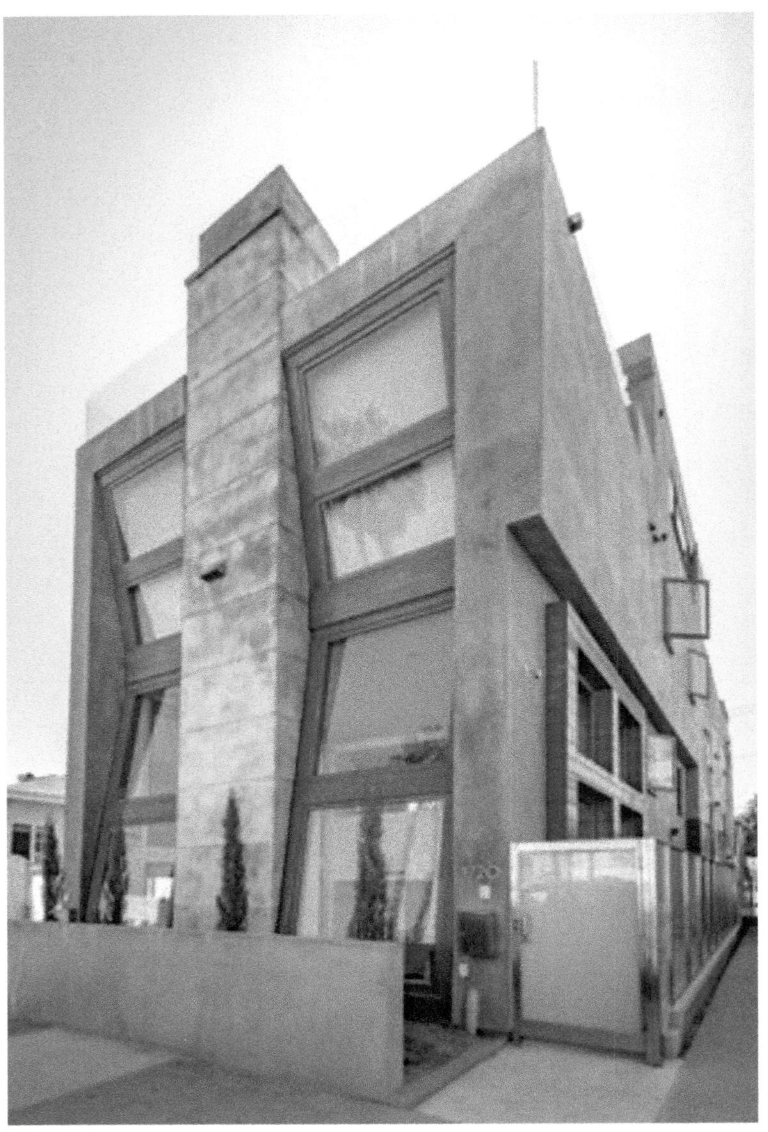

1720 Abbot Kinney Blvd. Los Angeles, CA 90291

Contact:

www.TheGeniusofFlexibility.com/contact/

Owner:

BobCooley@TheGeniusofFlexibility.com

LA Elite Resistance Flexibility Trainers:

LutherCowden@TheGeniusofFlexibility.com

NickWare@TheGeniusofFlexibility.com

ChrisRenfrow@TheGeniusofFlexibility.com

BonnieCrotzer@TheGeniusofFlexibility.com

PeterDonovan@TheGeniusofFlexibility.com

LA Resistance Flexibility Interns:

NoelChristensen@TheGeniusofFlexibility.com

KajHoffman@TheGeniusofFlexibility.com

SamuelCamburn@TheGeniusofFlexibility.com

KatConnorsLongo@TheGeniusofFlexibility.com

KarenMason@TheGeniusofFlexibility.com

PatrickGregston@TheGeniusofFlexibility.com

JohnBagasarian@TheGeniusofFlexibility.com

ChrisPearsall@TheGeniusofFlexibility.com

AlexNolte@TheGeniusofFlexibility.com

EthanDupuis@TheGeniusofFlexibility.com

RichardGregston@TheGeniusofFlexibility.com

BrianMay@TheGeniusofFlexibility.com

THE GENIUS OF FLEXIBILITY NY NY

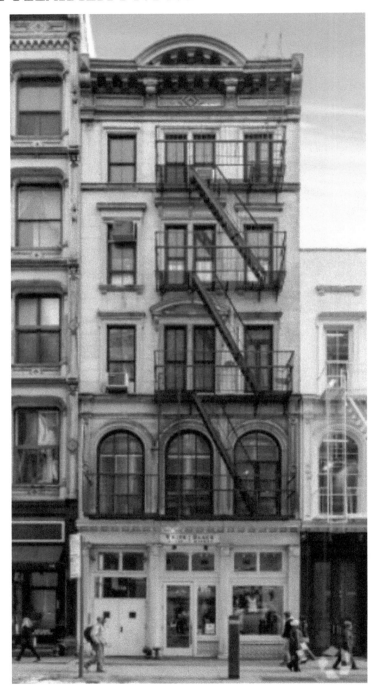

508 Broadway 2nd Floor NY, NY 10012
Contact:
www.TheGeniusofFlexibility.com/contact/
Owner:
BobCooley@TheGeniusofFlexibility.com

<u>NY Elite Resistance Flexibility Trainers:</u>

JohnKelly@TheGeniusofFlexibility.com

BerylHagenburg@TheGeniusofFlexibility.com

LutherCowden@TheGeniusofFlexibility.com

BonnieCrotzer@TheGeniusofFlexibility.com

<u>NY Resistance Flexibility Interns:</u>

KateRabinowitz@TheGeniusofFlexibility.com

EricDermont@TheGeniusofFlexibility.com

THE GENIUS OF FLEXIBILITY BOSTON

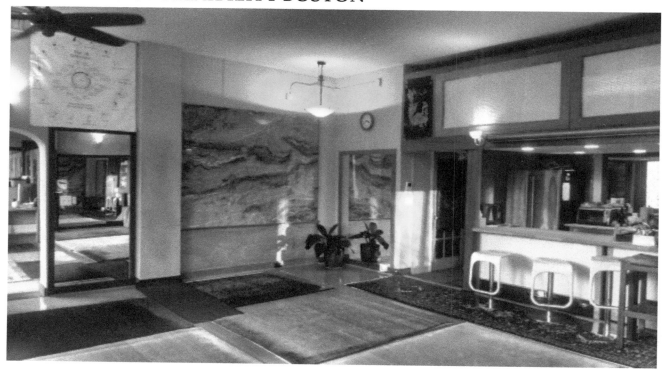

561 Boylston St 2nd Floor Boston, MA 02115
<u>Contact:</u>
www.TheGeniusofFlexibility.com/contact/
<u>Owner:</u>
BobCooley@TheGeniusofFlexibility.com

<u>Boston Elite Resistance Flexibility Trainers:</u>

ChrisRenfrow@TheGeniusofFlexibility.com

EricBeutner@TheGeniusofFlexibility.com

Resistance Flexibility Intern

RobObrien@TheGeniusofFlexibility.com

ZakOrme@TheGeniusofFlexibility.com

STRETCHWORKS—AFFILATE CENTER

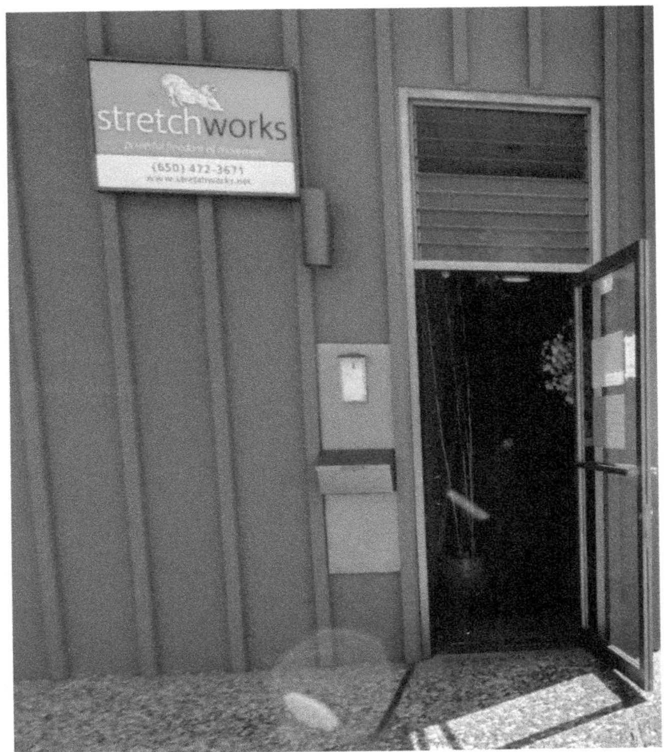

3636 Florence Street
Redwood City, CA 94063

<u>Contact:</u>

1-650-472-3671

<u>Owner:</u>

TomLongo@TheGeniusofFlexibility.com

<u>Elite Trainer:</u>

TomLongo@TheGeniusofFlexibility.com

<u>Resistance Flexibility Intern:</u>

NicholasRoby@TheGeniusofFlexibility.com

THE GENIUS OF FLEXIBILITY CENTER—SANTA BARBARA

A totally green center in the heart of Santa Barbara

Santa Barbara Contractors Association, Built Green Santa Barbara, the Santa Barbara Trust for Historic Preservation, and California Department of Parks and Recreation

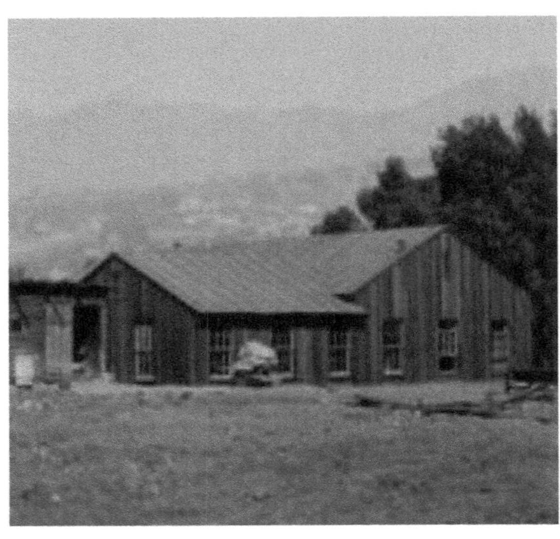

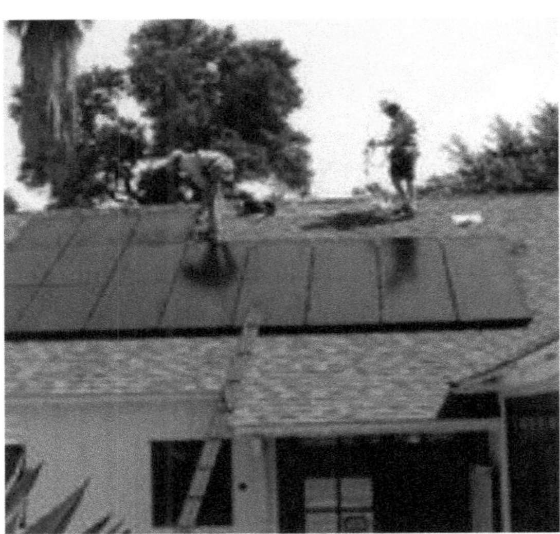

Originally part of the Santa Barbara School of the Arts, the building is a rehabilitated historic structure using state of the art green building practices. Green building practices go beyond energy and water conservation to incorporate environment sensitive site planning, resource efficient building materials and superior indoor air quality, and examination of life cycle costs, transportation energy and embodied energy.

SBCA member contractors will install FSC wood throughout, breathable membranes and specialized vapor shields, drainage planes, foam insulation, high performance architectural replacement windows, heat pump technology, low flow and waterless plumbing fixtures, tankless water heater, ultra high efficiency lights, solar water heating, photo voltaic electric generation panels, improved indoor air quality and site water control.

SANTA BARBARA TRUST FOR HISTORIC PRESERVATION

805-965-0093

SANTA BARBARA CONTRACTORS ASSOCIATION

805-884-1100

BUILT GREEN SANTA BARBARA

805-884-1100

CHAPTER 14

RESISTANCE FLEXIBILITY THEORY

Putting theory into practice

There are several important principles that compose the theory of Resistance Flexibility. Each is a discovery of itself and often a paradigm changer.

Resistance Flexibility is not the same as excessive eccentric loading. In Resistance Flexibility Training the end range of motion is determined and limited to the capacity of the target muscles groups capacity to shorten. This principle is not currently considered in EEL research design. Potential injury can result from EEL if this principle and practice is not considered.

• The Principle of True Flexibility

You've discovered that a muscle is only truly flexible to the point where it can continue to maximally resist while being lengthened. When a muscle can no longer contract maximally, it is being over-stretched and is subject to injury. Increased flexibility translates into increased biomechanical efficiency as well as increases in power, speed, and acceleration. Flexible muscles are much less likely to be injured and stay youthful longer. A muscle is not flexible if it cannot contract at any point while being elongated regardless of range.

• The Principle of Limitations

You've discovered that a muscle's ability to shorten is inversely proportional to its ability to lengthen. Limited flexibility results in a proportionately limited shortening ability of your muscles. A muscle can only shorten maximally if it has achieved optimal flexibility. Optimal flexibility translates into optimal performance. Flexibility is the highest correlating factor for athletic success.

• The Principle of Concomitance

There exists an exact association between distinct muscle groups and organ/tissue and genetic personality types. Predictable benefits can occur based on this concomitance.

• Principle of Natural Posture

It takes no mental gymnastics to have good posture. If you remove ADFST, then your body naturally forms into wonderful posture. Attempts to control or improve one's posture through mental control lead to joint distress.

• The Principle of Equivalency

The four equivalent parts are instinct, knowledge, being and perspective respectively of the physical, thinking, emotional, and spiritual worldviews. Everything inside is reflected in everything outside.

• The Principle of Balancing Muscles

You've discovered that muscles directly across from one another through the center of that body part are called Balancing Muscles. For example, the balancing muscles of the target muscles being stretched need to be flexible enough so that they can contract sufficiently to move you through the stretch movement to stretch your target muscles. It is not usually the muscle that you are trying to stretch that is limiting you but its balancing muscle group that cannot shorten sufficiently to allow you to move into the stretch. Balancing muscles need to be close to equal in strength and flexibility.

When the muscle on one side of your body is short and inflexible the balancing muscles on the other side of your body is also short and inflexible.

• The Principle of Opposing Muscle Groups

You've discovered that muscles perpendicular to one another are called the counter-balancing muscle groups. An example of counter-balancing muscle groups would be your central quads and hamstrings, and your central adductors and central abductors. Another example would be your anterior-lateral muscle groups and posterior-medial muscle groups, and your anterior-medial muscle groups and your posterior-lateral muscle groups. Note there are only four pairs of counterbalancing muscle groups in either your legs or arms. If your target muscle being stretched does not release tension by stretching its balancing muscle group, then you'll need to stretch the counter-balancing muscle groups.

• The Principle of Strength and Flexibility

You've discovered that because a muscle must contract strongly (even maximally) while stretching, that muscle will need to have sufficient strength while stretching in order to be capable of stretching. Strengthen a muscle before you stretch it, to insure your success when stretching it. Flexibility training also results in a 15% increase in strength, as well as strength training resulting in a 15% increase in flexibility. It takes twice the force to stretch a muscle as to strengthen it. The flexibility and strength of a muscle are balanced only if the muscle's strength equals half of the resistance force when it is being stretched.

• The Principle of Five Conscious Choices

There are five choices everyone needs to make when stretching or being assisted: Starting and Stopping, Speed, Range, Direction, Force.

• Arm Dominance

Obviously everyone is mostly leg or arm dominant, and therefore it is important to develop whichever one is not dominant. It requires both the legs and arms to develop true flexibility when either self stretching or assisted stretching.

• The Spiral Pattern for Joint Distress

Because the affect of gravity on the body is a spiral, the pattern of dysfunction occurs in alternating joints on the two side of the body. For example, if a person has a hip girdle problem on the left side of their body, this also results in distress in the right hip joint, the left knee, and the right ankle and foot. The same pattern occurs in the upper body. For example, if a person has distress in their left shoulder girdle, then this results in distress in the right should joint, the left elbow, and the right wrist and hand.

• The Four *types* of Body Patterns of Distress

There are four form patterns of distress with concomitant *types* of concerns. If a person has a discernable difference between the upper and lower parts of their body, then they may have one of four of the physical *types* as their major problem. If they have most of their biomechanical concerns on one side their body compared to the other, then they can have one of four of the thinking types as their major problem. If they have a marked front and back body discrepancy then they may have one of the four emotional *types* as their major concern. And if a person has one arm and one leg on opposite sides of their body as their major concern, then they may have one of four of the spiritual *types* as their major problem.

• The Principle of Aerobic and Flexibility

You've discovered that because it takes many repeats to stretch a muscle, when you have the aerobic capacity necessary to do the necessary repetitions, then your flexibility training is successful. Aerobically train muscles before you stretch them. Good aerobic capacity is highly predictive of the *rate* you can increase your flexibility.

• The Principle of Nutrient Rich Food and Flexibility

You have discovered that your ability to increase your flexibility is significantly improved by having great nutritional habits. The quality of the food and water you have ingested throughout your entire life reflects in the health of your tissues. The only way to become more flexible is by constantly improving your diet. In many people, detoxing old bad food residues from your body is necessary before any increases in flexibility can occur.

• The Principle of Concomitance

You've discovered that there exists an exact association between distinct muscle groups and physiological and psychological benefits that can be produced by increasing the flexibility and strength of on each of the different 16 groups of muscles. Knowing in advance what specific benefits can be derived from different types of stretches allows you to self-diagnosis and then decides which stretches you wish to work on.

• The Principle of Reflection

Stretching teaches you that your body and your life reflect each other. When a musical note is played, everything resonates with that note. Both your life and your body reverberate one another. Therefore improve your body and your life will be moved to improve. You've discovered this explicit connection between what is happening in your life and where those things reflect within you. The ways you know how to *be* reflect in your body in predictable muscle groups. The healthier your behavior the more flexible those concomitant muscle groups become. By changing yourself internally or externally produces a change in the other change yourself inside and your life changes, or change your life and your insides change. The same applies for emotional and psychological changes.

• The Principle of Genius

Your true self reflects through your genius. Being capable of connecting with the genius in others connects you to the genius in yourself. This way of being brings forth compassion, unconditional love, integrity, and acceptance to everyone.

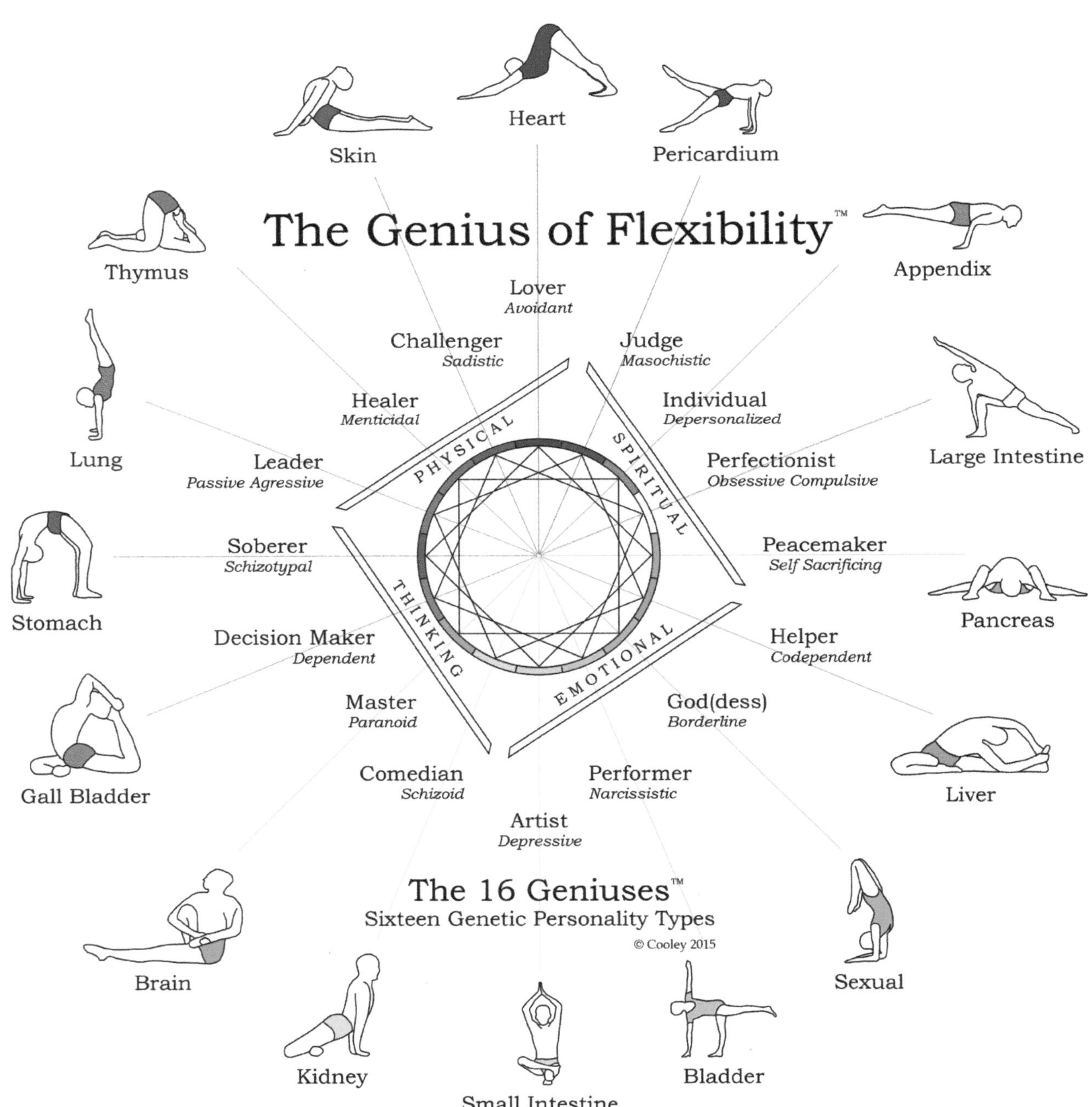

Four Parts of Cooley's Yoga & Resistance Flexibility

Physical, Thinking, Emotional, and Spiritual

PHYSICAL

POSITIONING AND MOVING

Deferring to your body. Let your body show you how to position, reposition, and move to obtain the best stretch instead of just habitually moving.

THINKING

ATTENTION AND IDENTIFICATION

Deferring to your mind. You decide what idea you want to do and then the idea directs you to what to pay attention to - things either inside or out yourself, so you can learn how to do the thing you decided to do. Sensing what exactly is being stretched and the effect of the stretch instead of controlling your attention.

EMOTIONAL

USE OF TENSION AND RELAXATION

Deferring to your breathing. The muscles naturally generate tension when stretching. A person can be aware of the tension necessary to stretch a particular part of their body and will have to either reduce the amount of tenseness that is already present or increase the tension appropriate to the stretch instead of controlling your breathing.

SPIRITUAL

USE OF RESISTANCE OR YIELDING

Deferring to your spirit. The body naturally resists when stretching. This resistance is created by the fascia. A person may either need to resist more or reduce their resistance in order to get a stretch instead of controlling their energy.

"The whole is greater than the sum of the parts. Your body knows how to use all four of these parts when stretching. Let all four parts happen naturally."

Concomitance of Resistance Flexibility with Traditional Chinese Medicine (TCM)

The binding association between different types of stretches and their ability to access and produce specific benefits is an example of *concomitance*. A concomitant relationship between two things explicitly demands that one thing always **bring** with it the other…they have an inseparable relationship, *not* a casual relationship!

When one thing is inseparably connected or associated to another thing, there is said to be a ***concomitance*** *between those two things.*

Perhaps the most important concomitance with TCM organs and meridian muscle groups is the 'body part' or tissue association with each organ.

Organ	Tissue / Body Part	System
GB	Ligaments	Digestive (Fat Metabolism)
LV	Tendons	Digestive, Detoxification
LU	Oxygenation	Respiratory, Cardiovascular
LI	Venous Blood Flow	Digestive, Waste Elimination, Cardiovascular
ST	Muscles	Muscular, Digestive, Metabolism
PA	Fascia	Digestive (Enzyme Catalysts)
HE	Blood Volume	Arterial Circulation
SI	Cerebrospinal Fluid	Craniosacral
BR	Nerves	Central & Peripheral Nervous
SE	Hormones	Endocrine and Reproductive
PE	Arterial Blood Flow	Peritoneal
SK	Skin	External Immune (Integumentary)
BL	Bones	Skeletal
KI	Joints	Urinary
AP	Cartilage	Digestive, Elimination of Toxins
TH	Lymph Nodes	Internal Immune

Maximum Flexibility = Maximum Contraction

If the resting length of a muscle is this long:

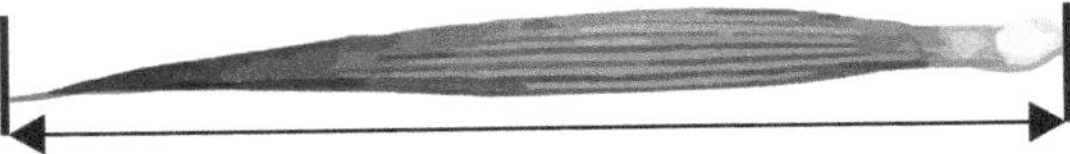

And if maximal flexibility length can be achieved:

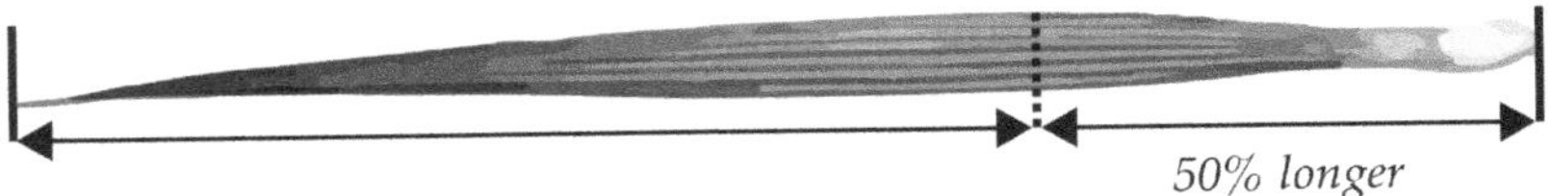

Then this contraction shortening length is possible:

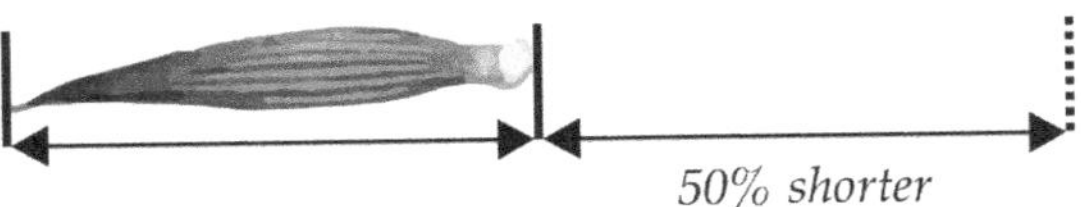

BUT,

Again, if the resting length of a muscle is this long:

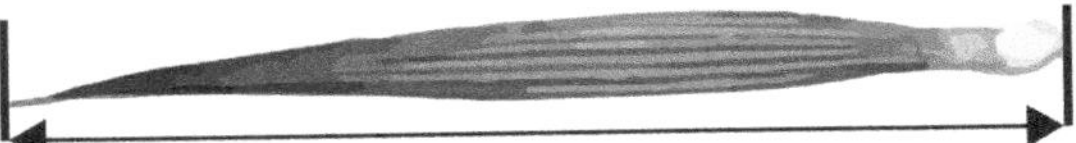

And sub-maximal flexibility is only 25% greater than resting length:

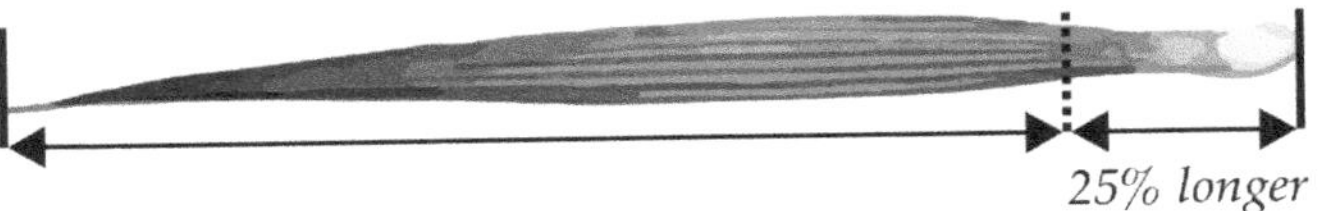

Then only 25% shortening can occur:

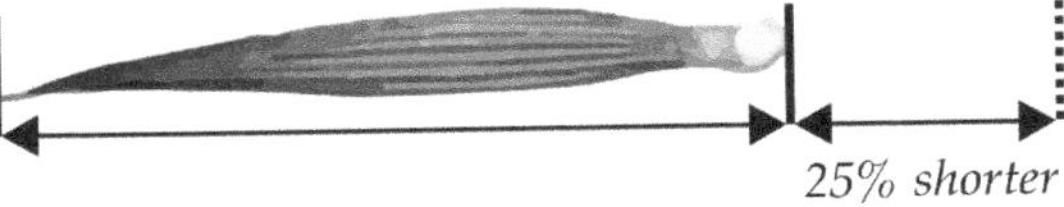

TRADITIONAL CHINESE MERIDIAN LINES
(See www.TheGeniusofFlexibility.com/TrainingArchive for details)

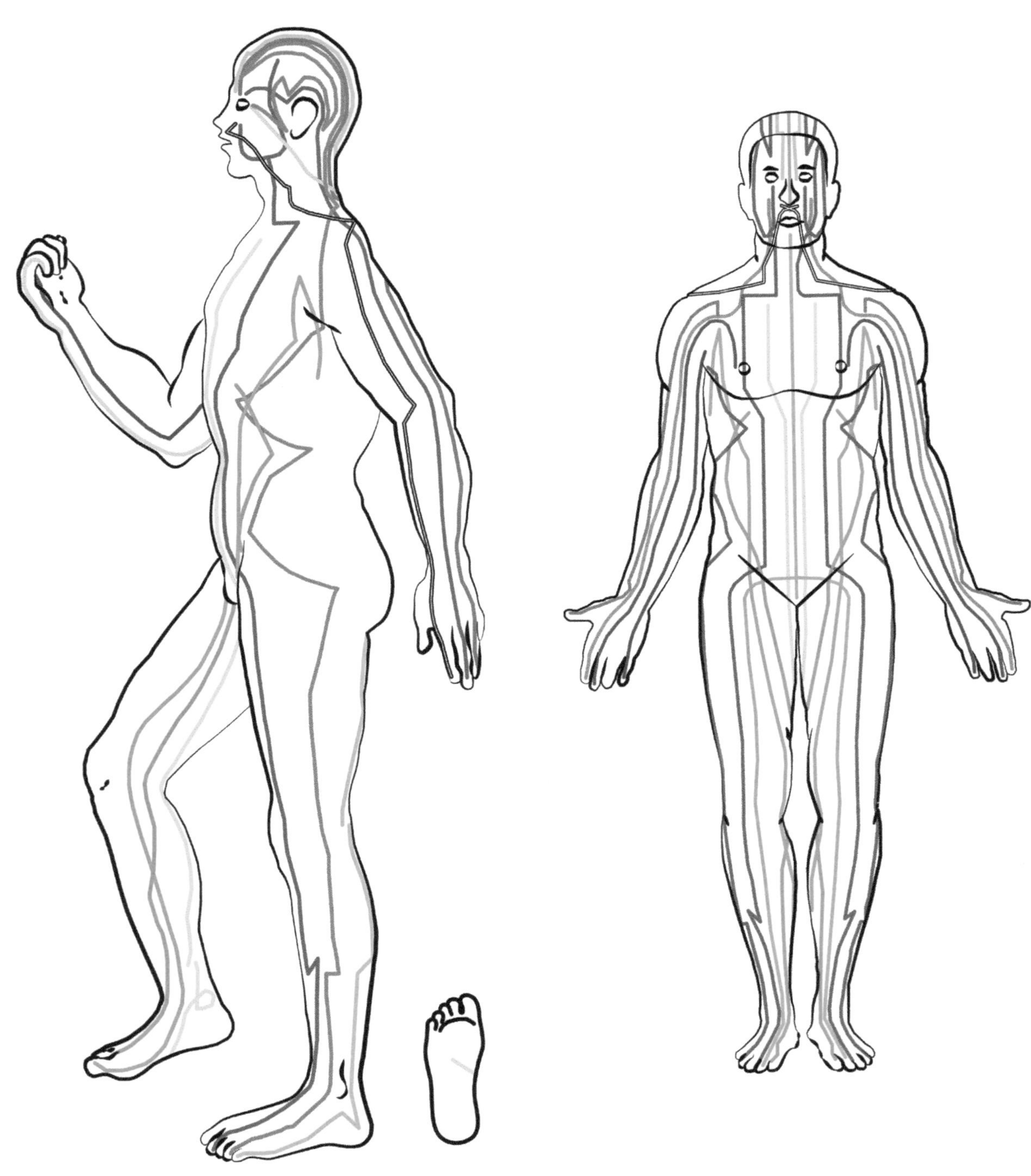

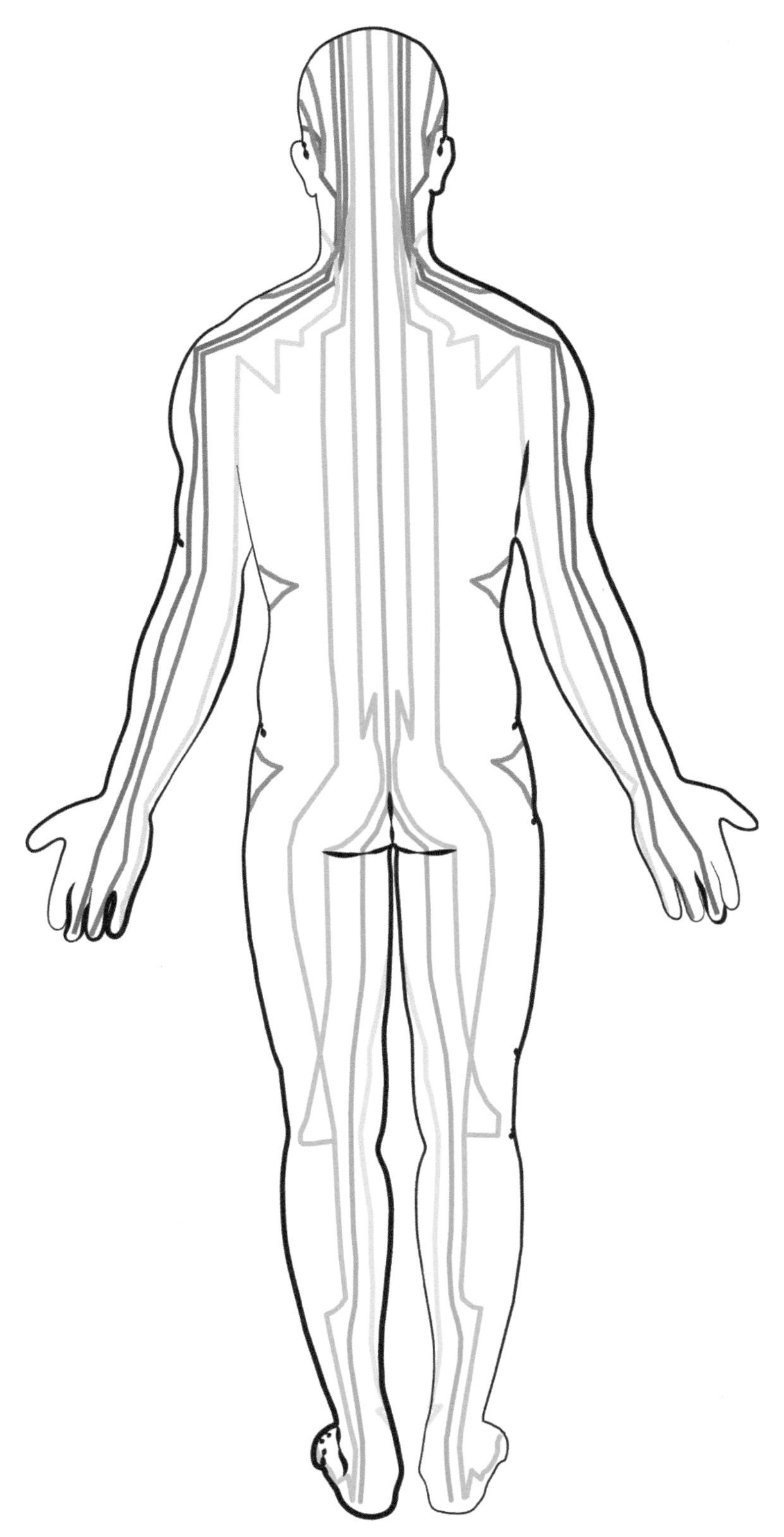

CHAPTER 15

RESEARCH ON RESISTANCE FLEXIBILITY

Always more unknown than known…

RESEARCH HIGHLIGHTS

1. THE STRETCH REFLEX

The stretch reflex is displayed as pandiculation in all animals when they stretch. This is the basis of all flexibility. All animals instinctively contract muscles when stretching.

2. ENDOSCOPIC VIEWING OF RESISTANCE FLEXIBILITY AND FASCIA

Nick Ware and Bob Cooley participated with Jean Claude Guimberteau in Endoscopic Filming of Resistance Flexibility's affect on fascia compared to traditional strength training and traditional stretching.

3. ULTRASOUND VIEWING OF RF AND FASCIA

Nick Ware and Bob Cooley participated in Ultrasound Viewing of Resistance Flexibility affect on fascia and scar tissue.

4. INTERNATIONAL FASCIA CONGRESSES

Nick Ware and Bob Cooley presented their clinical trial of Resistance Flexibility's affect on flexibility at the 3rd International Congress on Fascia. Bob Cooley also gave nine submissions for presentations at the 4th International Congress on Fascia and four were accepted.

The following are the abstract submissions for the 3rd and 4th International Fascia Congresses. ("SEE APPENDIX FOR ABSTRACT SUMMARIES)

<u>3RD FASCIA CONGRESS ABSTRACT PRESENTATION</u>

1 DOES RF RESULT IN RAPID HAMSTRING LENGTH INCREASES AND ACCLELERATED RANGE OF MOTION INCREASES BECAUSE OF FASCIA CHANGES?

4TH FASCIA CONGRESS ABSTRACT SUBMISSION LIST

1 A TENSEGRITY IDEAL MODEL OF FASCIA™.docx

2 TRANSFIGURATION OF ACCUMULATED DENSE FASCIA AND SCAR TISSUE.docx

3 COOLEY 16 KINEMATIC PATTERN BIOMECHANIC MODEL™.docx

4 CONCOMITANCE OF TRADITIONAL CHINESE MEDICINE.docx

5 PSYCHOLOGICAL EFECTS FROM ACCUMULATED DENSE FASCIA AND SCAR TISSUE.docx

6 CONCOMITANCE OF GENETIC PERSONALITY TRAIT.docx

7 POTENTIAL LOW BACK PAIN ELIMINATION THROUGH RESISTANCE FLEXIBILITY™ OF BICEPS FEMORIS.docx

8 ROTATOR CUFF REHABILITATION AND PREVENTATION THROUGH RESISTANCE FLEXIBILITY™.docx

9 CONCUSSIONS, RF, and ADFST ELIMINATION.docx

5. EXCESSIVE ECCENTRIC LOADING ABSTRACTS

Resistance Flexibility is not the same as Excessive Eccentric Loading. During Resistance Flexibility the end range of motion is determined by the capacity of the balancing muscle group's ability to shorten. This protects the person from overstretching. This principle of end range being limited by the capacity of the balancing muscle group is not currently considered in Excessive Eccentric Loading training.

Hundreds of scientific studies have been conducted on Excessive Eccentric Loading. A short review of several articles follows:
The Use of Eccentrically Biased Resistance Exercise to Mitigate Muscle Impairments Following Anterior Cruciate Ligament Reconstruction: A Short Review
Sports Health: A Multidisciplinary Approach 2009; 1:31, Gerber JP, et al
"Compared to standard rehabilitation, adding an early 12-week eccentric resistance training program 3 weeks after ACL reconstruction safely and dramatically improves quadriceps and gluteus maximus volume strength, and hopping ability measured at 15 weeks and at 1 year following surgery."

Safety, Feasibility, and Efficacy of Negative Work Exercise via Eccentric Muscle Activity Following Anterior Cruciate Ligament Reconstruction
J Orthop Sport PhysTher 2007: 37(1): 10- 18, Gerber JP, et al
"Negative work exercise (via eccentric muscle activity) has the potential to be highly effective at producing large quadriceps size and strength gains early after ACL-R. Negative work

output increased systematically throughout training, while knee and thigh pain remained at relatively low levels. The addition of negative work exercise also induced superior short-term results in strength, performance, and activity level after surgery."

Effects of Early Progressive Eccentric Exercise on Muscle Structure After Following Anterior Cruciate Ligament Reconstruction
J. Bone Joint Surg Am 2007; 89:559-570, Gerber JP, et al
"Eccentric resistance training implemented three weeks after reconstruction of the anterior cruciate ligament can induce structural changes in the quadriceps and gluteus Maximus that greatly exceed those achieved with a standard rehabilitation protocol."
Muscle Damage and Muscle Remodeling: No Pain, No Gain?
J Experimental Biology 2011; 241:1-6, Flass KL, et al
"Increase in muscle size and strength can be achieved independent of any symptoms of damage...eccentric exercise regimes might be perfectly suited for these elderly exercise-intolerant individuals because of the low energy requirements and high force-production abilities of eccentric muscle contractions."

Eccentricergometry: increases in loco- motor muscle size and strength at low training intensities (08)
Am J Physiol Regulatory Integrative Comp Physiol: R1282-R1288, 2000, LaStayo PC, et al
"Many elderly individuals with cardiovascular disease cannot exercise at intensities sufficient to provoke improvement in skeletal muscle mass and function...(these patients) could, at the very least, maintain their muscle mass and perhaps even experience an increase in muscle size and strength using an eccentric biased exercise rehabilitation."

Chronic Eccentric Exercise: Improvements in Muscle Strength can Occur with Little Demand for Oxygen
Am. J. Physiol. 276 (Regulatory Integrative Comp. Physiol. 45): R611-R615, 1999, LaStayo PC, et al
"The strength enhancements with eccentric training in our study, with very mini- mal cardiac demand, may have profound clinical applications. The strength improvements....occurred despite the eccentric training requiring the same or less V02."

When Active Muscles Lengthen; Properties and Consequences of Eccentric Contrac- tions
News Physiol Sci 2001; 16:256-261, Lindstedt SL, et al
"Eccentric exercise, which requires minimal energy and thus oxygen support, may be ideally suited for an aging population for rehabilitation as well as increasing both strength and power in all individuals."

Elderly Patients and High Force Resistance Exercise—A Descriptive Report: Can an Anabolic Muscle Growth Response Occur Without Muscle Damage or Inflammation?
J Geriatric PhysTher 2007; 30(3):128-134, LaStayo P, et al
"Elderly individuals participate in resistance exercise to induce an anabolic response and grow muscle to help overcome functional deficits."It is important to note that resistance

exercise biased towards eccentric muscle contractions can induce high muscle forces while at low metabolic costs."

Increased Strength and Physical Performance with Eccentric Training in Women with Impaired Glucose Tolerance: A Pilot Study
J Women's Health 2009; 18(2):253-260, Marcus RL, et al
"Eccentric resistance exercise is an easily tolerated yet potent intervention that can potentially mitigate worsening physical function and mobility-related consequences of sarcopenia in aging women."

Comparison of Combined Aerobic and High-Force Eccentric Resistance Exercise With Aerobic Exercise Only for People With Type 2 Diabetes Mellitus
PhysTher 2008; 88(11):1345-1354, Marcus RL, et al
"Utilizing eccentric resistance exercise may be ideally suited to maximum lean tissue outcomes, at a fraction of the cardiovascular cost of concentric and isometric resistance exercise."

The Positive Effects of Negative Work: Increased Muscle Strength and Decreased Fall Risk in a Frail Elderly Population
Journal of Gerontology: MEDICAL SCIENCES 2003; 58A(5): 419-424, LaStayo PC, et al
"These data demonstrate that lower extremity resistance exercise can improve muscle structure and function in those with limited exercise tolerance. The greater strength increase following negative work training resulted in improved balance, stair descent, and fall risk only. Because low energy cost is coupled to high force production with eccentric exercise, this intervention may be useful for a number of patients that are otherwise unable to achieve high muscle forces with traditional resistance exercise."

High-Intensity Negative Work Reduces Bradykinesia while Improving Balance and Quality of Life in Persons with Parkinson's Disease
Journal of Neurologic PhysicalTherapy 2004; 28(4):173 Dibble LE, et al
"Persons with Parkinson's Disease demonstrate reduced bradykinesia and improvements in their balance function and physical components of quality of life as a result of high intensity lower extremity negative work."

CHAPTER 16

FIRST GLIMPSE INTO THE TYPES

Adding Light To Something Already Lit

Excerpt: THE 16 GENIUSES — *16 Genetic Personality Types 1.0 Cooley*
(Release: March 30, 2016)

The 16 Genetic Personality *Types*

More than two decades ago I discovered sixteen genetic personality *types*, I call them the *sixteen geniuses*. I have attempted to present the *types* to you by reproducing the exact words they use to describe themselves. As you read their words, your imagination can bring forth the inimitable lives, and intelligences of the *types*.

Once you know about types,

for the rest of your life,

anytime you meet anyone,

you will always think, and forever be unable not to think,

the indelible question:

"What type is this person?"

When the sperm fertilizes the egg, the genetic blueprint of your personality *type* is formed, and then your life shapes you but can never change your *type*.

You probably conceptualized that I discovered the *types* by being a paleontologist at a remote archeological dig or as an academic researcher stumbling into rare scrolls in an ancient library, but nothing could be further from the truth. I originally and somewhat unintentionally discovered the *types* from within my own body, while attempting to rehabilitate myself from a tragic pedestrian automobile accident.

What was I going to call these *types*? I decided to name each *type* by titling them with two of their most exceptional high personality traits. The *types* are geniuses because each *type* has salient, differentiable, and perquisite high intuitive traits, each with their own *type* of intelligence.

To know which *type* you are, you'll need to know about all the *types*. I'm wondering…which one of the 16 *types* are you?

The Genius of Decision Making and Devotion

The Genius of Freedom and Humility

The Genius of Power and Truth

The Genius of Completion and Perfection

The Genius of Sobriety and Self-Knowing

The Genius of Communication and Peace

The Genius of Right Action and Unconditional Love

The Genius of Creativity and Affirmation

The Genius of Problem Solving and Mastery

The Genius of Intimacy and Will

The Genius of Openness and Judiciousness

The Genius of Challenges and Community

The Genius of Hope and Diversity

The Genius of Understanding and Humor

The Genius of Change and Integrity

The Genius of Healing and Soul

The Accidental Discovery of the *Types*

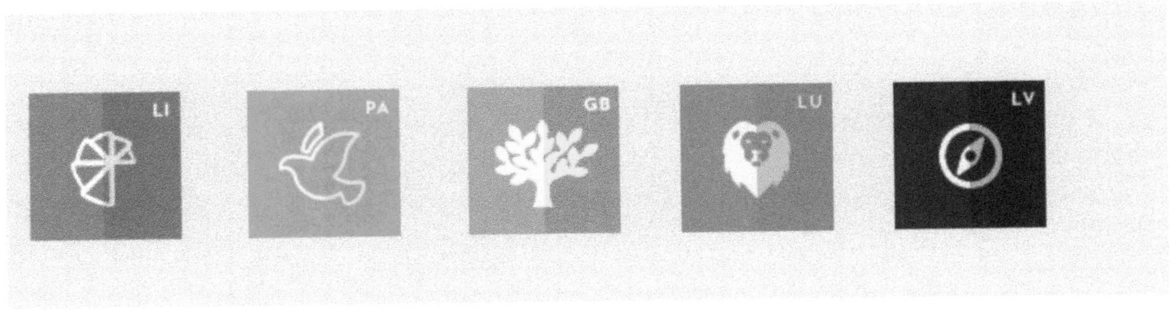

I remember when everyone became not just who they are,

but also a type.

The discovery of the *types* happened as a result of a sequence of explorations and revelations that occurred while I was attempting to rehabilitate my body from our pedestrian automobile accident. The discoveries I made resulted in me improving physically, next my physiological health increased, then my psychological health developed, and finally I was reconnected back with my life. I was unknowing before I discovered *types* that any of these concomitances existed or were possible.

The discovery story goes something like this…

First, in order to increase my flexibility I discovered that muscles naturally contract when being stretched. This 'stretch reflex contraction' results in the muscles tensing and resisting when being elongated during a stretch, and as long as you don't interfere with this reflex tension, muscles naturally tense and stretch. I later coined this Resistance Flexibility™. I then created sixteen different *types* of Resistance Flexibility™ exercises for each of the different muscle group that would move us in all eight directions for both my lower and upper body—16 total.

Secondly, after spending several months successfully upgrading my posture and movements by Resistance Flexibility exercises, unexpectedly I couldn't help but notice that by stretching each of those different muscle groups I was getting dramatic improvements in my physiological health, and even more unexpectedly that the different muscle groups I was stretching, each positively affecting a different organ's physiological health, corresponded exactly with the same muscles/organ correspondence in Traditional Chinese Medicine (TCM).

Thirdly, as if all this wasn't already unbelievable enough, I discovered when Resistance Flexibility™ training each of the different muscle groups besides each upgrading me biomechanically and physiologically, each different *type* of stretch also improved my psychological functioning in specific and predictable ways. Those concomitant changes in my psychological health turned into a theory of sixteen personality *types*. This is how the genesis of types began.

So quite unexpectedly while practicing sixteen different *types* of Resistance Flexibility exercises, I experienced that not just my body, but also my personality was being altered. I wasn't even looking to know about *types* at the time, and I didn't know I wanted to know about them even as it was happening. I learned over time that I was more closed minded about the very idea of *types* than anyone I have ever since met. I just wanted my life back.

Oh… I always wanted to know why other people behaved

in many ways that I found myself disconnected from.

To me, people simply seemed worlds apart.

Sure I could do some things other people couldn't do,

but also I wanted to be able to do what I saw others doing that I couldn't.

So the *types* were accidentally unearthed while I spent an extreme number of hours each day practicing these different *types* of Resistance Flexibility exercises, observing not only how the stretches targeted specific improvements in my physical and physiological health, but also how they psychologically affected me in predictable ways. I experienced my perception of the world and myself being reconfigured with each *type* of stretch—16 totally different ways of being, universal *types* engulfed me, morphing my consciousness. The sixteen different *types* of stretches had plugging me into a pansophy on *types.*

For me, types needed to be discovered

from within myself and from a solid physical experience,

thus establishing a physical foundation for the theory of types.

This physical foundation was essential

because the mental nature of knowing types needs grounding;

for without this grounding,

no footing into this new concept of types

could endure the passage of time.

Your Body Holds the Key to Knowing *Types*

Everyone that attempts the 16 different types of stretches,

uses exactly the same words to describe

how they feel, and perceive the world

when they do each different type of stretch

And everyone uses the same words to describe the types,

everyone.

I had to know if other people would have the same experiences of the *types* from stretching their bodies as I did. So, I had many different *types* of people practice the same stretches at the same time, and yes, everyone began to experience not the same physical and physiological changes as I had, but also everyone began to exhibit the same personality *type's* behaviors from the same *types* of stretches.

But this is how each type feels everyday since the moment they were born,

and how they will feel for the rest of their lives.

I traveled to many different countries and had people from different nationalities, cultures, religious preferences, socio-economic backgrounds and educations, etc. do the same *types* of stretches, but regardless of any of their differences or preferences, everyone always used the exact same words to describe the personality traits brought forth by different *types* of stretches.

Apparently the body is the way to identify types,

to experience the types from within yourself.

Your body gives you access to a universal language that each type

uses to describe themselves.

Several years after discovering the *types,* I did uncover ancient texts that referred to what I called *types.* One source calling them sixteen Gods or Goddesses, and another text calling them sixteen Masters. Then in the past several years, I began developing the science to validate the existence of these genetic *types* on the genome, as well as technology to allow everyone to know everyone's *type* using the Internet or phone App.

Nature Versus Nurture—Genetic Personality Types (GPT)

There was only one question that remained:

Were types created from conditioning or were they genetic?

Mothers know that her children are born and will remain very different from one another regardless of how similarly they are raised. They probably do not know about the idea of *types* yet, but they know that their children are different "somethings." It seems that mothers have known this forever; every mother I ask does, while many psychologists still seem more or less clueless on the idea that people are born *types*. However, people that are the same *type* are like identical twins that were raised by different parents, in different parts of the world, having had innumerable different events occur to them etc., but they exhibit the identical behaviors because they are the same *type*.

I reasoned that the only way I could determine if personality *types* were created by conditioning or by genetics was to find pairs of identical twins who where separated at birth for a good amount of time since birth. So I tested in simple double blind studies different pairs of twins, to see what *type* they were. They thought they were being measured for a flexibility analysis but they were really being tested to see what *type* they were. They not only had identical patterns of flexibility and inflexibility compared to different personality *types* but they were most definitely the same personality *type* as each other, and they knew they were the same *type*, they just didn't know their personalities were a *type*.

Leave it to this unique group of identical twins

that were separated at birth for many years

to demonstrate that types were genetic and not nurture based.

When the sperm touches the egg, everyone's *type* is set for life (perhaps even before that). And after that it's kind 'an up to you to become the *person* you want to be. You can grow and change but not into another *type*; you are hard wired your whole lifetime as a particular *type*—that is why they are called *genetic personality types*. Your parent's *types* do not determine what *type* you are, for *types* are born more or less random regardless of the parent's *type*. Surprisingly you can be more similar to someone you are not related to, that is the same *type* as you, than members of your own family.

The Geniuses Reveal Themselves Through 'The Trade'

Any time someone benefited from what I knew,

they'd offer some piece of the puzzle that was necessary for my healing.

After I had learned that different stretches could morph me into different *types*, I started seeing people differently. In particular I found that when I would teach people something that was specifically valuable to them that I had learned from my self-stretching, they would suddenly share something that was specifically valuable to me. I was constantly surprised at how unassumingly and non-chalantly people would tell me the exact thing that I needed to know, at the exact moment I needed to know it. I ended up calling this *type* of synchronicity— the *trade.*

How did they know exactly what I needed to know?

I was learning to heal myself through healing others,

intuitively we knew what each other needed.

I somehow found a way to perceive the real person,

if and only if their essence experienced me listening to them.

I learned to listen to the voice behind the words.

The real person inside of everyone

kept telling me exactly what I needed to know.

If I argued, disconnected, dissociated or otherwise

diminished the value in what they were telling me,

then the real person inside them would stop speaking to me.

I was looking not just at the outside person, but at the inside person—

through their skin…at their Genius.

Their Genius was healing me.

I found good information in books and classrooms, but nowhere could I find what I was now *experiencing* through people telling me what I needed to know. What I learned was emerging organically—with real people confronting real problems. Each individual problem became an opportunity to learn many things that no one ever knew before. People were allowing me to be their guide as I honored their authority to be their own true and unique genius—a spirited, energetic self that had countless incredible gems to teach—exactly what everyone needs to know!

So what I had always needed the most to know about,

those things that are so obvious to everyone else but so clueless for me,

I could now learn from different types of people.

I am eternally humbled by the wisdom that each type of person is capable of,

and who offer freely this information to anyone that knows to listen.

A crystal formed in my mind around the idea of the 16 types of people.

Balancing/Unconscious *Types*

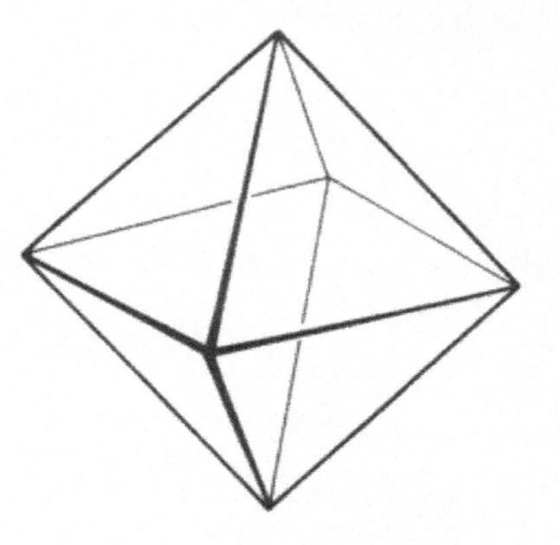

A decade later,

I understood that what one type is conscious of,

their balancing type is unconscious of.

and that your unconscious is the other gender.

The final piece of the puzzle about *types* showed up again because of physical reasons. When I would stretch one muscle group, the muscle group on the opposite side of the body would need to shorten. I discovered that the capacity of a muscle to shorten was directly proportional to its ability to stretch. So when I wanted to stretch a particular group of muscles, I have to make sure the muscles on the other side of the body were flexible enough to shorten. In Western anatomy they call these muscles agonist and antagonists, but in Chinese anatomy they call them balancing muscles.

Well because I had already discovered that specific muscle groups developed one of the *type's* traits within me, I decided to call those *types* on either side of the body—balancing *types*. And just like the muscular actions of balancing *types* are complimentary, so are their high/low traits. A person initially only sees half of the pixels as they look at the world. The entire other half of reality can only be seen when the unconscious part of them is in full operation. Access to this second half is the balancing part of a person and this part sees the world in the way the *balancing type* sees the world.

And, the balancing types are

the best pairing for long-term intimate relationships

because they are within each other.

I'd rather be with someone that doesn't need me to be someone else.

A New Body—Mind Psychology Based on *Types*

It takes a lot to know someone,

but only a moment to type them.

Strangely and unexpectedly when I wanted to know more about a particular *type*, that *type* of person would contemporaneously show up at my doorstep. It was through a wave of almost unbelievable synchronicities like this that the information on *types* was developed and is still developing. And it was in this way, that a new theory of *types* was born: a theory that has a transcendental spirit, but an unshakeable rock-solid physical root and foundation. Jung stated: "What are the bodily correlatives of a given psychic condition? Unfortunately we are not yet far enough advanced to give even an approximate answer." Is it too audacious to say this has now been accomplished?

At this point I realized

that it might be almost totally impossible

for most anyone to believe how and what I discovered

about the types.

I had initially discovered the types from nothing other than self

physical flexibility exercises,

and not from books, not from a dig, from nothing…but myself.

Yet the evidence was apodictic.

Because I discovered the *types* through the rehabilitation and upgrading of my body, this is a new body-mind psychology, a psychology that everyone can generate from within their own body. This *type* concept lays a new foundation for psychology while providing what is already known in the field of psychology with a telamon, and thus a new organizational wholeness and insaturation. This *type*-based psychology also emphasizes a way to have a greater aliveness and positive spirit in psychology, a psycho-spiritual approach to understanding everyone, a truly positive psychology.

This is a new unified psychology,

where instead of having a problem-centered approach,

work is instead directed to develop the person

in just those ways they were never developed

that were the reasons why they had those specific problems.

This new twenty first century *type* approach to psychology explores human consciousness from a wellness perspective in addition to the traditional illness categorization. I have enormous respect for the elite historical psychological figures that drove psychology before me, while myself having come from a different background and perspective. This is my ken of *types*—a fractal psychology that takes the abstruse study of psychology and gives it a real physical foundation. A psychology based on balancing/unconscious *types.*

New ideas about types,

innumerable and unfathomable in their effect,

ideas almost wholly unknown to most,

were initially discovered by consequences and later by intention,

are revealed in this book.

Everyone already knows a lot about personalities,

but knowing <u>types</u> coalesces everyone's ideas.

That is why I like to say knowing types is like

adding light to something already lit.

APPENDIX—ABSTRACTS

COOLEY'S TENSEGRITY FASCIA MODEL™

Robert Cooley BS Eric Beutner LMT
The Genius of Flexibility Center—Research
914 A Santa Barbara St Santa Barbara, California 93101
email: BobCooley@TheGeniusofFlexibility.com

BACKGROUND Cooley's tensegrity fascia model™ is a polyhedron with fully triangulated surfaces including only four compressed struts (repulsion), and with prestressed tension members (attraction) with a right handed twist. This tensegrity model is formed because of the requirement of the fascia to be able to move three dimensionally with six degrees of freedom whose eight permutations established Cooley's 16 Kinematic Patterns™ for the lower and upper body.
METHODS Cooley's 16 Kinematic Patterns™ is used for the biomechanical analysis of human motion for Resistance Flexibility (RF) training and rehabilitation. Cooley's 16 Kinematic Patterns™ for the lower and upper body are: FL/AD/IN, FL/AD/OU, FL/AB/IN, FL/AB/OU and the complimentary patterns of EX/AB/OU, EX/AB/IN, EX/AD/OU, EX/AD/IN.
RESULTS Cooley's tensegrity fascia model™ reflects the basis for the myofascial training and rehabilitative therapeutic modality called Resistance Flexibility™ that addresses the three dimensional 8 permutational kinematic patterns for the lower and upper body. The model demonstrates biomechanical principles for balancing and opposing muscle groups, and bilateral symmetrical balancing of muscles groups.
CONCLUSIONS Identification of the eight permutation patterns possible from the six degrees of motion elegantly displays into Cooley's tensegrity fascia model and satisfies Euler's Formula. This elastic model helps to explain the otherwise current chaotic description of fascia movement with a placable functioning unit for movement in eight directions. Vertices, tension elements, or compression elements may be shared so that this tensegrity unit can connect and create a chain of tensegrity units allowing for an infinite variety of shapes all acting as one in the myofascialskeletal system of contiguous muscle groups. DISCLOSURES Research supported by The Genius of Flexibility 501(c)(3) Non-Profit Corporation.

REFERENCES

Fuller, R.B (1975). *Synergetics, Explorations in the Geometry of Thinking.* Macmillian. Donald E. Ingber, Journal of Body Works and Movement Therory. 2008 Jul; 12(3): 198–200. Tensegrity and mechanotransduction

Cooley RD and Ware NM. *"Does Resistance Flexibility result in rapid hamstring length increases and accelerated range of motion increases because of fascial* changes?" Poster Presentation March 2012, 3rd International Fascia Research Congress, Vancouver, B.C.

TRANSFIGURATION OF ACCUMULATED DENSE FASCIA AND SCAR TISSUE (ADFST) BY RESISTANCE FLEXIBILITY™

Robert Cooley BS

The Genius of Flexibility Center—Research

914 A Santa Barbara St Santa Barbara, California 93101

email: BobCooley@TheGeniusofFlexibility.com

BACKGROUND Resistance Flexibility™ (RF) involves the use of tension and resistance while self or assisted flexibility training compared to traditional methods of stretching that simply use elongation. The resistive forces created by naturally tensing and resisting during RF are two to six times the maximum force produced when strength training the same muscle groups yet no pain is experienced.

METHODS Based on international clinical cases, the Biceps Femoris and the Triceps characteristically house the greatest amount of accumulated dense fascia and scar tissue (ADFST). A Lafayette muscle testing dynamometer was used to measure the differences in maximum forces generated during strength training compared to RF training and a Lafayette Acumar goniometer was used to measure increases in ROM, and shortening capacity in Biceps Femoris and Triceps in individuals ranging in age from 16 to 65.

RESULTS RF™ Significant increases in flexibility with parallel increases in the capacity of the muscles to shorten, and the rate and acceleration of shortening were noted compared to traditional stretching and deep tissue massage techniques.

CONCLUSIONS The forces necessary to cause significant positive changes in fascia structures that result in increases in flexibility and strength can be produced with zero pain during self or assisted RF. Best method to measure increases in flexibility is by measuring the capacity of the muscle to shorten not simply ROM. Removing ADFST also eliminates biomechanical limitations and substitutions, and as well as postural deformations of sway back, lumbar lordosis, thoracic kyphosis, and forward tilt. Further research is warranted.

DISCLOSURE Research supported by The Genius of Flexibility 501(c)(3) Non-Profit Corporation.

REFERENCES

M. R. Pull and C. Ranson. Physical Therapy in Sport, 8 (2007), 88-97,

P.C. LaStayo, J.M. Woolf, M.D. Lewek, L. Snyder-Mackler, T. Reich, and S.L.Lindstedt. "Eccentric muscle contractions: their contribution to injury, prevention, rehabilitation, and sport" Journal of Orthopaedic & Sports Physical Therapy, 2003; 33:557-571.

Cooley RD and Ware NM. "Does Resistance Flexibility result in rapid hamstring length increases and accelerated range of motion increases because of fascial changes?" Poster Presentation March 2012, 3rd International Fascia Research Congress, Vancouver, B.C.

COOLEYS 16 KINEMATIC BIOMECHANIC PATTERNS™ FOR THE EVALUATION OF MYOFASCIA FLEXIBILITY AND STRENGTH

Robert Cooley BS

The Genius of Flexibility Center—Research

914 A Santa Barbara St Santa Barbara, California 93101

email: BobCooley@TheGeniusofFlexibility.com

BACKGROUND Traditional measures of joint ROM are from the neutral anatomical norm positions. Cooley's 16 Kinematic Biomechanical Patterns™ uses six degrees of freedom: flexion/extension, adduction/abduction, and outward/inward rotation to create 16 kinematic permutation patterns. The eight permutation kinematic patterns are FL/AD/IN, FL/AD/OU, FL/AB/IN, FL/AB/OU, and their complimentary patterns of EX/AD/IN, EX/AD/OU, EX/AB/IN, EX/AB/OU each for the lower and upper body. Each of the eight patterns encompasses a 45-degree arch to complete the 180 degrees of movement possible in the lower and upper body. Because myofascial structures present through 8 directions of movement, only Resistance Flexibility (RF) uses the 16 three-dimensional directional kinematic patterns as the model for evaluation, development, and rehabilitation. Balancing and opposing muscles groups, and bilateral symmetry balancing are included in this biomechanical evaluation.

METHODS Thirty individuals ranging in age from 16–66 were measured with a goniometer for hip and shoulder joint ROM and maximal shortening capacity on three consecutive days using Cooley's 16 Kinematic Patterns™. Balancing and opposing muscle groups of the hip and shoulder joint were also evaluated.

RESULTS Mean values for optimal ROM were created for the 8 Kinematic Patterns for the hip and shoulder joint and myofascial characteristics. ADFST usually occurs in the lateral and posterior muscle groups while chronic tenseness occurs in the anterior and medial. Best method to measure of true flexibility is not to measure ROM but to measure the capacity of the muscle to shorten.

CONCLUSIONS Current methods of evaluating ROM based on anatomical norm positions lack sufficient permutational analysis for human movement. Cooley's 16 Kinematic Patterns presents a new model for flexibility and strength evaluation that includes myofascial analysis for ADFST. The capacity of a muscle to shorten is dependent and directly proportional to the capacity of the muscle to shorten. Further research is warranted.

DISCLOSURE Research supported by The Genius of Flexibility 501(c)(3) Non-Profit Corporation.

REFERENCES

Cooley RD and Ware NM."Does Resistance Flexibility result in rapid hamstring length increases and accelerated range of motion increases because of fascial changes? Poster Presentation March 2012, 3rd International Fascia Research Congress, Vancouver, B.C.

CONCOMITANCE OF TRADITIONAL CHINESE MEDICINE (TCM) MERIDIANS AND FASCIAL PATTERNS

Robert Cooley BS Chris Renfow MAOM

The Genius of Flexibility Center—Research

914 A Santa Barbara St Santa Barbara, California 93101

email: BobCooley@TheGeniusofFlexibility.com

BACKGROUND Cooley's 16 Kinematic Biomechanical Patterns™ of the lower and upper body are concomitant with the myofacial pathways of contiguous muscle/organ/meridian groups in TCM. TCM explicitly states a concomitance with specific contiguous muscle group pathways and organ and tissue health. Accumulated dense fascia and scar tissue (ADFST) is characteristically found in the yang muscle groups while the yin muscle groups retain chronic tenseness. The Energy Cycle in TCM also forms an orderly progressive arrangement for joint structure biomechanical evaluation for the lower and upper body as each pair of balancing meridian muscle groups corresponds to the exact sequencing of joints. Resistance Flexibility (RF) training of each of the 16 meridian pathways myofascia structures can positively affect the postural and movement biomechanics, and the physiological function of its respective organ and its body part or tissue association. Two new muscle meridian pathways were evaluated not currently identified in TCM.

METHODS Individuals ranging in age from 16 to 66 were evaluated for normal, accumulated dense fascia and/or scar tissue in Cooley's 16 Kinematic Patterns™. Correlation of TCM diagnosis with myofascia flexibility and strength was noted.

RESULTS There were significant correlations with ADFST in concomitant TCM meridian muscle groups with TCM evaluation of health conditions. Transfiguration, elimination, and renovation of ADFST correlated with reported health increases.

CONCLUSIONS Increases in ADFST in TCM meridian pathways correlates with evaluations in TCM. Fascia may prove to be the missing link between the myofascial structures of the body and the meridians of energy flow that are the basis of Traditional Chinese Medicine (TCM).

DISCLOSURES Research supported by The Genius of Flexibility 501(c)(3) Non-Profit Corporation.

REFERENCES

Bob Cooley Pacific College of Oriental Medicine Symposium 2009 *Traditional Chinese Medicine (TCM) and Resistance Flexibility and Strength Training—A flexibility Concomitance with Meridian Theory*

Cooley RD and Ware NM. "Does Resistance Flexibility result in rapid hamstring length increases and accelerated range of motion increases because of fascial changes?" Poster Presentation March 2012, 3rd International Fascia Research Congress, Vancouver, B.C.

PSYCHOLOGICAL EFECTS FROM ACCUMULATED DENSE FASCIA AND SCAR TISSUE (ADFST) CHANGES FROM RESISTANCE FLEXIBILITY™

Robert Cooley BS

The Genius of Flexibility Center—Research

914 A Santa Barbara St Santa Barbara, California 93101

email: BobCooley@TheGeniusofFlexibility.com

BACKGROUND Trauma results in accumulated dense fascia and scar tissue (ADFST) with the concomitant physiological distress, depersonalization, franticness, compulsive reenactment, menticide, lust, and toxicity replacing normal psychological and physiological health. Trauma can result from emotional (sexual), head, body, or life abuses. This research documents the significant positive psychological and physiological health upgrades that result from Resistance Flexibility (RF)™ training in Cooley's 16 Kinematic Pattern muscle groups. ADFST is explicitly connected to the past events, and holds that part of the person in a warped sense of time and space. Dramatic changes in the person's perception of time and space are reported as the myofascial flexibility and strength is upgraded through RF, and with concomitant predictable results in personality trait developments. While being RF trained either in self or assisted stretches, there is a commonly reported experience of being unable to sense the enormous amount of resistive force the person being stretched is generating while RF.

METHODS Thirty individuals ranging in age from 16 to 66 reported on their psychological developments after one month of assisted RF performed three times a week for one hour.

RESULTS Participants reported concomitant psychological benefits from removing ADFST in Cooley's 16 Kinematic Biomechanical Patterns for the lower and upper body consistent with Genetic Personality Type (GPT) theory. Traumatized myofascia tissues place a ceiling on athletic and artistic success, emotional maturation, and longevity. Removing of ADFST becomes a psychological freeing agent.

CONCLUSIONS Improvements in flexibility and strength in Cooley's 16 Kinematic Patterns muscle groups for the lower and upper body can result in dramatic psychological upgrades, and GPT trait development. Further research is warranted.

DISCLOSURES Research supported by The Genius of Flexibility 501(c)(3) Non-Profit Corporation.

REFERENCES

Callaghan P. (2004). Exercise: a neglected intervention in mental health care? Journal of Psychiatric and Mental Health Nursing, 11, 476-483.

Cooley RD and Ware NM. *Poster Presentation* March 2012, 3rd International Fascia Research Congress, Vancouver, B.C.

A THEORY OF 16 GENETIC PERSONALITY TYPES (GPT)™ CONCOMITANCE WITH SIXTEEN MYOFASCIAL KINEMATIC PATTERNS

Robert Cooley BS

The Genius of Flexibility Center—Research

914 A Santa Barbara St Santa Barbara, California 93101

email: BobCooley@TheGeniusofFlexibility.com

BACKGROUND Accumulated dense fascia and scar tissue (ADFST) is located in predictable muscle/meridian pathways in the myofascial structures concomitant with Cooley's 16 genetic personality types (GPT)™. Cooley's sixteen genetic personality types (GPT)™ trait identification and differentiation parallels the myofascia flexibility and strength in Cooley's 16 Kinematic Patterns™ of the lower and upper body. The 16 genetic personality types are concomitant with predictable differentiable bone rotational interrelationships (BRI) of the lower or upper body for each type. A physically based and derived psychology was theorized based on personality types whose traits identification and development were concomitant with 16 kinematic permutations of the body and TCM meridian/organ pathways. GPT theory adds a positive psychology theory that designates equivalent high trait development to current personality theory and practice that defines only dysfunctional traits. 16 types of physiological concomitances of the organs and meridian pathways in Traditional Chinese Medicine and GPT form the basis of a new psychological theory that can be used for an individual assessment that correlated the genetic type and its relationship to myofascia dysfunction, and physiological health and disease.

METHODS Thirty-two individuals ranging in age from 16 to 66 were typed and evaluated for ADFST in Cooley's 16 Kinematic Patterns™ for both the lower and upper body. Types were identified from their BRI patterns of the 16 GPT.

RESULTS Significant correlation with myofascia health and sixteen personality high/low trait evaluation.

CONCLUSIONS Elimination, transfiguration, and renovation of ADFST in Cooley's 8 kinematic patterns can correlate with the development of predictable increases in the high personality traits/values of the 16 GPT. This is an ever-increasing psychological data base. Further research is warranted.

DISCLOSURES Research supported by The Genius of Flexibility 501(c)(3) Non-Profit Corporation.

REFERENCES

Bob Cooley Pacific College of Oriental Medicine Symposium 2009 Traditional Chinese Medicine (TCM) and 16 Genetic Personality Types

Cooley, Bob. The 16 Geniuses—Sixteen Genetic Personality Types (release Fall 2015)

POTENTIAL LOW BACK PAIN ELIMINATION THROUGH RESISTANCE FLEXIBILITY™ OF THE BICEPS FEMORIS

Robert Cooley BS

The Genius of Flexibility Center—Research

914 A Santa Barbara St Santa Barbara, California 93101

email: BobCooley@TheGeniusofFlexibility.com

BACKGROUND Resistance Flexibility™ (RF) involves the use of tension and resistance while self or assisted stretching compared to traditional methods of stretching that simply use elongation. The resistive forces created by tensing and resisting during RF are two to six times the maximum force produced when strength training yet no pain is experienced. Based on extensive international clinical experiences, the Biceps Femoris has the largest amount of accumulated dense fascia and scar tissue (ADFST) compared to all other muscles. Elimination, transfiguration, and renovation of the ADFST in this lateral hamstring has shown to eliminate low back pain. Increases in flexibility from RF parallel proportional increases in the capacity of the Biceps Femoris to shortening, and the rate and acceleration of shortening for the kinetic pattern of jumping.

METHODS Thirty random individuals ranging in age from 16 to 65 who reported a history of low back pain but with non-significant pathology of the low back, performed assisted RF training for three sets of ten repetitions of Biceps Femoris bilaterally, and for the TFL/IT band for three alternating days over a three week period. Participants self-reporting of low back pain results.

RESULTS Reported elimination of low back from RF training of the Biceps Femoris and TFL/IT band after a three week training trial with a three month follow up evaluation. Increases in ROM and shortening capacity in the Biceps Femoris and TFL are consistent with reported low back pain reduction or elimination. All statistical analysis was performed with $p \leq 0.05$.

CONCLUSIONS RF™ can be utilized for the possible elimination of low back pain in individuals with previously evaluated non-pathological conditions in the low back. Further research is warranted.

DISCLOSURES Research supported by The Genius of Flexibility 501(c)(3) Non-Profit Corporation.

REFERENCES

C.L. Brockett, D.L. Morgan, U. Proske. *Human hamstring muscles adapt to eccentric exercise by changing optimum length.* Medicine and science in sports and exercise, 2001;33:783-790

Cooley RD and Ware NM."Does Resistance Flexibility result in rapid hamstring length increases and accelerated range of motion increases because of fascial changes? March 2012, 3rd International Fascia Research Congress, Vancouver, B.C.

ROTATOR CUFF REHABILITATION AND PREVENTATION THROUGH RESISTANCE FLEXIBILITY™

Robert Cooley BS

The Genius of Flexibility Center—Research

914 A Santa Barbara St Santa Barbara, California 93101

email: BobCooley@TheGeniusofFlexibility.com

BACKGROUND Rotator cuff rehabilitation can be facilitated by identifying and removing accumulated dense fascia and scar tissue (ADFST) in Cooley's 16 Kinematic Patterns™ of specific myofascial muscle groups of the upper extremity. ADFST in the Infraspinatus is the source/target muscle for rotator cuff dysfunction because it is primarily responsible for the external rotation of the humerus during flexion. Resistance Flexibility™ (RF) involves the use of tension and resistance while self or assisted stretching compared to traditional methods of stretching that simply use elongation. The resistive forces created by naturally tensing and resisting during RF are two to six times the maximum force produced when strength training yet no pain is experienced. Increases in flexibility from RF paralleled proportional increases in the capacity of the muscles to shortening, and the rate and acceleration of shortening.

METHODS A Lafayette dynamometer was used to measure the differences in maximum forces generated during strength training compared to RF training in in the rotator cuff muscles: Infraspinatus, Triceps Brachii, Biceps, and Supraspinatus, in 30 random individuals ranging in age from 16 to 65. A Lafayette goniometer was used to measure increases in ROM, and shortening capacity after three sets of ten repetitions of RF on those muscles over a three consecutive days of training.

RESULTS RF™ results in significant increases in flexibility with parallel capacity increases in the muscles to shorten, and the rate and acceleration of shortening of the Infraspinatus, Triceps Brachii, Biceps, and Supraspinatus resulting in increase in shoulder joint Flexion/Add or Abd/Outward rotation.

CONCLUSIONS The forces necessary to cause significant changes in fascia structures that result in increases in flexibility and strength can be produced with zero pain during self or assisted RF. Removing ADFST also eliminates biomechanical limitations and substitutions and postural deformations.

DISCLOSURES Research supported by The Genius of Flexibility 501(c)(3) Non-Profit Corporation.

REFERENCES

P. Jonsson, P. Wahlstrom, L. Ohberg, H. Alfredson. *Eccentric Training in chronic painful impingement syndrome of the shoulder; results of a pilot study.* Knee Surgery, Sports Traumatology, Arthroscopy. 2006; 14:76-81|

Cooley RD and Ware NM."Does Resistance Flexibility result in rapid hamstring length increases and accelerated range of motion increases because of fascial changes?" March 2012, 3rd International Fascia Research Congress, Vancouver, B.C.

TRAMATIC BRAIN INJURY (TBI) AND CHRONIC TRAUMATIC ENCEPHALOPATHY (CTE) HEALING THROUGH ELIMINATION OFACCUMULATED DENSE FASCIA AND SCAR TISSUE (ADFST) BY RESISTANCE FLEXIBILITY™ (RF)

Robert Cooley BS
The Genius of Flexibility Center—Research
914 A Santa Barbara St Santa Barbara, California 93101
email: BobCooley@TheGeniusofFlexibility.com

BACKGROUND Individuals with Traumatic Brain Injury (TBI) and Chronic Traumatic Encephalopathy (CTE) commonly report chronic head aches, diminished cognition, memory loss, limitations in concentration, digestive disorders, depression, depersonalization, movement impairment, skull and face deformations, impaired intimacy, lust, speech impairment, thwarted spiritual development, toxicity, shock, NDE, disturbing dream content, and anger management sometimes resulting in murder and/or suicide. Resistance Flexibility™ (RF) can be used to significantly upgrade the myofascial structures targeting those muscle groups that are concomitant with these specific physical, physiological and psychological concerns.

METHODS Individuals with Traumatic Brain Injury (TBI) and Chronic Traumatic Encephalopathy (CTE) were Resistance Flexibility™ (RF) trained in specifically targeted myofacial muscles groups of Cooley's 16 Kinematic Patterns™ including the Upper Trapezius, Supraspinatus, Infraspinatus, Pectoralis Minor, Latisimus Dorsi, Teres Major and Minor, Subscapular, and the Psoas Major, Semitendinosus, and the Biceps Femoris.

RESULTS Immediately after RF training individuals reported: elimination in chronic headache; increased cognition, memory and concentration; postural and dynamic movement improvement. After a month of RF training individuals reported: digestive improvements; brain health; heightened mental function exceeding pre-concussion abilities; increases in auditory acuity; relief of chronic pain; increased consciousness of desire, perspective, and personal ambition; elimination of chronic discomfort, pain, and lifelessness; increase in judgment and discernment; and increase in intimacy, and inter/intrapersonalness.

CONCLUSIONS RF training with individuals with TBI and CTE reported significant physiological and psychological benefits. Future research is needed.

DISCLOSURE Research supported by The Genius of Flexibility 501(c)(3) Non-Profit Corporation

REFERENCES

Bob Cooley, Laurent Robinson, Andrea Kramer NFL Network Super Bowl Sunday 2013 *Concussions and RFST*

Cooley RD and Ware NM.*"Does Resistance Flexibility result in rapid hamstring length increases and accelerated range of motion increases because of fascial changes?"* March 2012, 3rd International Fascia Research Congress, Vancouver, B.C.

EEL ABSTRACT REVIEWS

The Use of Eccentrically Biased Resistance Exercise to Mitigate Muscle Impairments Following Anterior Cruciate Ligament Reconstruction: A Short Review

Sports Health: A Multidisciplinary Approach 2009; 1:31, Gerber JP, et al

"Compared to standard rehabilitation, adding an early 12-week eccentric resistance training program 3 weeks after ACL reconstruction safely and dramatically improves quadriceps and gluteus maximus volume strength, and hopping ability measured at 15 weeks and at 1 year following surgery."

Safety, Feasibility, and Efficacy of Negative Work Exercise via Eccentric Muscle Activity Following Anterior Cruciate Ligament Reconstruction

J Orthop Sport PhysTher 2007: 37(1): 10- 18, Gerber JP, et al

"Negative work exercise (via eccentric muscle activity) has the potential to be highly effective at producing large quadriceps size and strength gains early after ACL-R. Negative work output increased systematically throughout training, while knee and thigh pain remained at relatively low levels. The addition of negative work exercise also induced superior short-term results in strength, performance, and activity level after surgery."

Effects of Early Progressive Eccentric Exer- cise on Muscle Structure After Following Anterior Cruciate Ligament Reconstruction

J. Bone Joint Surg Am 2007; 89:559-570, Gerber JP, et al

"Eccentric resistance training implemented three weeks after reconstruction of the anterior cruciate ligament can induce structural changes in the quadriceps and gluteus maximus that greatly exceed those achieved with a standard rehabilitation protocol."

Muscle Damage and Muscle Remodeling: No Pain, No Gain?

J Experimental Biology 2011; 241:1-6, Flass KL, et al

"Increase in muscle size and strength can be achieved independent of any symptoms of damage...eccentric exercise regimes might be perfectly suited for these elderly exercise-intolerant individuals because of the low energy requirements and high force-production abilities of eccentric muscle contractions."

Eccentricergometry: increases in loco- motor muscle size and strength at low training intensities (08)

Am J Physiol Regulatory Integrative Comp Physiol: R1282-R1288, 2000, LaStayo PC, et al

"Many elderly individuals with cardiovascular disease cannot exercise at intensities sufficient to provoke improvement in skeletal muscle mass and function...(these patients) could, at the very least, maintain their muscle mass and perhaps even experience an increase in muscle size and strength using an eccentric biased exercise rehabilitation."

Chronic Eccentric Exercise: Improvements in Muscle Strength can Occur with Little Demand for Oxygen

Am. J. Physiol. 276 (Regulatory Integrative Comp. Physiol. 45): R611-R615, 1999, LaStayo PC, et al

"The strength enhancements with eccentric training in our study, with very minimal cardiac demand, may have profound clinical applications. The strength improvements....occurred despite the eccentric training requiring the same or less V02."

When Active Muscles Lengthen; Properties and Consequences of Eccentric Contractions

News Physiol Sci 2001; 16:256-261, Lindstedt SL, et al

"Eccentric exercise, which requires minimal energy and thus oxygen support, may be ideally suited for an aging population for rehabilitation as well as increasing both strength and power in all individuals."

Elderly Patients and High Force Resistance Exercise—A Descriptive Report: Can an Anabolic Muscle Growth Response Occur Without Muscle Damage or Inflammation?

J Geriatric PhysTher 2007; 30(3):128-134, LaStayo P, et al

"Elderly individuals participate in resistance exercise to induce an anabolic response and grow muscle to help overcome functional deficits."It is important to note that resistance exercise biased towards eccentric muscle contractions can induce high muscle forces while at low metabolic costs."

Increased Strength and Physical Performance with Eccentric Training in Women with Impaired Glucose Tolerance: A Pilot Study

J Women's Health 2009; 18(2):253-260, Marcus RL, et al

"Eccentric resistance exercise is an easily tolerated yet potent intervention that can potentially mitigate worsening physical function and mobility-related consequences of sarcopenia in aging women."

Comparison of Combined Aerobic and High-Force Eccentric Resistance Exercise With Aerobic Exercise Only for People With Type 2 Diabetes Mellitus

PhysTher 2008; 88(11):1345-1354, Marcus RL, et al

"Utilizing eccentric resistance exercise may be ideally suited to maximum lean tissue outcomes, at a fraction of the cardiovascular cost of concentric and isometric resistance exercise."

The Positive Effects of Negative Work: Increased Muscle Strength and Decreased Fall Risk in a Frail Elderly Population

Journal of Gerontology: MEDICAL SCIENCES 2003; 58A(5): 419-424, LaStayo PC, et al

"These data demonstrate that lower extremity resistance exercise can improve muscle structure and function in those with limited exercise tolerance. The greater strength increase following negative work training resulted in improved balance, stair descent, and fall risk only. Because low energy cost is coupled to high force production with eccentric exercise, this intervention may be useful for a number of patients that are otherwise unable to achieve high muscle forces with traditional resistance exercise."

High-Intensity Negative Work Reduces Bradykinesia while Improving Balance and Quality of Life in Persons with Parkinson's Disease

Journal of Neurologic PhysicalTherapy 2004; 28(4):173 Dibble LE, et al

"Persons with Parkinson's Disease demonstrate reduced bradykinesia and improvements in their balance function and physical components of quality of life as a result of high intensity lower extremity negative work."

The Safety and Feasibility of High-Force Eccentric Resistance Exercise in Person with Parkinson's Disease

Arch Phys Med Rehabil 2006; 87:1280-2, Dibble LE, et al

"Persons with mild to moderate PD can safely and feasibly participate in high-force eccentric resistance training."This type of exercise….may be ideally suited for subjects with PD because high levels of muscle force are generated with low metabolic demands."

High-Intensity Resistance Training Amplifies Muscle Hypertrophy and Functional Gains in Persons with Parkinson's Disease

Movement Disorders 2006; 21(9): 1444- 1452, Dibble LE, et al

"Persons with Parkinson's Disease in this study who performed high-force eccentric resistance training demonstrated…increases in muscle volume (that) appears to be important in improving muscle force and mobility in persons with PD."

INDEX

Lightning Source UK Ltd.
Milton Keynes UK
UKHW050713040419
340474UK00001B/8/P